PERFECTION

PERFECTION

400 YEARS OF WOMEN'S QUEST FOR BEAUTY

Margarette Lincoln

YALE UNIVERSITY PRESS
NEW HAVEN AND LONDON

For information about this and other Yale University Press publications, please contact:
U.S. Office: sales.press@yale.edu   yalebooks.com
Europe Office: sales@yaleup.co.uk   yalebooks.co.uk

Set in Adobe Garamond Pro by IDSUK (DataConnection) Ltd
Printed in Great Britain by Clays Ltd, Elcograf S.p.A

Library of Congress Control Number: 2024938421

ISBN 978-0-300-26458-6

A catalogue record for this book is available from the British Library.

10 9 8 7 6 5 4 3 2 1

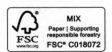

CONTENTS

ILLUSTRATIONS

PLATES

9. *An Officer in the Light Infantry, Driven by his Lady to Cox-Heath*, by John Collet, 1778. Yale Center for British Art, Paul Mellon Collection.

10. *Princess Amelia Sophia Eleonore of Great Britain*, by Thomas Hudson, *c.* 1745. Yale Center for British Art, Paul Mellon Collection.

11. English exercise chair, *c.* 1840–1900. © Science Museum Group.

12. *Cricket Match Played by the Countess of Derby and Other Ladies*, 1779.

13. *The Fair Toxophilites*, by William Powell Frith, 1872. IanDagnall Computing / Alamy.

14. Macfadden's *Physical Culture*, 1921. Pictorial Press Ltd / Alamy.

15. *Mrs Bennett, Afflicted with a Skin Disease*, *c.* 1818–21. Wellcome Collection.

16. *Pompadour at Her Toilette*, by François Boucher, 1750. Harvard Art Museums / Fogg Museum, Bequest of Charles E. Dunlap. © President and Fellows of Harvard College.

17. Box for rouge and patches, *c.* 1750–5. Metropolitan Museum of Art, Bequest of Kate Read Blacque, in memory of her husband, Valentine Alexander Blacque, 1937.

18. Chamois Face Leather packing box, early twentieth century. Photographed in the collection of the National Liberation Museum 1944–1945.

19. *Transplanting of Teeth*, by Thomas Rowlandson, 1787. Wellcome Collection.

20. *A French Dentist Shewing a Specimen of his Artificial Teeth and False Palates*, by Thomas Rowlandson, 1811. Wellcome Collection.

21. Upper set of vulcanite dentures with wooden box, 1850. British Dental Association Museum / Science Photo Library.

22. 'Reach for a Lucky Instead', advertisement, 1930. Stanford School of Medicine, Stanford Research into the Impact of Tobacco Advertising, CC BY-SA 4.0 DEED.

IN THE TEXT

NOTE ON CONVENTIONS

In quotations, original spelling, punctuation, and capitalisation have been retained throughout.

The pre-decimal currency in Britain consisted of pounds, shillings, and pence, indicated by the symbols £ s d. Under this system there were four farthings in a penny (d), twelve pennies in a shilling (s), and twenty shillings in a pound (£).

The Bank of England calculates that goods and services costing £1 in 1660 would have cost £1 17s 2d in 1800, £1 7s 9d in 1900, and £159.70 in 2021: see https://www.measuringworth.com/ukcompare.

Before decimalisation, Britain used imperial units of weight. There were sixteen ounces (oz) to the pound (lb), fourteen pounds to a stone, and eight stone to a hundredweight.

I use the term 'Black' to denote people of African descent, recognising that racial categories are mutable and that over the centuries Blackness has denoted many different ethnic groups. I have not capitalised 'white' when the term refers to an ethnic category, but I do make it clear that it is not a natural description of appearance and that 'whiteness' is socially constructed.

I am conscious of sizeism and have used the word 'fat' not 'overweight', although I occasionally resort to 'plump' for variety. I also use 'corpulence', favoured in the nineteenth century. The World Health Organization formally recognised obesity as a global epidemic in 1997, designating it a major public health problem. I use the term 'obesity' in that context.

PREFACE AND ACKNOWLEDGEMENTS

This book looks at how women's quest for perfection and social acceptance has dominated their lives over centuries, often at the cost of their health. It takes in the effect of household manuals, physicians, quacks, advertising, social media, and other influences on public opinion about the norms of health and beauty. It reflects a wide spectrum of women's experience, drawing on a variety of historical examples and on poignant accounts from diaries and personal letters. Sources are paramount. These evocative stories from the past inform the continuing critical debate about what it means to be a woman.

In the West, beauty topics and concerns about body shape and health continue to take up much space in all media. There are studies focusing on corsetry and makeup, but no one has looked in such detail at multiple aspects of the body in women's quest for health and beauty. No one has considered how a spectrum of beauty practices has developed over centuries. And no one has touched on the impact of these bodily treatments on gender definition, social and racial inequality, and the sense of ageing.

This is a study of women. Men may face similar pressures, but most communication about beauty, shaping how it is perceived and valued in society, is aimed squarely at women. The social demands of fashioning the body have long moulded the female experience of private and public life. This book tries to capture women's lived experience of consuming health and beauty products, of maintaining a desired weight, and the excitement, or trauma, of adopting the latest fashion trends.

In all countries, evolving definitions of beauty are part of national history, and still resonate today. Here, the focus is on British society, but there are extended comparisons to life in the United States, since British and American culture have long influenced each other. Britain and North America are notably multicultural, which broadens the inclusivity of this study. There are contextual references to Europe, especially to France, since British women were alert to French fashions and beauty trends. And examples are drawn from British colonies.

The starting point for this study is the mid-seventeenth century. Health and beauty manuals did circulate earlier, but by 1650 such works were part of a broader movement. Among the European elite, they were already coloured by luxury consumption, itself a marker of wealth and taste, and a spur to international trade.

This work is not an attempt to define beauty – never a static concept – although it does distinguish between beauty and fashion. It centres on women's quest to be considered attractive, giving their own viewpoint wherever possible. It covers the pursuit of health insofar as that relates to good looks and wellbeing, not the cure of specific illnesses. It includes personal exercise regimes but does not extend to the larger world of sport.

The approach is holistic: successive chapters cover not only cosmetics, skin, hair, corsets, diets, and the emulation of physical role models, but also dental health, hygiene, and spa retreats. There is much piquant and humorous detail, not least because the book also explores the lotions, deodorants, undergarments, spells, and beauty aids which have seduced users throughout the centuries. This coverage can be quixotic and entertaining, although sensational claims based on flimsy evidence – such as the notion that Victorian women consumed tapeworm eggs to lose weight – receive no credit. That said, this study shows that a great many beauty practices are bound up with the unfair treatment of women and with oppressive concepts of cultural deficiency.

Taken as a whole, the book reveals the socially constructed underpinnings of femininity, its constant state of flux, and the expression of gender identities beyond the binary framework of male and female. In the seventeenth century, for instance, fashionable women wore skintight, male riding coats above their skirts, to the discomfort of conservative male onlookers like Samuel Pepys. In the eighteenth century, the Chevalier d'Éon, a former captain of dragoons and an expert swordsman, spent the last thirty years of his life in female dress, even daring to fence in public wearing a petticoat.

Studies of health and beauty have generally focused on upper- and middle-class white women. This study strives to be much more inclusive, as far as sources allow, and captures women's voices from a wider social range. The pursuit of health and beauty inevitably also underscores issues of class and social inequality. Extreme fashion statements like the crinoline were prohibitively cumbersome for agricultural and industrial labourers, and often banned in factories, yet thousands of factory workers depended for their livelihoods on the manufacture of steel hoops to support wide skirts. A diverse workforce was reliant on the changing demands of health and beauty, not least because extensive industries grew up that both shaped and catered for social expectations. The book features blatant examples of conspicuous consumption and emulation but also includes fascinating insights into the role of technology in shaping the body.

A history of ideas of beauty cannot be separated from ideas about race or the history of colonialism; the realities and legacies of how women's beauty was treated in British colonies continue to affect British society today. The centrality of white women's history in Britain is in part a consequence of demography: West Indians only began to migrate to the United Kingdom in large numbers from the 1950s. Even so, the white person's experience should not be treated as normative. There is no absolute position from which ideas of beauty can be viewed or judged; these ideas are bound up with issues of identity, and different identities underwrite different values.

This study highlights the historical aspects of 'whiteness', the ways in which it has been socially constructed, and how it has functioned within the wider history of race and colonialism. The insights offered are incomplete and fallible but do help to contextualise contemporary debate about the ways in which gender, race, and class shape the lives of groups co-existing in Europe.[1] There is not the same extent of primary source material across the centuries for Black women in Britain as for white, owing to racism and inequities, even though historians have done considerable recovery work to reveal the experiences of Black women and women of colour in relation to beauty. Occasionally, I have referenced the African American experience to help fill gaps, despite there being only a partial overlap between the experiences of Black American and Black British women, since Black British cultures are specific. I have taken the advice of Black colleagues and experts in their field, and I hope that this book is a springboard for other, more detailed readings of this subject. We certainly should not assume that just because there are fewer historical sources for Black, working-class, or queer women, these marginalised figures were not active in all areas of beauty culture.

The book contributes to discussion about 'fashioning the body', as championed by feminist writers and cultural commentators. It extends beyond the subject of dress and fashion history. It touches on the role of moralists, but also looks at the development of consumer goods and the pressures of commercial society. It shows how the pursuit of beauty entails making the personal a public issue, how selling creates pressures of expectation, and how even attempts to reject such expectation can be commodified. It takes in debate about whether cosmetics contribute to female oppression or enable women to create their own identity, considers the role of technology and industry in self-presentation, and explores the influence of mass advertising and sport on perceptions of the body. It also looks at the effect of contemporary platforms, including social media, which offer fresh opportunities to explore gender and ethnic identity through self-presentation.

The scope of this book allows it to expose connections between fields often treated separately. And the 400-year time frame allows for an analysis of change and continuities. There are unifying themes, notably women's resilience and creativity in finding opportunities within the social constraints imposed on them. In addition, an emphasis on human stories allows readers to judge how past lives resonate with lived experience today. The result is an intriguing exploration of how women through the ages have come to terms with their looks and with the natural processes of growing old. Crucially, this book investigates topics that society continues to have strong opinions about, revealing anxieties about health in an era of pandemics, and thoughts about the pursuit of 'beauty' today.

I would like to thank my agent, Maggie Hanbury, and my editor, Julian Loose, for their support throughout. I am grateful to the expert team at Yale, especially to Frazer Martin for his close reading of the manuscript, to Rachael Lonsdale and to Lucy Buchan. I also owe a debt of thanks to the copyeditor, Hester Higton, and to Yale's anonymous reviewers, who did much to shape the proposal and who commented helpfully and in detail on the final draft.

The University of Portsmouth's Centre for Port Cities and Maritime Cultures has provided a stimulating intellectual environment for this project, while the Women's Studies Group 1558–1837 has offered a welcoming forum for the exchange of ideas. I am indebted to expert staff at the British Library, the Caird Library, the Institute of Historical Research, and the London Metropolitan Archives, and to Delia Gaze for the use of helpful source material.

Special thanks are due to Rose Sinclair, who gave up her time to read several draft chapters and who made vital suggestions; her support and critical eye have improved the manuscript considerably. I am fortunate to have benefited from Olivia Wyatt's insightful comments on the manuscript. She saved me from several errors, and her professional insights have proved invaluable. I am grateful to Roger Knight and to other members of the Cumberland Society who offered encouragement at a critical juncture. I would also like to thank hairstylist Shaan Amber, and Janice Knox-Goba and Olawa Mabayoje of JKG Organic Ltd, for sharing their expertise. As ever, my greatest thanks go to my family, especially to Annie, for the initial idea, and to my husband, Andrew, who has cheerfully read every word.

INTRODUCTION

From antiquity to modern times, people through the ages have been obsessed with health and beauty, and no wonder. Personal appearance has always been linked to power, status, morality, and self-identity. And yet perceptions of beauty depend on the eye of the beholder and vary with race, culture, sexual orientation, gender identity, class, and historical period.

This book looks at women's pursuit of health and beauty, chiefly in Britain, and at how this pursuit has evolved over the last four hundred years. The subject risks being dismissed as trifling, but it brings insights into the deeper realities of life. It shows women not just as consumers but as agents trying to determine their place in the world. It touches upon such varied topics as self-identity and the role of women, mostly white and well-to-do, in furthering trade and colonisation. And it shows how notions of beauty helped to marginalise other women, including those who were victims of colonisation.

Of course, women have always adorned and shaped their bodies according to personal preference and convention. Health and beauty tips circulated widely in oral culture and featured in household manuals long before the production of makeup and toiletries became mega-industries. But personal adornment is a form of communication; it can

1

signify social status and even political opinion. The subject of health and beauty also throws light on issues of gender identity, since the body is integral to our experience and performance of gender.

Health and beauty concerns are life-changing, which helps to explain why they are so often linked to wish-fulfilment stories and why beauty products routinely promise some fairy-tale transformation. This attractive possibility helps to explain the enduring popularity of the Cinderella story and the appeal of television makeover programmes. The story has been told in its present form since the seventeenth century, while adaptations for opera and film have encouraged gender-fluid interpretations, helping to keep it relevant. Even so, the ambiguity of the Cinderella tale reflects the ambivalence of many tips about health and beauty, which often fail to have any effect. Cinderella is usually defined in contrast to her 'ugly' or proud sisters but she is not necessarily pretty. What marks her out is the size of her foot, which few adults can alter. Her shoe size hints at an innate claim to higher status; even in Victorian times, small feet were taken to be a sign that the owner did not belong to 'the walking classes'.[1]

There is a dark side to this long-standing preoccupation with personal appearance. Some early makeup contained white lead and other dangerous ingredients that seared the skin; in extreme cases, wearing a corset and tight-lacing for a petite waist deformed the rib cage; the history of dental care has its own gallery of horrors. Women's quest for beauty holds dangers even today. Crazes such as CoolSculpting, or the freezing of unwanted fat cells, have led to disfigurement. Home treatments purchased online can also carry risks: Apetamin, a drug which promises weight gain and fashionable, Kardashian-type curves, has been linked to liver damage. But health and beauty advice has always mixed sensible tips with flavour-of-the-month panaceas. This book throws a spotlight on historic fads, and it produces surprising revelations. A spa town was often no health retreat but a glorious opportunity to indulge in a giddy round of entertainment. Sea bathing for the constitution prompted voyeurism on a startling scale. Men carried telescopes, not to look out to sea, but to train them on beach beauties. Even supposedly staid Victorian women clustered near bathing machines to watch men swimming naked.

Health and beauty topics are always newsworthy because we all have a body. Variations only add interest. We may be tall or short, have proportionally longer legs and arms, or a longer spine (which makes for a smaller waist). And we all change shape as we grow up and grow old. The relative plasticity of the body encourages us to think that with inclination and resolve we can mould it to whatever shape is the current ideal. And the growth of industries producing dietary supplements shows that health is understood to be integral to achieving the desired look. Just as our identity is formed through social interaction, so our body is shaped by social and cultural forces which motivate us to adapt it. In turn, the appearance and condition of our bodies influence our physical and emotional experience. We are always conscious of the effect our appearance has on others, which is why many of us like to edit selfies. The body is so firmly implicated in a range of power relations that personal appearance can be a source of anxiety, although women do take pleasure in beauty products and the opportunities they offer for self-expression. In short, individuals naturally desire to control their own bodies. To the extent that anyone can be bothered, the body can also be treated as an artwork. In the early twentieth century, artists associated with futurism did just that and wrote a manifesto about it.

Historically, women's bodies have been moulded in ways calculated to improve their life chances. This examination of women's pursuit of health and beauty over four hundred years illuminates their position in society, their role within the family, and changes over time. Beauty practices are inevitably connected to class because beauty is high-maintenance and takes time and money. A focus on health and beauty also illuminates a broader context of social, cultural, racial, economic, and political factors. In tracing how women presented themselves, we can gain insights into their experience of contemporary science and medicine, or of changing patterns of consumption with the growth of empire. Many white women mentioned in this book were Londoners when the capital was an imperial metropolis. Their lives offer opportunities to glimpse how empire was experienced 'at home', just when an ideal of female beauty was closely connected to Britain's sense of its 'civilising mission' in the colonies. Finally, the material culture relating to health and beauty reveals changing social values, especially regarding hygiene. To explore a history of health and beauty is to get a better understanding of how we have come to think about modernity.

It can be hard to find women's voices from the past. Only the elite could devote funds and leisure to their personal appearance, so it is even more difficult to trace opinions from the lower classes and women of colour. In some sources it helps to think about what is not being said. And since beauty is often treated as competitive, accounts can be intentionally unfair. Many of the examples included here are of elite white women who were knowingly on display and understood that their entire appearance conveyed a spectrum of meanings that would be assessed; but other voices feature wherever possible.

BEAUTY AND OPPRESSION

There is a long tradition of criticising women for enhancing their looks. For centuries, women of all classes were discouraged from the overt pursuit of beautification, which is one reason why it is hard to find them writing about it. Such censure can seem deeply misogynistic, as in Jonathan Swift's poem 'The Progress of Beauty' (1719), which describes how a young woman rises from her pillow a mass of dirt and sweat. She needs four whole hours at her dressing table before she can pass for a beautiful woman. The same theme was often rehearsed in satirical prints, as in Thomas Rowlandson's *Six Stages of Mending a Face* (1792), which shows an ageing woman transforming her appearance with a wig, a fake eye, false teeth, and cosmetics. Rowlandson's immediate target was Lady Archer, an aristocrat who hosted private gambling parties. These parties were technically illegal, and ladies who played for high stakes were eventually fined in 1797. While Archer happened to be a redhead, not a good look at the time, the chief cause of Rowlandson's disgust was the amount of makeup she wore. It indicated that she was basically ugly and had something to hide. Male criticism of women using fake hair and fake teeth resurfaced in the Victorian period, after progress in the manufacture of dentures lowered prices and brought them to the masses.[2] The fear of not being able to distinguish between true beauty and the artificial kind is a deep-seated one.

Makeup itself has long produced moral uncertainty. In some contexts, visible makeup was associated with prostitution; in others, it made women seem more respectable. There is a kind of ambivalence in the very process of making up, since, as soon as onlookers notice its effects, they become aware of a difference between the veneer of makeup and the face itself. After 1850, the anxiety surrounding women's use of cosmetics and what the habit said about their temperament was compounded by notorious court cases involving wives charged with poisoning their husbands. Arsenic was easily obtainable in the Victorian era; some white women ate it for a youthful pallor. Branded arsenic wafers (pills) and arsenical lotions to remove blemishes were openly marketed. They worked by poisoning the blood so that it carried fewer red blood cells to organs; anaemia then left the skin clear and pale. The body can tolerate a little arsenic but when husbands died in mysterious circumstances, wives were suspected of feeding them large quantities. The crime was hard to prove but in one notorious case Florence Maybrick was sentenced to life imprisonment in 1889 for murdering her husband with arsenic. Only an element of doubt saved her from being hanged.

Criticism of women's clandestine use of cosmetics was heightened by the controversy surrounding Madame Rachel Leverson, whose beauty treatments were not only fraudulent but also seemed to encourage her female customers to deceive men. She set up shop in London around 1860, selling exotic-sounding beauty products. Her business failed and she was sent to debtors' prison. On her release she tried again; this time, due to her flair for advertising, she began to prosper. The title of her marketing pamphlet was 'Beautiful for Ever' and it became her catchphrase. She targeted older women and special-ised in 'enamelling' the face and décolletage. This was a form of face painting. The skin was prepared with an alkaline wash, then painted with a semi-paste of whitening agents, which also helped to fill wrinkles and depressions. Well-to-do women visited Leverson's premises in secret, as the process was frowned upon. She soon dabbled in intimida-tion and fraud – blackmailing clients to pay her large sums for continued treatment and secrecy, even convincing one woman that she had gained the affections of an aristocrat.

Madame Rachel was tried for fraud in 1868, found guilty, and given a five-year sentence. She was prosecuted for the same offence in 1878, dying in prison two years later. At trial, she was depicted as an evil force, preying on the gullible. Some suspected she was also involved in an abortionist racket. Her harsh sentences reveal both racial prejudice (she was Jewish) and male opposition to successful businesswomen able to rise above their class at a time when the ideal woman was supposed to be in the home. The publicity surrounding her trials helped to give cosmetics a bad name. 'Beautiful for ever' became a Victorian tag line for false praise and blatant artificiality that disguised the truth. The successful music-hall performer and songwriter Arthur Lloyd even turned the Leverson case into a ditty, 'Mrs Mary Plucker Sparrowtail, or Beautiful for Ever'. It was an enormous hit, making female vanity and cosmetics an even greater topic of derision.

Body size is another area of discrimination and fat-shaming is by no means a recent phenomenon. In the past, elite women who happened to be unusually heavy were easy targets of satirical prints and private gossip. Albinia Hobart, made Countess of Buckinghamshire in 1793, grew increasingly fat with successive pregnancies. Her size was taken to be a sign of aristocratic luxury. Together with her gambling habit, it made her an object of ridicule, especially after the French Revolution, when many feared that the degenerate habits of the rich threatened social order. Some of the prints targeting her carried heavy sexual innu-endo, suggesting that her size was a bar to sexual relations. At the time,

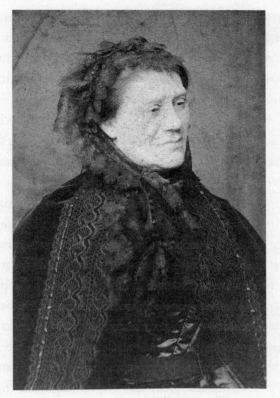

1. Madame Rachel (c. 1814–80) at the time of her first trial in 1868.

fat girls had difficulty finding husbands on the marriage market, as prospective in-laws feared that their bulk might make them infertile. This was true of the eldest sister of Louis XVI, nicknamed Gros-Madame. She had a pleasant enough face, but 'features . . . drowned in fat'.[3] She did eventually marry but remained childless, though subjected to the distressing infertility treatments of the age.

Ideals of female beauty are built around constructed racist as well as sexist boundaries. The concept of 'whiteness' is a social construct. White skin was early used as a marker to differentiate the rich from peasants forced to labour outdoors. In the colonial period it became racialised and was called into play to help maintain and justify cruel and oppressive power relations among different peoples. This study shows the growth of the concept of whiteness and racialised beauty. It extends to issues related to the health and beauty of Black and Asian women, but the complex area of the sexual objectification of Black women's bodies falls mostly outside its remit.

That said, it is impossible to pass over the outrageous exhibition of Sarah Baartman, a Khoikhoi woman from South Africa. Also known as Sara or Saartjie (the Afrikaans diminutive of Sarah), she was brought to Europe in 1810 and exhibited in freak shows in Britain and France. Derisively marketed as 'The Hottentot Venus', her protuberant buttocks were exposed to view for the titillation of male visitors and to satisfy lurid curiosity. After her death, in 1815, Baartman's dismembered and dissected body was kept in Paris until her remains were returned to South Africa for burial in 2002. Plaster casts of her body parts were used to help calibrate socially constructed differences between white and Black female beauty. Scrutinised according to Eurocentric tenets of scientific racism, her statistics were used to bolster arguments for white supremacy. She was held to be a naturally inferior example of humanity, from which Western biological advancement could be measured. Scientific racism has been totally discredited but it long influenced attitudes towards Black women, fostering myths such as the notion that they can better tolerate pain.

Baartman's story, now widely known, has assumed cultural significance as the epitome of both colonial exploitation and the fetishisation of the Black female body. She has become an icon to women who have experienced discrimination. The rumour in 2016 that Beyoncé was about to finance and star in a film based on Baartman's story prompted outrage. Beyoncé was denounced as lacking in basic human dignity and accused of further exploiting Baartman in order to reinvent herself as a serious writer and actor.[4]

Baartman's tours were well publicised. The mockery prompted by her distinctive contours may have partly mirrored the policing of white women's bodies. As early as 1786 there was a print in circulation among elite circles of a naked white woman with gigantic breasts and huge buttocks. Entitled *A Modern Venus, or a Lady of the Present Fashion in the state of nature*, it was based on a drawing of 1785 made by the artist Mary Hoare, who had been trained by her father, William, a portraitist in Bath. The drawing seems to have been made for the amusement of female friends; it mocked the fashions of the time. But the writer and collector Horace Walpole at once saw its commercial potential and had it printed. The resemblance between this satirical image and later prints of Baartman is marked.

Representations of Black beauty long remained elusive. In 1800, Britain had a population of about 10.5 million, of which some 10,000 were Black according to historians, although contemporary reports put the figure at around 20,000.[5] But white people rarely encountered Black people outside ports and industrial towns, and in the paintings of white artists, Black figures were seldom the central focus; wealthy visitors to galleries and studios in Britain and Europe were thus able to disregard their presence in works of art. Few white scholars and artists admitted that ideals of feminine beauty were culturally relative.[6] From the later nineteenth century on, attempts to foster imperial pride in Britain had the effect of increasing condescension towards colonial peoples. This was evident in myriad forms of popular culture. For example, world festivals were organised for the British public which presented Africans as curiosities in mocked-up villages. In 1895, around eighty Somalians were displayed at Crystal Palace in traditional dress.

Dismissive representations of Black people, and educational projects involving demeaning human displays, helped to promote an ideology of racism. Favourable publicity surrounding key Black figures did little to counteract negative views. Queen Victoria's goddaughter Sara Forbes Bonetta, a princess of the Egbado clan of the Yorubas in West Africa, was much admired for her beauty and intelligence, and there were popular Black entertainers such as Elisabeth Welch. But Black looks were consistently undervalued, which helped to feed racial prejudice.

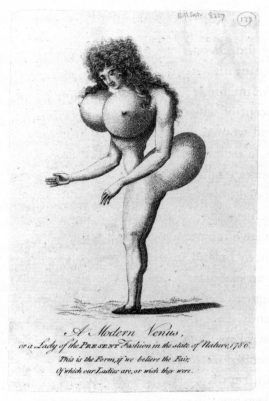

A Modern Venus,
or a Lady of the PRESENT Fashion in the state of Nature, 1786.
This is the Form, if we believe the Fair,
Of which our Ladies are, or wish they were.

2. A satire on the body shape needed to suit the extravagant fashions
of 1780s Britain.

Recently, the lack of representations of Black beauty in galleries has been addressed by such artists as Lynette Yiadom-Boakye. Her enigmatic portraits of fictitious women of colour are appropriately timeless, with minimal background detail assigning them to a particular period. But the ideology attached to the concept of whiteness still enables systemic racism today, feeding on racial oppression and contributing to it. In many social contexts where white people are in the majority, whiteness is so normalised as to be rendered invisible, and the notion of white privilege is hotly disputed. As this book shows, beauty standards are rooted in various forms of oppression.

ASPIRING TO BEAUTY

Women, heavily judged on their looks, may aspire to beauty for the status and opportunities it brings. On this front they are open to manipulation. An infamous example dates from around 1800 when the fashionable concept of white beauty mimicked the fatal symptoms of tuberculosis. Frail women were suddenly in vogue. Among the upper classes, thinness, a pallor that accentuated blue veins, sparkling eyes, and flushed cheeks (really all signs of a constant slight fever) were admired as the height of 'hectic beauty'. Healthy women endured self-deprivation to achieve the ghostly but feverish look.

Young girls were often prepared to withstand torments as martyrs to beauty. In southern Ireland in the 1780s, Dorothea Herbert and her friends evolved an elaborate routine to obtain pale skin and willowy frames. They went to bed wrapped up like greasy pomatum sticks in paper, 'Our Hands, Faces, and Chests were compleatly cover'd with Tallow and Brown Paper, made into various sorts of Ointments – Our Arms were Suspended in the Air by strong Ropes fastend to the Tester of the Bed – Our feet tied to the Valance to stretch our Legs and Make us grow tall.'[7] Sleep was difficult. When summer came, they wore thick linen veils to preserve the milky complexion achieved with such sacrifice.

It was commonly understood that pain was necessary to achieve beauty. Some Victorian women put up with daily discomfort to produce the fantastic bodily contours dictated by fashion. The moral expectations of women of the time, especially middle-class women, also involved restraint. Domestic handbooks preached selflessness, charity, and self-discipline. This mental rigour coloured women's domestic management. With the growing appreciation of the importance of hygiene, it became a woman's responsibility to maintain standards of domestic cleanliness. It was also her duty to preserve her youth and neat appearance. Some women appreciated that such standards afforded them a leadership role. Susan Cocroft, author of *The Duty of Beauty*

(1915), advised that it was women's privilege to cultivate a beautiful body and charming manners, 'because they educate, refine and uplift. Thus they are most potent agencies in usefulness; they "allure to brighter worlds and lead the way".'[8] From this viewpoint, the cultivation of beauty was not vanity but a noble route to uplifting the world and redeeming it from sordidness and gloom. Often the outcome was that women internalised subtle forms of control which then took on the character of benign self-discipline.

Some, like Madame Rachel, found opportunities to make a good living from the burgeoning beauty industry, and so became implicated in the commercial exploitation of female hopes and fears related to appearance. Commercial pressures intensified existing constraints related to class, race, moral convention, and sexuality. Today, women are bombarded with images of how they should look. In an image-conscious, consumer culture, women's bodies are increasingly commodified. Even when this development is laid bare, it is still hard to buck the trend. Women who do not 'beautify' themselves, or who choose to follow non-standard views of beauty, are judged accordingly.

Even so, women are not passive victims of oppressive male standards of beauty. They help to develop those standards through creative innovation and by expressing stylistic preferences. And this has always been the case, despite opposition. In 1930, one female columnist complained that women had only to wear a little waistcoat or shirt blouse for observers to complain that they were becoming totally unsexed and indistinguishable from men. Yet even she underestimated women's determination to innovate and dress as they pleased. She wrongly predicted that women of the future would never adopt as a fashion item anything so unflattering as trousers.[9]

Some argue that by engaging with the world of beauty, the cosmetics market, and works on fashion, women collude in their own oppression. But they can be followers of fashion and creative agents at the same time. This book shows that for centuries women's experiences have been framed by beauty culture, by bodily practices, and by the cultural meaning inherent in such rituals. Yet these same practices have also helped them to create and re-create individual identities. Rapid self-reinvention can be a source of pleasure. As early as 1890, one woman reviewed all the arguments for and against using cosmetics, and concluded, 'After all is said and done every woman will simply do as she likes – if she likes to powder she will do so, if she does not, mayhap she will leave it alone!'[10]

In the last thirty years, there has been a new medium for the discussion of beauty: the Internet, offering instant publication worldwide. It favours images, concise text, and topicality to foster immediate engagement. It enables self-publication and encourages apparently straight-shooting health and beauty directives such as 'Make this year your best running year yet!' At the same time, it offers an outlet that magnifies trivial anxieties: 'Does sitting make your butt flat?', 'Are you worried about runner's face?' Online content is larded with advertisements, and marketing ploys are often concealed, meaning that women must be ever more adept at evading forces that seek to exert power and control. On the plus side, social media is an unrivalled platform for passing on beauty tips and explaining how to achieve certain styles. Black people credit it with helping to advance the natural hair movement among young people, so that Afro hair is increasingly worn in traditional styles, although the trend is decades old. Young women who create content for these platforms build enormous influence online, perhaps at the expense of their privacy.

Beauty culture remains deeply controversial. This book shows how the obsession for perfection can dominate women's lives. It illustrates the making of modern women – not just the external aspects of how they presented themselves and were perceived, but also how they felt about the process of preparing themselves to be looked at, and the pressures such scrutiny placed on them. It explores women's lived experience, their resilience, and their creativity in finding opportunities within the social constraints placed on them. We are increasingly aware that physical health and beauty relate to mental health and wellbeing.

Regrettably, much writing on the topic, particularly that on social media, still seems designed to make women hate their bodies more.

If at one level this book is about women's search to make the most of their appearance and feel better about themselves, at another it explores the economic, political, social, and cultural aspects of that search. Chapters are devoted to specific themes, and work to build up an integrated picture of this wider context. Beginning with body shape, the book also considers diet and exercise, skin, makeup, hygiene, teeth, hair, and spas and sea bathing. Beauty can be policed in ways thought to uphold social stability, or owned and kept veiled, or treated as a currency and exploited for commercial gain. That said, to a greater or lesser extent all individuals project onto the body their ambitions, creativity, and sense of self. In Western societies, each woman, whatever her race, class, or background, uses health and beauty practices to help create a unique identity.

ৡ 1 ৢ

BODY SCULPTURE

We are used to iconic images of royal power that emphasise body shape: the square, padded figure of Henry VIII of England in fleshy middle age, feet planted apart, codpiece thrusting forward; the painfully conical torso of his daughter Elizabeth I, surrounded by an enormous farthingale, an embodiment of virginal majesty; the hand-on-hip pose of the ageing Louis XIV of France, exhibiting his shapely, silk-stockinged legs and thighs up to an alarming height. We relish stories about the excessive consumption of rulers and celebrities, and the agonies they endured afterwards to achieve a body shape that suited contemporary trends. Famously, Britain's George IV had a stomach that hung down to his knees by the time he reached his sixties. He was cruelly mocked and unable to silence critics. After all, his waist measured fifty inches even after he had squeezed into a tight corset.

But how did ordinary people sculpt their bodies? Women – and some men – have long worn garments to support and shape the body to match the vogues, morals, and cultural dynamics of the day. Any fashionable silhouette creates an intriguing interplay with idealised concepts of the human form. Nudes were rarely seen before the nineteenth century, other than in a few religious or mythical paintings. Greek statues had a key role in forming a culturally constructed, ideal body image. From about 1660, the upper classes encountered classical statues as part of their education, when the Grand Tour through France and Italy became a customary stage in the education of young men, and a few women. In Paris, they mingled with the elite to polish their manners; in Rome and Florence, they encountered the masterpieces of classical antiquity. For some, gazing at nude statues was an elite form of pornography. Happily, it also catered for same-sex attraction. The Venus de' Medici, a Hellenistic statue of the goddess of love, soon became the pattern of female beauty. It was much copied for stately homes and gardens, but Venus's unfettered limbs stood in uneasy juxtaposition with the corseted and padded body of the contemporary woman of fashion. These white statues were also deeply racialised. They made it easier for the powerful upper classes to take no account of the Black female body, and helped to prioritise whiteness within the colonial order.[1]

This chapter explores the devices used to alter women's body shapes and looks at why such garments were worn, how they influenced behaviour, and what meanings they held. Different eras have placed a premium on different parts of the female body. The monied classes in seventeenth-century western Europe commissioned flattering portraits that reveal the importance placed on white female bosoms. In later centuries, society was fixated on a tiny female waist. Undergarments for women have generally compressed the stomach, nipped in the waist, added curves to the hips, and lifted or sometimes flattened the breasts. Trendsetters have been wonderfully inventive: from the late seventeenth century, the female silhouette has been shaped by panniers (side hoops), stays, bum rolls, cork rumps, the crinoline cage, bustles, corsets, stomach belts, girdles, and push-up brassieres. These devices have provided the basic shape needed to set off outer clothes, themselves designed to express the wearer's sexuality, personality, class, and social status.

Body-shaping devices have always provoked conflicting opinions. Restrictive undergarments were early linked to female oppression.

When in 1717 Lady Mary Wortley Montagu travelled to Turkey with her ambassador husband, she visited a hammam. Turkish women, naked in the steam baths, urged her to join them, and she had to reveal her whaleboned stays to avoid undressing. The women sympathised at once, assuming that a jealous husband had locked her into some infernal 'machine'.[2] Their reaction caused Montagu to question her sense of self, as well as the social norms of her time. Yet women usually welcome some breast support, and many have viewed the shaping of their bodies as empowering and even creative. Are specific silhouettes largely imposed on them by men, or do they show women taking control of their own bodies? Opinion about this has long been divided and arguments in support of either view are mostly simplified and polarised.

BODICES AND STAYS

A kind of corset, called a bodice, was developed in renaissance Italy and introduced into the French court in the mid-sixteenth century. It was stiffened with whalebone, sometimes with metal or wood, and fastened by lacing. By some odd trick of fashion, it compressed female waists just when men were sporting doublets with a low, pointed waist and padded 'peascod belly' which made them look pregnant. But across Europe women soon adopted the bodice. In England it was often known as a 'pair of bodys' because it was made in two sections, usually laced in the front. This undergarment did not touch the skin; it was worn over a linen shift, which helped to keep it clean. It might also have detachable sleeves and be worn visibly, for show.

A well-fitting bodice supported the bosom and pinched in the waist, making the waist appear smaller in relation to the full skirts that women wore. It pushed the bust up but did not artificially separate it – male interest lay in the mounds of the breasts visible above the bodice. Given that the rest of the female body was well covered, breasts became the centre of erotic attraction. When Samuel Pepys caught sight of Nell Gwyn at the door of her lodgings in Drury Lane, it was her upper body that attracted him: 'In her smock-sleeves and bodice, looking upon one – she seemed a mighty pretty creature.'[3]

Women with money had their bodices made to measure and demanded comfort as well as a good fit. At the end of the seventeenth century, Dorothy Wood, a merchant's wife, made the sixteen-mile coach journey from their country estate into London just to purchase a new bodice. She complained in a letter to her husband that after three visits the bodice maker still had not got the shape right, so she would be late coming home.[4] Given the expense of a trip to London, her efforts show how important it was to have a well-fitting, flattering garment.

By the early eighteenth century, the term 'stays' had replaced 'bodice'. For a time, the two words were used interchangeably, but eventually 'bodice' was reserved for a bodice coat, worn over tight stays. Women also had the option of wearing 'jumps', the name given to stays that were lightly boned or not boned at all. Jumps, laced at the front, gave the bust light support but did not shape the torso. Some wearers thought them a healthy choice and wore them for leisure or during pregnancy. This gave rise to lewd banter: that a woman who loosened her stays might soon find she could barely squeeze into jumps.

A pair of stays signalled the wearer's status and there were minutely graded versions for different consumers. High-end garments could be elaborate and expensive, made of coloured silk or satin, embroidered in silver and gold, or decorated with gold and silver lace. For this reason, they were often stolen; clothes were easily turned into ready money at pawn shops. No wonder that some owners had their names embroidered into the shoulder straps so that their property could be identified.

Stays moulded the upper body but were not necessarily uncomfortable if laced just to fit snugly; stiff tabs at the lower edge eased out over the hips to support and give fullness to the petticoat. The wearer could not bend at the waist but, for labouring women, this helped to prevent back pain: they had no choice but to bend their legs and keep a straight back when lifting heavy loads. When they did need to lean over, they loosened their stays. Francis Place, a London tailor who grew up in the

1780s, remembered watching poor women hard at work over their washing tubs in the street, 'their leather stays half laced and as black as the door posts', their breasts exposed.[5] Even so, it was accepted that women would strive for an upright posture most of the time. A whalebone busk or stiffener made of wood, ivory, or metal could also be slotted down the front of the stays for a flatter shape and to prevent stays from wrinkling uncomfortably. Sailors on whaling ships carved busks from whalebone in their free time, as an intimate gift for their sweethearts, but long busks did make sitting difficult.

There were variations in the way stays were cut: French stays always had cachet and usually set the trend, but Italian stays were also popular. Then, in 1753, the artist William Hogarth set out his theory of aesthetics in his *Analysis of Beauty*, in which he argued that S-shaped, curved lines were more attractive than straight ones, illustrating his point with drawings of female stays and the curved calf of the male leg. His book prompted debate, but afterwards the pattern for stays did gain a more noticeable curve, emphasising the waist and the breasts. Some designs did not permit women to lift their arms above shoulder height – a sure indication of social class because wearers would have found hard labour impossible. Eighteenth-century stays were usually back-laced, another indication of status because wearers often needed help to dress – although most families (except for the very poor) had at least one maidservant.

There was obviously social pressure to sculpt the upper half of the female body. It was considered lax to appear in public without stays; only the most degraded class of women went without them. Francis Place remembered such women in his childhood, all habitually drunk. Their gowns were low round the neck and open at the front, and in warm weather they wore no handkerchiefs around their shoulders so that 'the breasts of many hung down in the most disgusting manner'.[6]

In contrast, firmly laced stays signalled self-control and therefore virtue as well as status. This was especially the case in Britain. An advert for a 'Good, Tight, Clean Chambermaid' in 1736 typically insisted that she should not wear 'Stays Low before' because she must set a modest example.[7] Outer appearance was held to be a sign of inner character. Since prostitutes were identified by their lack of stays and consequent 'Airiness of their Dress', fashionable ladies who went about town in loose morning gowns and padded waistcoats, rather than stays, risked being compared to whores.[8] Even the loosening of stays after a hearty dinner led to bawdy gossip: in Catholic France when one aristocratic lady took such measures, onlookers furtively debated whether she was swelled with the Holy Spirit or just suffering from wind.[9] Social convention, linked to assumptions about sexual behaviour, operated as a powerful incentive on women to lace up.

If a married woman received male visitors without being firmly laced in stays, it was taken as a sign of wantonness. Servants, always on the lookout for rumpled cushions, hair powder on sofas, disordered dress, and other signs of illicit affairs, readily volunteered such details if cases of adultery came to court. When Admiral Knowles accused his wife of sleeping with a naval captain who visited the house, a maidservant testified, 'My Mistress would often pull off her Stays against the usual time of the Captain's coming.'[10] The unlacing of stays was soon regarded as a metaphor for intercourse. The garment uniquely combined sexual allure and respectability. All the same, this effect did not routinely apply to the lower classes: a fat Wapping landlady was caricatured as a mere woolpack laced into stays, adorned with petticoats, and put on stilts.[11]

There were critics who railed against stays and women's obsession with achieving a 'fine shape'. Doctors warned women against lacing their corsets tightly during pregnancy. A British proposal to tax stays in 1775 claimed that these 'Diabolical Machines' hindered the 'natural Effects of Pregnancy' and weakened the progeny of the middling and upper classes so that 'imperfect Copies of Englishmen are produced to the World'.[12] But in an age when birth control was poorly understood and unreliable, and when women might be pregnant during most of their childbearing years, stays were often used to conceal pregnancy. In 1754, Sarah Jenkins wore a strong wooden busk, despite the pain it caused her, to hide the fact that she was about to give birth.[13] She had got pregnant while her husband was at sea and planned to do away with the child before his return.

Children also routinely wore stays. Some parents put boys and girls into stays to encourage straight growth, fearing deformity from rickets and other medical conditions which would limit a child's earnings or cost the family money. Some parents were concerned about status because gentility demanded good deportment. The pressure to put children into stays chiefly reflected anxieties about their prospects, not respectability, but many adults also believed that wearing stays encouraged moral as well as physical health. Body shaping started from birth, and staymakers often supplied childbed linen. Tight swaddling of babies had mostly disappeared by 1770, but mothers still used 'rollers' – linen bands wrapped two or three times around the baby's torso and over the navel. This loose swaddling continued into the nineteenth century and was thought so essential that a woman who smothered her bastard child and claimed it had been stillborn might still be believed and escape punishment if she had bought baby linen and seemed to have anticipated a happy birth.[14]

At the age of three or four, boys were encouraged to exercise, whereas girls were bound tighter around the upper body; even charity girls were issued with leather stays. Mothers who wanted their daughters to make good marriages believed it was better to mould figures young, since it was more trouble to achieve a fashionable shape and 'a good air' if lacing in stays was left to the teenage years.[15] Critics argued that stays deformed children instead of making them grow straight, and certainly some parents could not afford (or neglected to buy) new stays as their children grew.

Even when tight-lacing was postponed until young bodies were fully formed, some warned it was dangerous:

Yet will their strait Lacing, by pressing the waist, and squeezing in the Flesh within the Ribs, hinder the free Breathing of the Lungs, interrupt the Action of the Stomach, and stop the Circulation of the

21

Blood and Juices; which must in a little Time produce many dangerous Disorders. These must soon beget an irregular intermitting Pulse, great and frequent Giddinesses in the Head, and upon any Exercise, violent Palpitations of the Heart, and what is still worse, a Foulness of the Stomach, a Nauseating of Meat, Vomitings, Wind, Gripings, and all the agonies of the worst Cholick.[16]

The issue was a confusing one, not least because there were staymakers who advertised that they could disguise or correct deformities, while others specialised in steel trusses to straighten bones, the springy tensile strength of steel being good for shaping the body. In addition, staymakers exerted a degree of commercial pressure on their customers, which would become more forceful with industrialisation.

Throughout the eighteenth century, moralists continued to denounce the tight-laced female shape: 'We behold monsters half divided – half-grown – half-starved, and half ruined . . . a distorted, disfigured being'.[17] Such reproaches sat well with periodic attacks on an allegedly corrupt aristocracy, most likely to dress fashionably. Yet what may have disturbed critics, who were usually male, was the overt sexual display of the female form, not the apparent self-harm. Some women eagerly laced their stays tightly, either to outdo rivals or because they derived pleasure from the sensation; those who wore taut stays shared intimate physical details of the effects. After Fanny Burney narrowly escaped public identification as the author of a successful novel, she confided, 'My heart beat so quick against my stays that I almost panted with extreme agitation.'[18] Whatever the nuances of the practice, stays remained popular because they were firmly associated with beauty, youth, morality, and status. And though tight stays might deform women, compressing the rib shaft, they rarely led to early death.[19]

Another reason why British women wore stays was that they were increasingly linked to national identity, setting white British women apart from foreigners wearing 'loose misshapen Dress'.[20] In the Indian subcontinent, to where Westerners were travelling in greater numbers from the eighteenth century, British women clung to their stays even though Mughal women were surprised by their unnatural body shape and some British men noted that women from home were all crooked to some degree whereas they never saw crooked women in Africa or the East.[21] While Lady Mary Wortley Montagu had admired naked women in the hot Turkish baths, a later English visitor viewed them with clear racial prejudice: Lady Elizabeth Craven complained in the 1780s that she had never seen so many fat women and that their flesh looked boiled. She noted that they did put on a kind of corset which, 'melted down as these were, was perfectly necessary', but their unfettered bulk disgusted her.[22] After Britain's North American colonies won independence in 1783, a London newspaper reported that women in Philadelphia seldom wore stays in the summer heat, sharply differentiating them from respectable English women.[23] And in 1791 an English aristocrat commented that French women had no shape, 'as they never wear stays; they are an immense size, and a little French woman is quite as broad as she is long'.[24] In a few years, the fashion for not wearing stays would cross the Channel but, for now, British women were confident that their rigid torsos denoted a superior character.

The ritual of being fitted for stays – at least for the elite and middling sort who could afford to have them custom-made – helped to forge the status of the garment as being somehow crucial to female identity. All stays were sewn by hand until reliable sewing machines were manufactured in the 1850s. For most of the eighteenth century, staymakers were men. Baleen, also called whalebone, was the stiffener of choice; strength was needed to cut strips of uniform thickness, though the tedious job of stitching the narrow channels to hold the whalebone might be given to sewing women.[25] Staymakers often visited clients in their homes to measure and fit a new garment. For the elite, this might be every five months or so, though the middling sort might make their stays last two years, and the poor even longer. In rural areas, staymakers advertised that they would travel up to fourteen miles for a home visit, while those based in London would travel up to ten miles.[26]

Clearly home fitting was an important part of the service. There was some uneasiness about male staymakers adjusting such an intimate garment. One newspaper described a husband's discomfiture at finding a staymaker in his wife's dressing room. 'Lord, Sir!' the staymaker expostulated, 'I lace and unlace Ladies of the first Fashion every Day of my Life, and unmarried Ladies too.'[27] The ambiguous position of the staymaker gave ammunition to critics of tight-lacing. In time, modesty prevailed: by the early nineteenth century, staymakers were advertising that their clients could be measured by female assistants.[28] The lower classes usually bought secondhand or ready-made stays, leaving them at the mercy of swindlers who substituted wood for whalebone.

Although body-shaping undergarments emphasised sexual differences, people still found ways to create gender-fluid, non-binary silhouettes to express aspects of their identity. Skin-tight riding habits, worn over riding stays, allowed women to adopt 'masculine' styles. Pepys described this fashion in the seventeenth century. He saw the queen's ladies of honour 'dressed in their riding garbs, with coats and doublets with deep skirts, just for all the world like men, and buttoned their doublets up the breast, with perriwigs and with hats; so that, only for a long petticoat dragging under their men's coats, nobody could take them for women in any point whatever – which was an odde sight, and a sight did not please me'.[29]

Riding dress of heavy, weather-resistant fabric, cut in a masculine style, was a practical option for women travellers, and some later opted for military designs, pushing gender boundaries further. Reactions were again mixed: some men might admire women in tight-fitting costumes, but others criticised '*hermaphroditical* riding habits':

I would beg the Ladies to ask themselves, how they should like a young Fellow in a *Suit of Pinners*, a *Pair of Stays*, and a *Mantua*? And whether there would not be something *very shocking* in such a one *making Love* to them? If Men would be thus disgusting to the Ladies in the Habits of Women . . . how little agreeable must the Ladies appear to the Men in such *masculine Dresses*?[30]

Women in gender-fluid costumes drew more criticism during times of national crisis. For instance, after the American Revolutionary War (1775–83) began to go badly for Britain, a playful, tolerant attitude to the blurring of gender roles became unsustainable. Caricatures of British officers and their women implied that army officers were effeminate, while their wives or mistresses were unnaturally ready to wear the breeches.

The most notorious person in the eighteenth century to use body sculpture to make a statement about sexuality was the Chevalier d'Éon. In 1777, aged forty-nine, this former soldier, diplomat, and spy for Louis XV began to live as a woman. Eventually d'Éon was brought to court, formally declared a woman, and required to adopt female dress. Why the chevalier acquiesced and claimed that an earlier life had been lived disguised as a man cannot be known; political as well as personal motives may have come into play. But plainly d'Éon challenged gender boundaries of the time and would likely be considered transgender today. From 1785, he lived in London dressed as a woman. An exceptional fencer, d'Éon prompted consternation by sometimes performing in breath-taking sword matches wearing female clothes, stripping down to tightly laced stays before a bout; today some trans people continue to admire a corset's figure-sculpting effect.

HOOPS, RUMPS, AND BELLY PADS

The lower half of the female silhouette has also been constructed in various ways. From about 1707, hoop petticoats became fashionable. These were stiffened with split cane sewn into channels, and they replaced the crescent-shaped bum roll, formerly worn to bulk out full skirts. The fashion permitted tantalising glimpses of ankle or leg. Erotic interest then focused on that part of the body: 'Those pretty Legs so Taper, and so Smart, / By which Men guess at ev'ry other *Part*.'[31] Wide hoops helped to make waists look small and, by spreading and supporting luxurious fabrics, provided scope for an extravagant display of wealth. But if hoops were a mark of status at first, by mid-century

25

almost all women wore them in some form; there were different models to suit every purse. Lower-class women only left them off in situations where they were totally impractical – in fields and workshops. In Britain, it was never quite decent for the well-to-do to dispense with hoops altogether, as Italian women reportedly did in the summer heat.[32]

By the mid-1730s, domed skirts had mostly been replaced by oval-shaped ones, held out at the sides by panniers or side hoops. These false hips allowed for an extra drape of fabric at the back and gave elite women an imposing presence. Panniers were at their widest in the 1740s, when women did have to go through entrances sideways, but eventually panniers were fitted with hinges so that they could be compressed. Vast hoops led to collisions and were easily ridiculed but the elite continued to wear them; small differences in shape and construction signalled the latest fashion. In fact, hoops offered some freedom of movement as they took the weight of petticoats, whereas the pressure of a bum roll could aggravate a back condition. They also allotted women their own physical space, keeping men at a distance.

Wide hoops played a part in social ritual. The elite were always in the public eye and women's body shape, so often used to represent and reinforce cultural conventions, was an early means of exerting soft power. Court dress, for example, was highly politicised and implicated in displays of power and political support: if a woman wore new, extravagant clothes to a reception at court, it was a sign of her family's loyalty. Hoops had to be worn at formal events. The artist and letter-writer Mary Delany reported in 1747 that hoops at court were of such an enormous size women appeared 'like so many *blown bladders*'.[33] Delany, middle-aged and married to a clergyman, was careful to be neither too much in fashion nor wholly out of it. Large hoops were more suited to the aristocracy who had spacious houses. Modestly sized hoops signalled a rational mind, and they suited Delany, who was a keen botanist and had a reputation for botanical illustration.

By the early 1770s, hoops were losing popularity. The letter-writer Lady Mary Coke complained that 'a great hoop is a very troublesome affair at a great dinner'. But hoops were still associated with standards of morality and politeness. When Coke described her visit to the royal governess, she wrote crossly, 'I had put on a hoop to be very respectfull, which I was sorry for, as we walk'd all round the grounds in the rain, which, being dress'd, was not agreeable.'[34] Women were now replacing their hooped skirts with a horsehair quilted petticoat, which was slightly easier to manage.

Aristocratic white women actively used body shape to assert their views in a political arena that was largely closed to them. They enjoyed powers of patronage, and daring trendsetters manipulated the rules of fashion to amplify their notoriety before turning this to political advantage. Georgiana, Duchess of Devonshire was famous for fashion in the 1780s. Tightly compressed torsos were already going out of vogue, and a loose-fitting dress of expensive white muslin, with a sash at the waist, had just been introduced into England from France. It was an informal garment suited to the privacy of the home, but early adopters, including the duchess and the poet and novelist Mary Robinson, set a trend by wearing it in public. The billowy shape was artfully contrived by tying hip pads called rumps to the waist and bunching muslin around the bosom, but it was billed as a 'natural' look. The duchess exploited this look to the full when canvassing for the Whig party, which tended to draw support from industrialists and merchants.

The false rumps which replaced hoops in this latest silhouette were stuffed with cork fragments and horsehair, and often shaped like buttocks. Versions could be made at home but they were also sold in rump shops. Satirists found it easy to mock false rumps: they seemed at odds with the natural innocence wearers strived for and invited prurient curiosity about how the effect was achieved. By the mid-1790s, a slimmer neoclassical silhouette was fashionable. Women seem to have welcomed it. The influence of the Grand Tour had encouraged a neoclassical revival in Europe and upper-class white women found that they could be part of this movement by emulating classical statues in their dress. Women were mostly denied a classical education, but by adopting a willowy silhouette they could show their appreciation of the classics. Waistlines rose, and fluid folds of muslin gestured towards Greek and Roman drapery. Emma Hamilton, who would gain notoriety as Nelson's mistress, helped to popularise the look in her celebrated 'Attitudes': candlelit performances in which she wore fluid costume and posed as well-known classical heroines.

The lithe body shape was associated with radical politics; its apparent simplicity implied a rejection of the artifice associated with the aristocratic old order and a re-alignment with supposedly classical virtues. It could also signal support for democratic principles and enthusiasm for the French Revolution. British Tory politicians feared that revolutionary unrest would cross the Channel, so the new fashion got a mixed reception. Women who followed the trend were suspected of making a political, not just a moral statement. To add to the complexity of meanings linked to this new look, it had an imperial context as well as a neoclassical one. The dress was commonly worn with gold earrings, Indian shawls, and African ostrich feathers. These accessories, all highly valued, also demonstrated that the spoils of colonisation were reaching the metropolis. The look announced European ingenuity and superiority.

The modish silhouette could be loaded with meanings to suit both reformist and conservative agendas. In an odd development – perhaps to make the filmy dress seem less brazen by emphasising women's matronly role, or maybe just to make it hang better – women started to wear padding that falsely suggested pregnancy. It had been tried before in 1783, when the Duchess of Devonshire was pregnant and admirers sought to emulate her. Now the aristocrat Caroline Howe told a friend that the padding was due to the influence of Emma Hamilton:

Has anyone wrote to you a description of a new fashion this year, some of the young Ladies artless wearing something which makes them appear as if with child . . . I believe this fashion originates in wishing to look like Lady Hamilton when equiped for a statue – I am assured & believe it true; that people belonging to the shops provided with these same pads ask their customers whether they would have those of 3 months or six months gone.[35]

'Balloon Corsets' were available for those who wished to appear in an advanced state of pregnancy.[36] Yet if the intention was to emphasise women's domestic role, belly pads only increased the ambiguity of the costume, making young girls seem sexually aware and in need of control; some feared the pads could hide bastard pregnancies. The fashion was soon dropped.

All the same, Caroline of Brunswick, Princess of Wales, adopted the high-waisted, white muslin dress, so from the mid-1790s it was occasionally worn at court. To achieve a smooth contour, most women wore light, unboned stays called a 'corset', which had developed in France from the 1770s but became more popular after the Revolution. A few daring individuals discarded stays altogether. But if maternity was briefly fashionable, fatness was not. Plump matrons resorted to a range of corsets lightly stiffened with bones at the centre front and centre back, which allowed them to achieve the new shape, but which were advertised as good for health and comfort. These corsets supported the bust and prefigured the modern brassiere; some also included a pad at the rear to encourage the folds of the wearer's muslin dress to flow easily from the high waist. The desired effect was to look slender and graceful rather than stiffly elegant. Boned corsets were also a prudent choice because in Britain a conservative backlash after the French Revolution emphasised women's domestic, passive role. But these corsets still did not compress the waist; fashionable dress was loose, so there was no point.

Society continued to politicise dress. References to hoops – now only worn on very formal occasions – became a means to criticise upper-class morality. Mary Robinson mocked aristocrats for their artificial shape in a comedy deriding female gamesters in 1794, 'Hoops of stiff Cane, were certainly design'd – To hide deformity that stalk'd

29

behind!'[37] She was alluding to the common notion that hoops allowed women to hide crooked limbs from suitors, but she was also suggesting that stiff manners and artificial silhouettes hid corruption. Flowing contours were preferable. It was certainly true that the lower classes could gain a better idea of their partner's body shape before marriage, especially in rural areas where the custom of 'bundling' courting couples in bed together was still practised. But in 1794 Robinson's lines seemed dangerously democratic; the play was a disaster and closed after three performances.

Clearly, women had to be aware of the political nuances of their silhouette, as well as what it signalled about class and sexual attraction. When Louisa, wife of Colonel William Clinton, quartermaster general in Ireland, attended an assembly in Dublin Castle in 1806, she allowed herself to appear troubled by her hoop. The style was outmoded but still obligatory at formal functions, where it signalled approval for conservative, pre-revolutionary times. Her behaviour was 'marked as an offence against the Irish drawing-room' because all knew that Louisa must have been perfectly familiar with wearing a hoop at the English court.[38] Her careless insult was a political mistake at a time when Irish funding for the war against Napoleon was at a peak and the authorities were desperate to dampen the forces of radicalism in Ireland.

By the early nineteenth century, people looked back with pity on the 'wigs and hoops, the stiff curtseys and low bows' of their forebears.[39] The latest willowy body shape was an expression of modernity, not least because the shawls and feathers usually teamed with the muslin dress announced that well-to-do white women were part of an expanding commercial, consumer society. Not being able to 'drop the hoop' was used as a metaphor for stiff manners.[40] Yet body-shaping undergarments still encouraged women to sit up straight with shoulders tucked in; they did not slump into chairs. And when they walked, they remained conscious of posture. A graceful deportment indicated status, education, and the possession of good manners. This helps to explain the scene in *Pride and Prejudice* in which Darcy exclaims that women only choose to pass the evening walking around a drawing room to have their figures admired.[41] His comment about the female body is a carefully placed clue to his character.

In the Regency period, substantial corsets soon made a comeback. There were even corsets to be worn when sea bathing, a fashionable new health pursuit. British aristocratic ladies once more censured the French for slopping around all morning without stays. One court lady professed to be alarmed by the change in the Princess of Wales's figure when she discarded her corset, commenting acidly, 'She ought to be warned not to indulge in this practice; for it might give rise to reports exceedingly injurious to her character.'[42] Towards 1820, waistlines dropped, and corsets lengthened and became rather more boned, though still shaped to the body. By the end of that decade, the focus was back on a tiny waist, accentuated by padded sleeves and widened, stiffened skirts. Women were once more weighed down by clothing.

VICTORIAN CORSETS

Technological advances helped corset makers to come up with foundation garments that compressed the female silhouette with renewed rigour. Corsets, now often cut on the diagonal to prevent splitting, or steam-moulded, reduced the waist even before lacing. Metal eyelets had been introduced in France in 1828, allowing corsets to be laced much more tightly. This French fashion was followed in Britain and North America. By 1848, genuine 'Paris-wove corsets' in a supposedly new elastic material were advertised in London as producing a nineteen-inch waist. There was an economic incentive to strive for this waist measurement because each additional inch increased the price of a corset by sixpence. The following year, imported French corsets produced an eighteen-inch waist.[43]

The ingenuity that went into the design of corsets meant that some were proudly displayed in London's 1851 Great Exhibition. In previous centuries, stays had been credited with preserving women from knife attacks, but robust Victorian corsets could deflect bullets. In 1885, a seaman quarrelled with his mistress because she refused to give up prostitution and marry him. He shot her in the abdomen and would have faced a murder charge had not the bullet 'struck the steel of her corset'.[44] Some warned, not entirely fatuously, that a corset's steel busk, up to four inches wide by the 1890s, would kill the wearer in a lightning storm.

If advocates claimed that rigid corsets were essential for a good shape, critics focused on the cumulative damage they did to the body. Clearly, the corset worked in exactly the opposite direction to the natural shape of the rib cage, which, in some cases, it slowly deformed, pushing intestines and organs out of place. When new, baleen is comfortably flexible and it moulds to the body, but extreme stories circulated of strips of whalebone snapping and puncturing internal organs. Male doctors ascribed a terrifying range of ailments to tight corsets, including hysteria, liver displacement, dyspepsia, constipation, circulation problems, nausea, vomiting, and dropsy. They insisted that corsets described as 'scientific', 'hygienic', or 'anatomical' and able to be worn without injury were just as dangerous, while 'electric corsets', fitted with a magnetised steel busk and advertised as a cure for weak backs or sluggish constitutions, were the work of quacks.[45] Such critics exaggerated the physical damage caused by tightly laced corsets. They may have used the corset debate to inflate their own professional standing or to promote the sales of their own design of foundation garment. But corsets certainly encouraged constipation and indigestion; newspapers were full of advertisements for flatulence remedies and anti-bilious pills.

Some Victorian women were said to have achieved waists as small as fourteen inches, trained from youth by rigid corseting in schools or by socially ambitious mothers, keen to 'do their duty' and shape daughters for the marriage market. But extreme tight-lacing was a niche practice. Surviving corsets in museum collections are often well worn, indicating that they must have been comfortable enough for daily use, even if women kept tighter ones for special occasions. The norm seems to have been to reduce the waist by four inches.[46] That said, excessive corseting did cause the back and stomach muscles to atrophy so that, paradoxically, tight-lacers experienced pain if they did not wear a corset. Because of this, and to help preserve the hourglass figure gained by corseting all day, some women also wore corsets through the night. The domestic consequences of tight corseting began to be aired in newspapers, some even warning men not to marry corset wrecks: 'A lady laced so tightly that she can scarcely stand, in any walk of life is sure to make no progress. If she marries, she will always be a drag upon her husband.'[47]

The fashion for a wasp waist does seem to have been a factor in the declining birth rate among the aspiring middle classes. Genteel women used corsets to help construct their position in society and practised tight-lacing to a point that those who worked for a living could not possibly contemplate. Weakened backs and night corsets might have been a disincentive to intercourse, while the effects of severe constriction certainly led to difficult births. Some women, aware that pregnancy would curtail an amusing social life, compressed their waist in a corset to encourage miscarriage.[48] In any case, prudish middle-class matrons seem to have suppressed signs of pregnancy for as long as possible before resorting to an adjustable maternity corset. After the birth they could opt for a 'restoring corset' to flatten the stomach.

The selection of the correct corset was a matter of fine judgement but there were practical tricks to achieving a good shape. In magazines and journals, fat women shared explicit advice on how best to put it on: 'Remember, the flesh must go somewhere, and rather distribute it than throw it above or below the corset, where it must go if the wearer laces.'[49] Corsets, and the silhouette each type produced, were also constant reminders of a woman's life stages. If she gained weight in middle age, the corset once kept for best remained a memento of her former youthful figure.

The lower classes could not afford the best-fitting corsets. When 'rational' corsets fitted with natural-rubber elastic were introduced mid-century, moralists complained that the poorer sort always insisted on 'strength and unyielding solidity', even weighing corsets and buying the heaviest kind in a self-defeating attempt to ensure long wear and value for money.[50] But in London's East End, lower-class women also set up corset clubs to help them save up for elegant garments. A fine corset indicated that they belonged to the upper gradations of the working class and would mark them out from other women who did hard physical labour.[51]

In the United States, especially after emancipation in 1865, African Americans wore tight corsets. The racial caricature of the shapeless Black 'mammy', popularised across the West in food advertising and in Hollywood films like *Gone with the Wind*, was a distortion that bolstered white prejudice while easing guilt about the mistreatment of Black people. Nineteenth-century photographs show that as African Americans entered public life, whether advocating for their communities in churches, clubs, and societies, or working as journalists, clerks, and teachers, they dressed as all professional women did, in corsets and tightly buttoned, floor-length dresses. The same was true of Black women in Victorian Britain, who often worked in the public eye, in caring professions and in the world of entertainment.[52]

Why did women take such pains to achieve an hourglass figure? Some men doubtless found a handspan, virginal waist erotic but women also found their corseted looks pleasing. For some, the pain was linked to a pleasurable sensation, associated with control and personal identity; waist-reduction was empowering and even addictive. Teenage girls vied with each other to achieve ever smaller waist measurements which also helped to create the illusion of a developed bust; mothers claimed their daughters insisted on lacing their corsets tightly, although they pleaded with them not to do it. Painful lacing might have been part of a victimisation syndrome dimly appreciated at the time: corsets were 'a proud symbol of the martyr power of the Sex'.[53] Tight corsets also helped to construct Victorian femininity; as in the eighteenth century, a contoured torso indicated status and morality. And critics of extreme

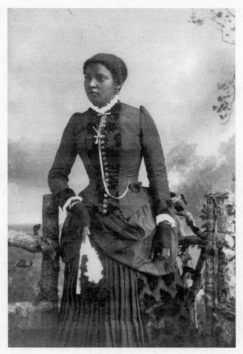

3. From a collection showing African American teachers, business owners, and community leaders in Florida, c. 1890.

tight-lacing may have been reacting to what they took to be the subversive aspects of a sensual, hourglass figure. In short, the physical and psychological effects of the corset combined with its social and cultural meanings to make it increasingly controversial.

The historic corset remains an obsession for some. The talented Mr Pearl, who designs corsets for celebrities today and who has trained his own waist to a mere eighteen inches by wearing a corset constantly except for bathing, praises the discipline imposed. He argues that the wearer cannot rush around, slouch, or eat immoderately, while the constant sensation of pressure on the body, and the enforced shallow breathing, can be harnessed for mental awareness.[54]

OUTRAGEOUS CRINOLINES AND
'RATIONAL DRESS'

If corsets were a contested topic, so was the crinoline, which became all
the rage in the mid-1850s, when a framework of steel hoops replaced
horsehair and linen petticoats. Before that, women had adopted various
measures to bulk out their skirts. In 1834, Jane Welsh Carlyle wrote to
her mother-in-law from London, 'the diameter of the fashionable
Ladies at present is about three yards; their *bustles* (false bottoms) are
the size of an ordinary sheep's fleece'.[55] She told the story of a maidservant who went out on Sundays with three kitchen dusters pinned
beneath her dress to create volume. Intellectual women like Carlyle
mocked such frivolities but emerging technologies were about to push
the diameter of skirts to extreme dimensions.

In 1856, the caged petticoat, made of steel hoops held by tape, was
patented in the United States, Britain, and France. The hoops sprang
back into shape after compression, but the key advance was that this
cage crinoline could be mass produced. It was hailed as a relief for
women because it was lighter, more hygienic, and freed the legs –
women no longer needed to kick out heavy petticoats as they walked.
The cage crinoline was therefore all about movement as well as static
shape. It affected how women walked and how they behaved: it enforced
a specific gait and bearing because, if skirts started to sway, women
showed too much leg. Some versions were five or six yards in circumfer-
ence, a mark of prestige in elite gatherings, but in most settings these
large crinolines took up too much room and by the late 1860s had
reduced in size.

Crinolines ruled out hard physical labour and announced, for the
well-to-do at least, that housework was performed by servants. Sara
Forbes Bonetta, whom Queen Victoria raised as her goddaughter in the
British middle class, wore a crinoline of carefully judged dimensions to
reflect her social degree. Yet versions of this latest fashionable silhouette
were within the reach of all classes because steel hoops were cheap to

purchase; maidservants were known to insist on their right to wear the style because it was a mark of status.

In the British West Indies, post-emancipation, many freed women adopted European styles of dress and Victorian concepts of feminine beauty. Motives varied. For some it was a style choice. Others saw it as a way to challenge perceived racial hierarchies and elevate their social standing when their African heritage was under attack. Even labouring women wore crinolines to the extent that this was possible and affordable, although some women preferred to combine African and European aesthetics in their dress.[56]

In Britain, while many young women enjoyed their crinolines, others were beginning to find them oppressive. The tilting crinoline was difficult to control and, in an age of open grates, a fire hazard; it

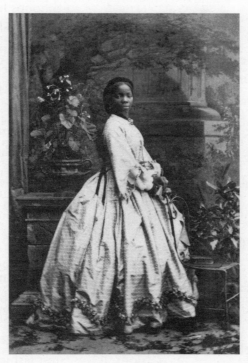

4. *Sara Forbes Bonetta in 1862, the year of her marriage to a wealthy Yoruba businessman, Captain Davies.*

was firmly discouraged in factories. Women campaigners for female suffrage, who began to meet in London in the 1850s, often abandoned them altogether for simpler clothes. From the 1870s, skirts were swept back into a bustle. Some bustles had springs and were designed to fold, but the sheer bulk of women's clothing remained burdensome: when women were fully dressed, their garments might weigh twenty-five pounds.[57] Contemporary advertisements indicate women's struggle to obtain voluminous skirts without extra weight: in 1886, an 'improver petticoat' was described as incorporating the softest, lightest 'French regulating mattress', which still sounds bulky.[58]

More middle-class women entered the workplace in the late nineteenth century as typewriters were introduced into offices. These women needed clothes that offered freedom of movement, not least on crowded public transport. And undergarments that shaped the female body became associated with the fight for female emancipation. Women who fought for the right to vote, property rights, and birth control denounced extreme corseting and argued for 'rational dress'. In 1881, the Rational Dress Society was formed in London. It campaigned against tight corsets, high heels, unwieldy skirts, and crinolines of any kind that impeded healthy exercise. The maximum weight of clothing (without shoes) that members would approve was seven pounds. These activists, mostly from the upper and upper middle classes, pointed out that corsets could not be left off if women were still expected to wear heavy folds and tight bodices, 'bands of skirts pulling in different direc-tions, and bones of bodices pricking and chafing here and there, cause an amount of discomfort not to be endured without the pressure of stays to deaden the sense of feeling'.[59] The Society called for a new atti-tude to body shaping, and sold daring active wear, such as divided skirts, at reasonable prices from its depot in Sloane Square.

In a reversal of women's earlier attitude to stays, the Rational Dress Society linked the acceptance of oppressive female dress to the deca-dence of the age. It predicted the end of Britain's greatness unless women themselves led the way to natural comfort. Members were acutely conscious that American campaigners were ahead of them. In the United States, activists involved in the temperance and anti-slavery movements, as well as in the campaign for women's rights, had called for dress reform since the mid-century. Some had taken to wearing long pantaloons called bloomers after their publicist, Amelia Bloomer. But this garment, worn under a short skirt, was controversial and mostly ridiculed.

The 'Corset Wars' heightened in the 1880s and 1890s. Critics of the corset calculated that the garment could exert a pressure of up to eighty pounds per square inch.[60] They conducted experiments on monkeys to show that this pressure could break ribs, although women who loved their corsets retorted that the poor monkeys had been subjected to a sudden shock, whereas they, accustomed to tightly laced corsets from a young age, were more resilient.[61] From 1894, the Anti-Corset League stepped up the campaign against tight-lacing. Male doctors, active in the movement, helped to bring forward convincing arguments. For example, they conducted school trials, comparing the performance of girls running races in corsets and out of them. Unsurprisingly, the girls without corsets ran faster: their heartbeats were twenty beats a minute slower, and their rate of respiration was half that of the corseted girls.[62] This was also the age of the bicycle, a form of transport that the independently minded 'New Woman' eagerly adopted. To ride safely, women needed shorter skirts or knee-length bloomers, as well as corsets that gave some freedom of movement. Yet bifurcated garments for women remained contentious. Caricatures depicted white women in bloomers as ugly, cigarette-smoking viragos; they were openly jeered at in the streets.

Clearly, some women, whether sympathetic to the cause of female suffrage or not, still favoured rigid corseting for the social advantages or erotic pleasure it might bring. Yet the media stoked up the Corset Wars, sharply defining two opposing camps, so that divided opinion about shaping the female body worked to fracture support for women's emancipation. Anti-feminists could even use corseting to justify female inequality, since they could claim that damaging oneself for an hourglass figure was irrational. Men who vaunted their common sense now mocked women for wanting to look like egg timers, although some admitted that they would not wish to be seen in public with an unfashionable woman.[63] Most reformers wanted moderate lacing, not a complete ban of the corset.

Late in the century, doctors promoted a straight-fronted, so-called health corset that supported rather than depressed the abdominal cavity. The new corset allowed more room in the waist area; the French stage star Sarah Bernhardt was an early adopter and from 1898 helped to make it popular. Yet women still laced the corset tightly, producing the voluptuous 'S' shape that thrust the bosom forward and the hips back. It was an era of rapid change and perhaps women found reassurance in retaining the custom of lacing. That said, the 'S' curve of the modish silhouette placed a strain on the back.

In North America and Canada from the 1890s, the 'S' curve was linked to the 'Gibson Girl', a feminine ideal named after the artist Charles Dana Gibson, whose illustrations did most to promote it. The 'Gibson Girl' was white, breezy, and athletic. She was essentially apolitical, so more socially acceptable than the New Woman in Britain. But the 'S' curve was another obvious distortion of the female body; in the early twentieth century, it slowly gave way to a more upright shape. After all, healthy, streamlined contours were suited to an age character-ised by mobility, speed, and change. But ironically, by 1904, the sinuous, flowing outline then in vogue required such long corsets that the wearer could hardly sit.

Despite the controversy surrounding restrictive female clothing, corsets remained firmly linked to British imperial identity. As early as 1814, elite 'Ladies of rank' in Bath had been invited to try the New Imperial Corset, 'the happiest invention yet discovered' for producing an elegant figure. Retailers continued to recommend durable corsets adapted to tropical climates for white women going to British colonies, although it was known that the women of South Asia wore no restric-tive garments to alter their body shape, while critics of the corset maintained that Turkish, Spanish, and Syrian women were beautiful without it.[64] British advertisements for corsets alluded to imperial superiority into the 1890s. For example, E. Izod & Son Ltd proudly declared that their corsets were sold 'in every country in the civilised world'; their trademark, a sloping anchor, referenced British sea power.[65]

Criticism of the corset therefore became linked to criticism of empire; missionaries were even accused of depopulating New Zealand by introducing corsets to Māori women.[66] Meanwhile, Western women were strong advocates of ending the Chinese tradition of binding women's feet, deemed uncivilised. This painful process reduced the length of the foot to about four and a half inches. But, like the corset, foot binding was a sign of status and helped girls secure marriage partners. It continued until the early twentieth century.

MASS PRODUCTION AND THE FEMALE SILHOUETTE

The Edwardian age was one of massive expenditure on dress. An upper-class woman might make five or six changes to her costume a day. Middle-class women seized every social opportunity to view the fashionable contours they should aspire to. By 1900, they were eating out in public as they had not done even a decade earlier; they wanted to see how the smart set lived and to emulate how they looked. Britain and the United States were now importing millions of pounds worth of silks, ribbons, corsets, feathers, and other dress trimmings from France each year. And before any gown was purchased or ordered, women were advised to make the right choice of corset to mould the body into the shape of the day. The implicit message was that somehow the female outline was flawed.

With the rise of mass production in the early twentieth century, the shaping of the female body supported ever greater numbers of workers. The trend had been evident earlier; the demise of the crinoline had been devastating for those involved in its production. Factories, chiefly in Yorkshire, had been making fifty tons of crinoline wire a week, while the largest crinoline factory in London, Thomson's, had employed over 1,000 women turning out between 3,000 and 4,000 crinolines daily.[67] Corset manufacture was also big business, and British firms kept a keen eye on international competition. In 1856, for example, the London press reported that Stuttgart's corset industry employed 1,800 workers producing 300,000 corsets annually.[68] From the 1870s, it was in North America that corset manufacturers developed into large-scale industrial organisations. By the 1890s, American corset firms had developed sewing machines with up to twelve needles, sewing parallel lines of stitching to hold stiffeners. In 1910, the Strouse, Adler factory in New Haven, Connecticut, was producing over two million units a year.[69] In Britain, meanwhile, corset factories started up in areas where there were pools of female labour. In 1899, for example, Vollers established a factory in Portsmouth; there women headed up naval families while husbands were at sea. Even so, the sweated system of home working continued to supply corsetry. In the early 1900s, poor women in London's East End were paid 3¾d a gross for sewing the steel strips into corsets.[70]

The development of basic designs that could support numerous variations was essential to factory production. Manufacturers then exploited economies of scale while responding to minor changes in fashion and pushing new lines. Mass production brought a choice of corsets to women at most levels of society. As manufacturers settled on a range of body types and produced sizes to fit, they boasted that everyone could buy a corset that would make people think it was made to measure. Nevertheless, there was still room in the market for smaller businesses. For example, Mrs Adair of Bond Street specialised in silk and elastic corsets that might stretch to fit. She also sold a range of rubber devices to address problem areas: chin straps to reduce double chins, forehead straps to lessen wrinkles, and the 'Ganesh Scrimmage Binder' to hold protruding ears in place – customers were assured that it bore some resemblance to a cap, so it could be worn day and night.

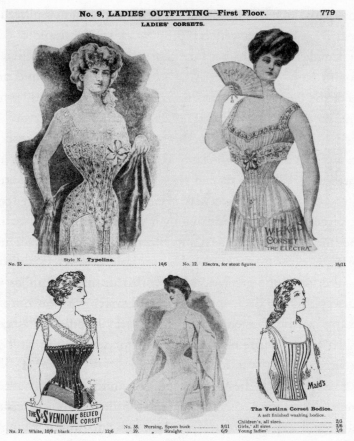

No. 9, LADIES' OUTFITTING—First Floor. 779

LADIES' CORSETS.

Style K. **Typoline.**

No. 23 .... 14/6

No. 12. Electra, for stout figures 15/11

THE S & S VENDOME BELTED CORSET

No. 17. White, 10/9 ; black 12/6

No. 38. Nursing, Spoon busk 8/11
No. 39. " Straight 6/9

The Vestina Corset Bodice.
A soft finished washing bodice.

Children's, all sizes.................	2/3
Girls,' all sizes.....................	2/6
Young ladies'........................	3/9

5. *Ladies' corsets from the Army & Navy Stores, 1907. By then the company had
branches in India and England.*

The development of new materials had a big impact on body
sculpture. As whalebone became scarce in the 1880s, American manufacturers developed 'Coraline' stiffeners from plant fibres. In the 1890s,
they started to use flexible spring steel; fortunately, it was resistant to
rust from perspiration. Rubber brought new possibilities. The S-shaped
corset, for example, offered little support to the bosom. Women who
found themselves deficient in that area resorted to rubber inflatable
breasts, although cotton padding was always an option.[71] After all,

43

throughout the nineteenth century women had achieved a fashionable silhouette by padding as well as tightly lacing their corsets.

The female silhouette became more than ever controlled by the market and targeted by advertising campaigns. For example, towards the end of the First World War, one London corset company promoted its 'Jurna' model in a high-end art magazine as the key to 'poise', which it defined as distinction, stateliness, and grace in society.[72] Poster advertising now fixed images of the latest corset firmly in the mind; photography was especially effective in these campaigns, and photographers for posters sometimes also worked on early films. Their images could be overtly sexual, featuring white women in their underclothes in intimate, bedroom settings; the sexuality of women in corsets was harnessed for profit.

Women's developing relationship with the market can be judged from changes in the process of buying a corset. Whereas once it had been common for women of the upper and middling classes to be custom fitted, by the late nineteenth century, as standard sizing became more reliable, there was a thriving ready-to-wear market. Women unable to get their size from local drapers could order from illustrated catalogues or respond directly to mail order advertisements. The well-to-do still expected their purchases to incorporate a satisfying experience. When William Whiteley, who created London's first department store in Bayswater from the 1860s, opened new premises in 1911 after a fire, he made sure that his corset, underwear, and baby linen departments were expensively fitted out in French walnut. Expert corset fitters were always in attendance, even though made-to-measure corsets were often adaptations of basic patterns. This became the norm in other department stores. Between the 1920s and 1950s, the lingerie department in any store was usually the most profitable.[73]

During the First World War, when British women took on jobs usually carried out by men, they opted for a less restricted body shape. Some had jettisoned stiff corsets already. After the war, there was a conservative reaction to this trend, depicted as a dangerously radical fad. From the viewpoint of corset manufacturers, it was bad for business. They hit back strongly, warning that not wearing a corset risked premature ageing and 'ballooning' of the waist and hips. Dr Jan Schoemaker, a Dutch surgeon writing in 1921 for the trade journal *Corsets & Lingerie*, even introduced offensive racialised and homophobic objections to going corset-free: 'The woman with a tight-muscled tense abdominal wall, flat hips, mannish chest, is usually to be pitied. She is unfortunate. If she has been produced and admired in quantities in England . . . it is not because the English are producing any healthier race, but because the number of biological mistakes among females are increasing.' Schoemaker claimed that feminists demanding sex equality were often of the type he thought objectionable, but that traditional gender roles would prevail since 'women who imitate men are not the kind that Nature selects to mother the next generation'.[74]

As part of the process of enticing women back to corsets, retailers insisted that it was best to have them fitted, or at least selected with the help of expert advice. In the United States, department stores began sending employees to corset fitting schools where they were trained in sales technique. For instance, they were taught never to recommend a corset as something they would wear themselves, for what customer wanted to wear the same model as a shop girl? The buying process was framed as an exercise in choice, and, up until the 1930s, London's larger department stores held corset parades over a period of one or two weeks to display their range. Now that waist training was no longer familiar to young girls, retailers understood that customers had to find the purchase of their first corset a reassuring and pleasurable rite of passage so that they became lifelong wearers. They renamed the old-fashioned corset a 'girdle', although at first the term applied only to lighter models. They even claimed that girdles were needed to correct the damage that corsets had caused. Advertisements therefore encouraged a sense of progress and optimism that women's figures could be moulded afresh thanks to scientific advances.

In the 1920s, the ideal silhouette had natural suppleness and ease of movement, essential for the fast-paced, energetic dances which were all the rage. Slim young women now slumped in wrap-on, almost boneless corsets. This rebellious slouch led an older generation to complain that they lacked deportment: 'Not one woman out of ten knows how to walk properly', exclaimed one matron, returning from Oxford Street. 'The only good walkers, who can carry their head erect and *wear* their clothes, are older women, of the Edwardian and late Victorian eras.'[75] But the youthful silhouette on trend was firmly associated with female independence. Paradoxically, the desire for a flat, boyish figure meant that stout individuals were encased in a corset from armpits to thighs. But most women of the interwar period looked back on Victorian corsetry with the same sense of liberation that Regency women had felt when they considered the wigs and stays of their grandparents. All the same, the corseted age evoked nostalgia; the traditional corset was increasingly fetishised and surrounded in mystique.

UPLIFT AND REDUCTION

During the Second World War, pin-up iconography directed male attention towards women's breasts, not least because the brassiere had developed into a garment that could produce a marked uplift. Women increasingly dressed in trousers, so prominent breasts were a key indication of gender difference. Dropped busts had been of little concern in the Edwardian age when the pigeon breast created by low corsets derived only minimal support from the bust bodice that women wore. From 1914, busty women resorted to reducing brassieres to obtain the cylindrical silhouette in fashion. But, in the 1930s, the brassiere was promoted as an essential item to counteract the harmful effects of compressing the breasts during the previous decade. Once again, the contours of a woman's body became medicalised.

Increasing numbers of women bought brassieres. The system of fixed cup sizes, devised in the United States in 1935, made it easier to choose the right size. Innovations in design and fabric selection helped to separate as well as lift the breasts, in styles which were marketed as more youthful-looking, although there was nothing natural in the pointy effect created by circle-stitched cups from the late 1930s. A woman's bust size could even help define her sense of self, not least because some critics associated large breasts with a lack of intelligence. Today women can buy padded, push-up, or breast-reducing bras. To some extent, contours can be adapted at will to achieve the glamourous power associated with large breasts or a flatter profile for exercise.

Although tight-lacing was outmoded in the twentieth century, women still desired to reduce their waists. One innovation was the rubber 'reducing' garment, which promised not just to mould the figure but to reduce the flesh. Rubber corsets were first advertised as medical appliances but, from the late 1920s, perforated latex roll-on girdles were developed as a popular garment. The claim that they could reduce weight was not entirely false, since they did encourage copious perspiration. Some even came with a matching latex brassiere, which must have been torture in hot weather. A shortage of rubber during the Second World War meant that it was reserved for military use, and the clammy, weight-reducing corset went into decline. Instead, Harvey Nichols recommended an all-in-one bra, girdle, and pantie, with a zip-fastened side that could be 'donned in a trice' during air raids.[76] But after the war Playtex revived rubber foundation garments; Dior's New Look, with its nipped waist and long, full skirt, drove women back to restrictive girdles.

The New Look was heavily promoted, not least because it was designed to restore the prominence of Parisian fashions in peacetime and to kick-start textile industries. Women of all classes may have been more compliant with new restrictions to their waist size because the ultra-feminine outline was associated with a return to normal life. And corsetry was still associated with self-discipline and respectability: in the 1959 box-office hit *Anatomy of a Murder*, when the defending attorney (James Stewart) needs to demonstrate that his client (Lee Remick) is of unblemished character, he tells her bluntly to wear a girdle for her court appearance. But women's demand for comfort proved a powerful trend. Playtex introduced its 18-Hour range in the sixties, including its Five Pounds Thinner girdle with 'fingertip' panels to flatten the stomach. Made from patterned elastic, the girdle was sold in a tube to emphasise how flexible it was, and women were assured it could be worn without discomfort for eighteen hours at a stretch. Hollywood stars promoted the Playtex girdle, just as famous stars had helped to publicise the straight-fronted corset earlier in the century, and it sold widely in Britain, North America, and France. The corsetry of an earlier era was mostly reserved for tailored swimsuits, bought by wealthy women of a certain age for luxury holidays.

With the advent of second-wave feminism, which condemned male-dominated practices throughout society, and which coincided with mini-skirts and the introduction of tights, restrictive girdles for everyday wear went into terminal decline. For some women, tight jeans helped to preserve a trim outline, though they might have to lie down to zip them up. Those still wearing corsets in the 1970s were gently mocked: an article in *Doctor*, the general practitioner's magazine, claimed that an increasing number of women were collapsing on high-flying aircraft. Allegedly, they had squeezed into corsets that were too tight and, 'like balloons released from the ground, the higher these well-proportioned ladies fly the more they expand'.[77] The claim was reported humorously in *Country Life*, but evidently social pressures still demanded slimness.

In today's multicultural Western societies, the promotion of a single, ideal female shape is unviable, but body sculpture is by no means a thing of the past. Discrete 'shapewear' in the latest high-tech materials delivers comfort as well as a svelte outline. Since the 1980s, cosmetic surgery has become increasingly popular as women strive to retain youth and to emulate role models. In recent years, iconic Black celebrities like Beyoncé and Rihanna have influenced surgical body shaping. Their toned, hourglass figures have helped them to become cultural icons; some white women now opt for procedures that make them appear to be of African heritage, or just more curvaceous. Kim

Kardashian, of Armenian heritage herself and an advocate of the waist trainer, has helped to spread the idea that it is possible to present as Black without being Black, a trend that the journalist Wanna Thompson denounces as 'blackfishing'.[78]

Yet contemporary attitudes to beauty are increasingly open to diversity, so cosmetic treatments, especially for the gender-fluid, may work to promote a sense of belonging rather than any ideal appearance. The latest synthetic materials offer transgender people opportunities that were not easily attained in the past. Transgender men can find purpose-built garments that flatten the breasts, perhaps while waiting for 'top surgery'. Chest-binding also helps non-binary people to reduce gender dysphoria and is popular with lesbians and cross-dressers. Chest binders are generally safe when fitted correctly, and medical websites give good advice about how they can be worn without complications. But, like all body-moulding devices throughout the centuries, they prompt debate.

Corsets and then bras have been regarded as symbols of oppression and unwarranted male control over the female body. Yet women have found empowerment in the reshaping of their bodies to construct an identity or to claim social status. The two viewpoints have co-existed since at least Victorian times; the corset and crinoline still linger in bridal wear, as some wish to appear ultra-feminine on their wedding day. And body shape is firmly linked to social opportunity. In the nineteenth century, wearing a tightly laced corset may have been a way for middle-class women, frustrated by limited prospects, to exert control. When society offered them more employment outside the home, they were free to exercise a degree of self-determination by insisting on rational dress instead. Body sculpture can even be a creative form of self-expression: when Madonna chose a Jean Paul Gaultier corset as outerwear during her 1990 world tour, it became an overt symbol of sexual empowerment. Paradoxically, as society combats a so-called obesity epidemic today, the trend towards wearing no corset at all has led to a new kind of tyranny: a lifestyle dominated by intense exercise to maintain the figure.

☙ 2 ❧

DIET AND EXERCISE

In 1758, a London newspaper carried a striking piece to help raise money for an asylum to house penitent prostitutes. The Magdalen Hospital would provide a refuge for 'ruined outcasts' who had been seduced and might otherwise be forced into sex work. The supporter of this scheme claimed, 'Want and hunger pinch hard . . . numberless, unhappy sufferers, of this sort . . . crowd our streets.'[1] The appeal reminds us that for many people the problem was not how to lose weight but how to get enough food for themselves and their family.

Women of the lower classes were physically active – as street hawkers, washerwomen, market women, and servants. Work in the home was physically exhausting, not least because water and coals had to be carried up and down stairs in heavy tubs. Few in this class set out to lose weight. Even the word 'diet' had a different meaning. When speaking of food, it meant people's daily allowance of provisions, or their customary fare. Doctors did sometimes prescribe a restricted diet but mostly for sickness rather than fatness. Only in the late nineteenth century did the word 'diet' immediately conjure up the aim of losing weight, and only from the 1960s was the term applied to food with a reduced calorie content. Physical exercise for women, if mentioned at all, was recommended as beneficial to health, rather than essential to keep a trim figure.

Does the altered meaning of the word 'diet' signal a change in our attitude to food? How has Western understanding of an 'acceptable' diet, or an 'appropriate' level of exercise, developed over time? How much exercise did women take in the past, and when did they first begin to exercise for health and beauty? And what role does exercise play in women's lives today? The answers to these questions say a lot about women's self-image and how they perceive their role in society.

A temperate, balanced diet has long been associated with health. This is because, from classical times until the mid-nineteenth century and the advent of germ theory, people believed that the body was driven by four fluids or 'humours' that had to be in balance. These fluids were blood, choler (or yellow bile), phlegm, and black bile. A person became ill if one fluid diminished or built up to cause an obstruction. This medical theory is implicit in seventeenth-century household manuals offering remedies for common ailments and recipes to keep the body in order, including concoctions to make the body fat or lean. It was entrenched until the late eighteenth century. When Admiral Boscawen's wife, Frances, bought a diary in 1763, it was pre-printed with rules for health typical of the age. Under the heading 'Of Repletion and Evacuation' it read, 'the whole art of preserving health may properly enough be said to consist in filling up what is deficient, and emptying what is redundant, that so the body may be habitually kept in its natural state . . . Repletion, for instance, from eating or drinking, requires a puke or abstinence.'[2] Nothing could be simpler.

Doctors recommended specific diets to correct an imbalance in bodily fluids and to improve medical conditions. There were diets for kidney stones, gout, and scurvy. Remedies called 'diet-drinks' were said to cure sores or clear the blood. From the late seventeenth century, a diet-drink was touted as a cure for syphilis. The remedy was promoted well into the 1790s, meaning that for nearly a hundred years the word 'diet' was tainted by an association with venereal disease. Patients under a doctor's care for syphilis were often prescribed exercise and a restricted diet, but the afflicted mostly wanted to hide their condition, not advertise it by keeping to a strict regimen. Their desire for secrecy encouraged the sale of quack remedies that promised a speedy cure. Doctors might also prescribe a 'low' vegetable diet just to maintain health. This regime was thought particularly effective in summer. Whenever George III felt indisposed, he put himself on a diet of water and potatoes. A 'milk diet' was reserved for severe, lingering illnesses like tuberculosis. In 1738, British newspapers reported that the French Queen Marie, wife of Louis XV, had visited a spa to drink the waters and then adopted a milk diet. She had been advised that another pregnancy might kill her and made a show of extreme ill health before banning the king from her bedroom for the rest of their marriage.

The first fad weight-loss diet is credited to George Cheyne, an affable Scottish physician. He enjoyed socialising and ate and drank so much that by the time he reached late middle age, in the 1720s, he weighed more than thirty-two stone. He was so short of breath that, if he heaved himself into his carriage too quickly, he felt dizzy and his face turned black. In desperation, he put himself on a prolonged vegetable and milk diet, successfully reducing his weight by a third. Afterwards he wrote books on diet and exercise based on experience, which were influential for the rest of the century.

Women across the class spectrum were easily seduced into self-medication for social and economic reasons. In seventeenth-century Britain, the mistress of a house was expected to keep a manual of remedies for common diseases so that she could care for her family. Then, in 1724, Dr John Maubray published *The Female Physician*, a manual on midwifery in which he advised a special diet for women who had just given birth. This was an important step because the diet was calculated to meet a perceived female need, not an illness. Four years later, an anonymous physician published *The Ladies Physical Directory*, giving the symptoms of a range of female complaints and their cures. He wrote in plain English so that literate women of all classes could understand and treat their disorders. They rushed to buy the book, which had gone through six editions by 1736.

But there was a nagging worry that British women, self-medicating for conditions alleged to be specific to their sex, were in fact becoming used to tippling all day long. Many of the syrups and cordials taken as remedies were alcoholic. In the first half of the eighteenth century, London was in the grip of the Gin Craze. And if the poor deadened their sorrows with cheap gin, commentators worried that well-to-do women were fast becoming addicted to luxury imported health drinks: 'Many a good woman, who would start at the mention of Strong Waters, cannot conceive there can be any harm in a Cordial . . . The ladies perhaps may not be aware that every time they have recourse to their Hartshorn or Lavender Drops, to drive away the vapours, they in effect take a Dram.'[3] In the 1780s, the wine Tokay de España was imported as having extraordinary powers to cure disorders of the stomach and bowels, even when laudanum, a tincture of opium, had failed. It was particularly recommended to women in childbed.

Such routine additions to the diet support the view that, in the past, European populations were more or less permanently drugged, or at least habituated to opiates and strong alcohol from an early age. It helps to explain Admiral Codrington's sharp reaction to the remedy his wife adopted for a cough and pain in her side when he was at sea during the Napoleonic Wars. 'The ale you take by way of support', he wrote, 'would be well exchanged for a quick done beefsteak or muttin chop'; he worried that her cough might be tubercular, recollecting 'a hectic beauty' they both knew who had the disease, and concluded rather clumsily, 'though you may be as fat as she is lean, I cannot be quite at ease'.[4]

Rude health, it seems, was more reassuring than delicate beauty. And yet fasting was particularly associated with women. Elizabeth I had used abstinence to help create her royal image, presiding over enormous ritual feasts but hardly touching the food. In the sixteenth and seventeenth centuries, self-starvation was a means for women to demonstrate a range of conditions including grief and penance. Not eating made some women seem exceptional: in the 1760s, a woman was said to have lived nearly four years on water alone.[5] Of course, regular fasting was part of the church year, and some believed that this penance had useful health benefits, helping to cleanse the blood and balance the body. In her younger days, Frances Boscawen fasted every Monday, although it may have been a response to acute anxiety while her husband was at sea because she did not do it in later life.[6]

Noticeable fatness, with associated diabetes, only emerged as a common problem among the gouty rich in the late eighteenth century. Hitherto, extremely large women were regarded as oddities. People would pay to see them at fairs and coffee houses. The death of Mrs Cousins, keeper of the sluice house near Hornsey and 'one of the fattest women of the age', was even reported in 1777 as a newsworthy event: her demise was occasioned by eating some eggs 'which were boiled too hard for her digestion'.[7] Yet, among the elite, overeating already drew criticism. It indicated a lack of self-control and prompted warnings that gluttony and too little exercise would shorten life.

Such advice usually emphasised the importance of preserving health, not beauty; after all, from the cradle Christian women were instructed to shun vanity and to mind their virtue more than their looks. That said a 1760 book of grooming tips for women stated baldly that 'too much fatness spoils beauty', and explicitly linked fatness with sloth and stupidity.[8] To keep a good figure, the author recommended less sleep, eating more meat than bread, and walking in the heat of the day to encourage perspiration. The diary of Anna Seward, a poet whose smooth verses earned her the title of 'the Swan of Litchfield', reveals how easily upper-class white women could gain weight. She claimed to have been a slim teenager until she paid a long visit to a wealthy relation:

Mrs C—n fed me up in that fatal month, like a porker, with choco-late, drank in bed at eight; a nap till ten; tea and hot-rolls at eleven; pease soup at one; a luxurious dinner at four; and an hot and splendid supper at midnight – the day-light intervals filled up with slow airings in the old coach, along the dusty roads, for it was in the heats of a blazing summer; and with lying on a couch.[9]

The weight she gained proved impossible to shift in adult life.

In eighteenth-century Britain, to the extent that people had money to choose their food at all, cultural pressures militated against a balanced diet. The population's ability to raise and eat large quantities of beef was linked to national identity. It was held to be the basis of British valour. The French, traditional enemies, were scorned for eating delicate *fricassées* if they had money, and frogs, snails, and 'weeds' if poor. British commentators claimed that the Portuguese hardly ever ate 'solid Animal Food' and implied that this was the case in the rest of Europe.[10]

Inasmuch as the British thought about a healthy diet at all, they worried about adulterated food: bread bulked up with alum, meal thickened with calcined bones, powdered pepper laced with hellebore, a toxic plant. Towards the end of the century, they did begin to see the value of balanced meals, shipping out fresh vegetables to the fleet during the wars against Revolutionary France. Criticism of the wealthy, their tables loaded with luxury fare, was always harsher in wartime, but fashionable women in the 1790s deflected criticism of their pampered diet by asserting that temperance and moderation were as common among the elite as among the lower classes. They claimed that 'costly materials were not necessary to constitute a debauch, nor profligacy less frequent under a thatched roof than under a lofty ceiling'.[11] Yet all the while, British involvement in the transatlantic slave trade and imperialism were encouraging widespread sugar addiction, helping to lay the foundations of what the World Health Organization terms a 'global obesity epidemic'.

EXERCISE IN PETTICOATS

Physicians did observe that exercise was essential for health. Dr Cheyne had been a great advocate of horse riding to 'shake the whole *Machine*', and around 1740 someone invented the 'chamber horse', a kind of leather seat on springs so that users could bounce vigorously up and down whenever the weather was too bad to ride out.[12] The invention was a precursor to the Chair of Health, devised at the end of the century for the gouty and rheumatic. This used electricity to massage the muscles and exercise the limbs. Dr Buchan, whose *Domestic Medicine* proved one of the most popular medical texts in Europe, was a firm advocate of exercise. His work, published in 1769, was aimed at ordinary people and offered preventative advice as well as cures. 'Nothing but exercise and open air can brace and strengthen the nerves', he wrote, insisting that fresh morning air was as good as a cold bath.[13] He railed against coaches, sedan chairs, and lolling in bed in the morning. He explained that inactive patients were always complaining of 'pains of the stomach, flatulencies, indigestions', but exercise would prevent ailments which medicine could not cure. He did think that women could better tolerate a sedentary life than men but reasoned that this only meant that lighter occupations should be reserved for women, so that they had less cause to resort to prostitution. It was never his view that women should be inactive.

Gentlemen were already exercising with dumbbells in the early eighteenth century. The early dumbbell may have been an apparatus similar to the kind used for swinging a church bell; it made no noise when 'rung' because the clapper was removed. Dumbbells made of wood or iron soon developed into the familiar shape of a bar weighted at each end, easily swung in the hand. Benjamin Franklin credited his long life to exercising with them every day. The growing craze for exercise brought opportunities to London's entrepreneurs. In the 1770s, Abraham Buzaglo set up a gym in the Strand opposite Somerset House. His apparatus included a system of bags and poles attached to a wall, and he promised a programme of exercises that would suffuse the body with warmth even when there was a hard frost. In the 1790s, the master clockmaker John Joseph Merlin built an early carousel or 'Aerial cavalcade' near Hanover Square, claiming that it offered ladies and gentlemen healthy exercise and entertainment. It whirled them around on wooden horses at fifteen or twenty miles an hour.[14]

The well-publicised benefits of exercise led to accusations that elite white women were indolent. They were said to avoid brisk open-air exercise in case it 'destroyed the delicate texture of their skin'; they deluded themselves that 'an idle lounge under the name of a walk' was enough to preserve health.[15] For many well-to-do females, exercise did just mean a walk to church, weather permitting, or a stroll in the park on Sunday afternoons. Yet British women had more freedom to walk the streets unaccompanied than their sisters on the Continent. In Portugal, for example, it was reported that 'no woman goes out of doors without permission of her husband or parents'.[16] Upper-class young Italian women were chaperoned into the 1890s, and even young married women were not allowed out alone.[17]

Even so, exercise was linked to the accomplishments that elite women needed to become marriageable. They were taught dancing by dance masters, either at home or in schools; their performances at balls helped them to fashion their status as ladies. Some also learned swordsmanship, since dancing and fencing were often taught together. Women might go riding, especially in the countryside, although major towns boasted indoor facilities and public riding schools. In London, upper-class women went to the refined riding-house in Pimlico, where they perfected a graceful seat on horseback. There was never any doubt of women's innate ability for physical exercise, since many performed as rope-dancers or daredevil riders in circuses, but social convention restricted what a genteel woman might do.

It is less well known that, in the eighteenth century, British women from the lower classes competed in energetic sports. On village fete days they ran races for smocks and other items of clothing, and even fought in prize boxing matches. They rode in horse races and played cricket – the first recorded women's game was in 1745 between the Surrey villages of Bramley and Hambledon. Few aristocratic women played cricket, although we do know that, in 1777, the fashionable Countess of Derby arranged a match with other women of her class at The Oaks, the earl's estate in Surrey; they must have played the game before. Noblewomen were strongly attracted to archery, which had links to the classical goddess Diana and could be performed with decorum in corsets and petticoats.

GROWING INTEREST IN DIET AND EXERCISE

In the late eighteenth century, doctors began to adopt a scientific approach to eating habits and exercise. They observed that the same regime operated differently on different constitutions, plumping up some and reducing others. Their objective was to come up with advice for a long healthy life and, since health was their object, they now began to classify fatness as a disease – a kind of oily dropsy rather than a watery one.[18] Dr William Wadd, who published a book on corpulence in 1810, noted that, although it was often hereditary, it chiefly afflicted the rich, who did not have to do manual labour to enjoy life's comforts.[19] Only now did the elite start to weigh themselves regularly on a cumbersome hanging balance. The practice became a modish novelty in Regency times, when sportsmen and celebrities including Beau Brummel and Lord Byron used the weighing apparatus at Berry Bros. & Rudd, a wine merchants in St James's. Byron's fight to stay fashionably slim is well documented. He purged, wore wool to sweat off the pounds, and resorted to one meal a day (potatoes and vinegar or biscuits and soda water).

Fat women tried various remedies to lose weight. Acids like vinegar were popular. Another option was Castile soap dissolved in water, which acted as a mild diuretic. Family doctors continued to urge a vegetable diet, abstinence, and exercise as the only safe measures. Dr Wadd noted the willingness of higher-weight people to resort to desperate measures that promised quick results, and their difficulty in keeping to any strict regime without moral support. He recorded the case of an unmarried woman, aged twenty-three, who was so fat she could not cross her apartment without getting out of breath. He told her to take the waters at Scarborough and to follow a strict diet. She began to lose weight, but her friends persuaded her that she had no need to be so hard on herself. She died aged just twenty-seven.

Public interest in fatness grew. In 1816, Wadd enlarged the third edition of his work with more examples and the latest medical observations. Current understanding of food values was limited but Wadd did note that a largely plant-based diet could not guarantee weight loss since beer and sugar were fattening. He drew comparisons between nations: the number of fat people in Britain, he claimed, far exceeded that in France or Spain, while non-Western cultures preferred women to be plump and even fattened them up before marriage. In this way he aligned himself with other European authors who were beginning to see fatness through a colonial lens, as Lady Craven did in the Turkish baths, and to associate it with those peoples they deemed less cultivated.[20] His warnings about corpulence were laced with alarming case histories in which he linked excess fat to a range of fatal conditions. Remarkably, these included spontaneous human combustion: 'A very fat woman, twenty-eight years of age . . . was found on fire in her Chamber, where nothing else was burning. The neighbours heard a noise of something like frying, and when the body was removed it left a layer of black grease.'[21] Wadd's descriptions of autopsies and investigations into the processes of digestion did much to evoke revulsion at the notion of fatty matter, although his original intention seems to have been to reassure the stout that it was within their power to lose weight.

Around this time, in an important development, temperance and exercise became firmly linked to beauty and not just health. In 1811, a lady at the British court confided to her diary: 'The Princess Charlotte is above the middle height, extremely spread for her age; her bosom full, but finely shaped; her shoulders large, and her whole person voluptuous; but of a nature to become soon spoiled, and without much care and exercise she will shortly lose all beauty in fat and clumsiness.'[22] In the same year, *The Lady's Magazine* advised readers that the secret of preserving beauty lay in a temperate diet, exercise, and cleanliness; a young woman given to overeating, much alcohol, and late hours would soon lose her charms. The magazine was particularly critical of *hot* bread and butter for breakfast, which, 'when taken constantly, are hostile to health and female delicacy. The heated grease, which is their principal ingredient, deranges the stomach.'[23] During the depression after the Napoleonic Wars, lasting into the 1820s, criticism of gluttony in Britain reached fever pitch. Fatness was a clear signal of indolence and the absence of willpower; it was branded a moral failing.

Doctors advised that prevention was better than cure, but genteel white women of the middling sort typically led restricted lives. Many now encouraged each other to take regular exercise, preferably in the open air, not least to banish melancholy. The writer and actor Frances Anne Kemble, better known as Fanny Kemble, wrote: 'Taking exercise has become, instead of a pleasure, a sometimes rather irksome duty to me; a lonely ride upon a disagreeable horse not being a great enjoyment; but I know that my health has its reward, and I persevere.'[24] She married an American and lived for a time in Philadelphia. There she noted that the women of New England easily lost their looks. In part, she imputed this to lack of exercise; they huddled in over-heated, ill-ventilated rooms during the long winter, and pinched their feet into such tight shoes they could hardly walk anyway. Indigenous women seemed much healthier. In the same vein, the Irish novelist Lady Sydney Morgan, married to a sedentary philosopher and surgeon, complained in 1832, 'I am suffering beyond all conception from want of air and exercise.'[25] The need for genteel women to have access to fresh air and exercise became axiomatic. The Poet Laureate Robert Southey wrote in 1834, 'We have ordered a pony-carriage; it is to be a light two-wheeled affair of the plainest kind, to carry two persons . . . I count upon it as one means of improving my wife's health, and, therewith, her spirits.'[26]

Given that middle-class women were largely confined to the house in the nineteenth century, indoor exercise equipment caught on. Lola Montez, a dancer and courtesan who wrote a guidebook on women's health and beauty in the 1850s, advised exercising with dumbbells in the open air to develop 'a handsome form', but women soon started to use them in the home.[27] Jane Welsh Carlyle strained her arm by two or three days' overzealous practice with dumbbells.[28] The irrepressible George Eliot had rather more success with racquet sports: 'We supply the want of regular lawn tennis by in-door battledore and shuttlecock, at which I am becoming an expert with both right and left hand. One advantage of our high drawing-room is its fitness for this exercise, which warms one better, and exercises more muscles, than walking.'[29] For once, the high-ceilinged, chilly Victorian drawing room was an asset.

Callisthenics for girls became popular in continental Europe during the 1820s. The exercise spread to schools for young ladies in Britain and the United States as people began to appreciate its health benefits. Exercise systems were published so that women could get fit in the family home, and physical drills were marketed as an aid to beauty as well as health. Douglas Walker published his *Exercises for Ladies Calculated to Preserve and Improve Beauty* in 1836, promising that they would prevent deformity and develop the muscles needed for 'a correct form'. Walker was a great proponent of 'Indian Exercises' using a kind of weighted 'Indian club'. These juggling-club-shaped wooden clubs were swung in patterns to build up strength. The British Army had already recognised the value of this form of exercise. Walker masked the link with Indian virility; he adapted the wooden club for white women and called it a 'sceptre'.[30] In London only his publisher and a callisthenics teacher in Regent Street stocked the sceptres, but Walker glibly assured readers that any carpenter could make one, weighting the knobbed end with two to four pounds of lead. He claimed that sceptres were an advance on dumbbells and that his exercise system combined military principles with grace.

Rigidly applied, Walker's precepts introduced another form of tyranny over well-to-do women. He discouraged riding on the grounds that side-saddles gave a twist to the whole body, while the loud tones needed when talking to companions on horseback yielded a coarse voice. He found fault with the way women stood, claiming that they raised one shoulder when writing, and inclined to one side when drawing with the arm elevated. His diagrams gave the correct position they should be taught to adopt. His rules were hard to reject outright because he also insisted that proper deportment was evidence of a good education and a complement to intellectual attainment.

By the 1880s, fresh air, cold baths, and exercise were the norm in British and North American schools. In French state schools for girls, gymnastics based on the English or German model was introduced in the 1880s. Novice teachers might find such lessons a trial, one woman writing, 'I always dread them more than anything. They give such scope for disorder', which may explain why callisthenics was often reserved for the end of the school day.[31] But in the United States, higher education colleges for women set up departments of physical training and employed specialist staff. One student wrote home excitedly:

> The gymnasium is to be newly fitted up with clubs, *ladders*, bars, and apparatus this week, and soon we are to begin to practice regularly. The regular classes only practice two periods of twenty minutes a week, but there are to be special classes for those who have any special trouble, such as round shoulders, weak back or ankles, or turned-in toes, and these are to have special exercises.[32]

By the 1890s, some women's colleges required students to devote three hours weekly to gymnasium practice throughout the whole of their course. The system pioneered in Sweden by Pehr Ling, based on anatomy, was especially popular.

Women who wished to teach physical education could take a two-year course, giving them new career opportunities. Gymnastics was thought to have a moral influence on the young as well as a health benefit, teaching them to move with exactness in unison. Sports had a role to play in colonisation. British dignitaries in Canada in the 1890s toured schools where uniformed children were instructed in physical drill, 'dumb-bells, Indian Clubs – marching, running & various exercises', and admired how well the lessons were conducted.[33] Female gymnastics was included in the 1908 Olympic Games, which did much to encourage nationalistic pride in the physical development and grace of women's teams.

Certain types of female exercise continued to evoke disapproval. In the nineteenth century, some feared that waltzing for hours in the stale air of a ballroom was a danger to health as well as to morals. Tuberculosis, which often seemed to afflict young girls, would surely follow.[34] But there were no such objections to skating, single-sex classes at a public gymnasium, golf, fencing, or cricket (though women were warned not to play in heels, and male commentators remarked that few women had the nerve to withstand the approach of a swift ball).[35] An additional attraction for upwardly mobile women was that many such activities were not only on trend but also excused luxury purchases or a new outfit. Tight-fitting silk combinations were worn for exercise. Some purchased a special costume just for walking, made to clear the ground by two and a half inches; it advertised their commitment to the healthy open air.

Magazines for women and teenage girls proliferated in the nineteenth century, thanks to advances in printing technology. They increasingly carried welcome advice about diet and exercise, but fads remained. In North America, a mechanical camel was invented in 1899, replicating the movements of a real 'ship of the desert' to give the female rider a slender figure. Some thought it would be better to suppress sweet factories; New York alone was already producing $10,000,000 worth of bonbons a year.[36] Exercise also became a means to signal great wealth. At the turn of the century, society women in New York were spending vast sums on private home gymnasiums, while plans for luxury new houses in the city routinely included exercise rooms. The middling sort were targeted by advertisements for more modest home exercise regimes, which guaranteed to make the body symmetrical without drugs or dieting in just a few minutes a day.

DIET AND HAPPINESS

Diet and a good digestion were firmly linked to health and happiness in the public mind by the 1840s. Dyspepsia was one of the great afflictions of the nineteenth century. Its prevalence even cast doubt on the progress of civilisation, since the pace of modern life, polluted cities, and pampered lifestyles seem to have combined to weaken the stomach. The process of digestion, still imperfectly understood, was fertile ground for speculation. Anxious dyspeptics obsessed over bodily functions and worried about the effect on their constitutions of certain foods. The Carlyles' health suffered greatly when their doctor advised them to avoid vegetables, which, as their letters recount, worsened their constipation. George Eliot urged her ailing friend Elma Stuart 'to avoid fruits, sweets, wines, and all *acid*-making foods, to keep your blood as free from acid as you can by baths, rubbings, exercise, and *diet*'.[37] Mrs Stuart became committed to the Salisbury diet, consisting of pints of hot water and minced steak, on which she subsisted exclusively for eleven years before declaring herself perfectly cured of what doctors now believe to have been chronic fatigue syndrome. She extolled the benefits of this diet in her book *What Must I Do to Get Well? And How Can I Keep So?*, which she dedicated to the memory of George Eliot. Published in the late 1880s, it saw twenty-five editions in ten years, was translated into French and German, and produced a cult following.

Feminists have argued that social pressure on women to diet and mould their bodies into some arbitrary standard of beauty is a ploy to distract them from public life and to safeguard male political power.[38] But dieting was at first a male preserve. It indicated manly self-control, respectable ambition, and a patriotic desire to be a useful citizen. Women were not credited with the same moral fibre and self-discipline needed to reduce their food intake and lose weight.[39]

This manly endeavour took root in Victorian Britain before crossing the Atlantic to the United States. In 1863, William Banting, an eminent London undertaker, published his *Letter on Corpulence*, describing a trail-blazing, low-carbohydrate diet with which he had personally conquered fatness. He claimed to write only for the public good but specifically addressed men. His diet did appeal to men, favouring foods associated with masculinity and wealth such as red meat and claret. His modest tone was endearing, and he was candid about his experience of being fat:

> Although no very great size or weight, still I could not stoop to tie my shoe, so to speak, nor attend to the little offices humanity requires without considerable pain and difficulty, which only the corpulent can understand; I have been compelled to go down stairs slowly backwards, to save the jar of increased weight upon the ancle and knee joint, and been obliged to puff and blow with every slight exertion.[40]

Banting insisted that weight reduction was a rational procedure and a sign of strength, in no way linked to feminine self-denial and sacrifice. After 1864, editions of his book included a height–weight table from a life insurance company, used to assess policy applicants. Medical opinion about the relationship between weight and health was inconsistent, and reliable data scarce, but such tables did encourage readers to weigh themselves and chart their progress.

Banting's work also pandered to class prejudice, since he implied that fatness was a problem for the nouveau riche who had not learned the self-control of the established elite. In contrast, his diet would nurture strong, disciplined men needed to build and maintain an empire. The book was a roaring success, particularly among the middle classes who appear to have been the target audience. In North America, the Banting diet encouraged discrimination against bulkier nationalities and races, increasingly regarded as unfit for power. The anti-fat bias among the white elite encouraged unfounded generalisations and had a strong racial element. When Bantingism was imported into India, it helped to bolster colonial rule by encouraging the English to think of themselves as disciplined empire builders. Dieting enabled English men and women to differentiate themselves from the native population.[41]

Yet dieting became popular with women only some twenty-five years after it had been taken up by men. Until then, the Venus de' Medici was still touted as a model of female beauty. The ideal woman was well rounded, and soft female contours signalled wealth and grace. One young white debutante recorded being fortified and fattened for the 1869 London season on 'an incalculable amount of nasty iron and porridge'; meagre women were advised to pour olive oil over each meal.[42] Only towards the end of the century was Banting's 'meat diet' promoted by women's rights activists, not least because it was associated with self-control, social responsibility, and class status. Meat four times a day was beyond the means of the poor, but the diet became popular with some New Women cyclists, keen to maintain a trim, athletic figure.

Women quickly saw that overt control of their bodies would signal their ability to manage independence. A regular, healthy lifestyle became central to the women's rights movement, which focused on such issues as birth control and divorce. The leader of the movement in the United States, Elizabeth Cady Stanton, offered this tip for public speaking, 'Dress loose, take a great deal of exercise, & be particular about your diet & sleep sound enough, the body has a great effect on the mind.'[43] Stanton lived in Britain for some five years in the 1880s and early 1890s, aligning herself with radical suffragism.

As more women were admitted to higher education, a slender, fit body became associated with intellectual achievement, reinforcing existing associations between fatness, stupidity, and laziness. The slim ideal became a means to discipline middle-class white women. There were few Black women in Britain until after the Second World War, but African American newspapers indicate that aspiring Black women similarly began to watch their weight in the 1880s, some taking long walks to offset any tendency to fatness.[44] Certainly, by the early twentieth century these newspapers were advising readers to practise self-denial and take outdoor exercise, but significantly only to regain 'normal lines' and a 'normal weight' if larger-bodied.[45]

By 1913, when very low-cut necklines became fashionable in London and Paris, upper-class women were all set to reveal considerably more soft tissue. The *Illustrated London News* gushed, 'modern women have learnt to take such care of themselves, have become such experts in the question of diet, and so Spartan in carrying out the needful self-denial . . . that a beautiful throat is the rule and not the exception at any gathering of Society women'.[46] By this time, weight reduction was firmly coupled with beauty as well as health. In Britain, Banting's regime had triggered a proliferation of public weighing machines at railway stations and chemists. These were mostly used by men, but women soon followed suit. The social reformer Beatrice Webb weighed herself each week at Charing Cross station, luxuriating over the loss of each half-ounce. Virginia Woolf, hardly plump herself, carped in 1918 that Webb was 'as bare as a bone'.[47]

TOWARDS A DIET INDUSTRY

Dieting was not at first promoted by the fashion trade or by eager doctors and businessmen selling diet foods. Arguably, it took hold in Western society from the 1890s as a response to the wealth and materialism of the elite, which was creating a sense of unease. And it seems that women dieted in private before weight watching was marketed in the press; after all, it was increasingly stylish to be slender. In affluent North America, snacking was already a problem, 'The sweetmeat habit, the nibbling habit, the starving habit, the stuffing habit, are about equally undesirable', warned one mentor in 1901, claiming to address girls at boarding school. 'If there is one practice more disastrous than another to the school-girl's health, I think it is the eating and drinking between meals.'[48] Starving to remain slight and eating chalk to produce an interesting pallor were both absurd, she continued, offering an alarming insight into contemporary practices. Lack of self-control when eating was to be avoided above all.

Diets to cure portliness in women and girls began to appear towards the end of the nineteenth century. They may have produced results if less was eaten, but some contained a great deal of misinformation despite ongoing advances in food science. Authors claimed that all sugary, starchy, and fatty foods were bad, that biscuits and toast were preferable to bread, and that even water was fattening.[49] The attraction of self-help guides to health and beauty was that they seemed to give women control. The Western woman's ability to choose her regime was hailed as a social advance and compared to practices such as Chinese foot binding, still used as an example of female oppression. But many doctors of the time failed to treat dieting women seriously. Plumpness was commonly ascribed to biological differences between men and women and therefore something women had to accept. Even so, by the early twentieth century the ideal physique for all people was athletic and lean. And since dress reformers who denounced the corset still valued a slim waist, a Western woman's 'natural' figure had to be sylph-like. The circulation of height–weight tables and the growing stand-ardisation of the female figure, thanks to ready-made clothing industries, put more pressure on women to conform to acceptable contours. This opened the door to quack therapies.

Most cures for stoutness promised quick results. One New York doctor who bluntly addressed his advertisement to 'Fat People' prom-ised that his 'correct scientific treatment' would give a weight loss of two to five pounds a week: 'No tight bandages to press your vital organs and cause serious complications, no purgatives that reduce strength with weight and cause stomach disorders also, no radical diet system to make you feel that life isn't worth living, no sickening treatment that leaves your skin wrinkled and flabby.'[50] Instead, his personalised, confi-dential home therapy, a correspondence course, offered weight loss without pain. Many such treatments were shrouded in mystery. In London, Madame Elvira advertised: 'Have you a double chin, large bust, large hips, large waist, and a large abdomen? Flesh hanging over your corsets at the back, adding years to your age?' If so, she had a 'wonderful discovery', guaranteed to remove all superfluous flesh by a simple and harmless method, never known to fail.[51] Higher-weight people were often swindled; fat-shaming and the prize of a slender figure persuaded many to part with their money.

The increasing availability of ready-made foodstuffs, such as Bird's custard powder, biscuits, and Bovril, lured consumers into purchasing modified foods that claimed to improve health. Just as some eighteenth-century doctors had recommended a vegetable diet in summer, so, in the late nineteenth century, Dr Tibbles' Vi-Cocoa, a mixture of malt, hops, cola, and cocoa, was touted as especially adapted to hot weather, providing vitality without overloading the digestive system. Dietetic Cocoa was advertised as good for dyspeptics and those with delicate constitutions. Such products led to confusion and slippage between slimming 'tonics' and new health foods like 'Frame Food' Jelly, allegedly as nutritious as malt extract and as delicious as jam, packed with 'bone and brain-forming' natural phosphates.[52] Or Tropon, a 'natural pure albumen', tasteless and odourless but 'the only real food for the healthy and invalids' alike.[53]

Advertisements targeted at women who wanted to lose weight offered similar-sounding products that could be bought from chemists or by mail order. Vogeler's Curative Compound, 'the formula of an eminent West-End London physician', was hyped in a persuasive advert describing a woman who became the envy of her friends for health and beauty: 'She used to suffer from indigestion, sick headache, constipation, torpid liver, sluggish kidneys, nervousness, want of vitality, sudden faintness and female weakness, and very often eruptions on her face and neck, but they are all evils of the past since she has taken her favourite medicine; and now she has perfect health.'[54] Mr F. Cecil Russell, a self-proclaimed specialist in fatness, promoted 'a pure vegetable product, without any admixture of the mineral poisons', offering consumers the 'delightful experience' of losing unnecessary and dangerous fat at the rate of many pounds per week. At the same time, it acted as a tonic and sharpened the appetite. Russell claimed that users could indulge this appetite because, as they returned to health, increasing brain and digestive activity naturally required more food.[55] He promised that patients would quickly and permanently reduce to shapely proportions without fasting or extreme exercise. His treatment was popular for at least a decade from the mid-1890s.

Other home treatments included Antipon, which also promised to cure 'obstinate cases of long-standing obesity' without drugs, dieting, or gymnastics, and Biomalz, a German tonic food, which undertook to strengthen muscle and remove flab at the same time.[56] Manufacturers played on fears of adulterated food by marketing 'pure' nutrients like Victoria Date Vinegar, advertised as good for digestion and the only vinegar guaranteed not to injure health. (Doctors had long warned of the dangers of drinking vinegar to get slim.) Although sensible advice about weight loss was increasingly available from doctors, it lacked the allure of these seductive products, promoted with illustrations in popular magazines.

Meanwhile, the American Bernarr Macfadden (born Bernard McFadden: he altered his name to what seemed a more virile form) helped to create an image of the powerful woman. In influential publications that promoted his bodybuilding, health, and nutrition theories, Macfadden explained how women could perfect their physique and attain beauty and health though exercise and judicious fasting. He had a large following in Britain as well as the United States, thanks to the body culture movement which spread from Europe in the nineteenth century. Some thought him an eccentric and others a fanatic, but his views anticipated later feminist arguments that women should regain control of their bodies. Macfadden railed against corsets and overeating, but also denounced prudery and sexual ignorance. His health magazine, *Physical Culture*, founded in 1899, supported female suffrage, and his many publications show how diet and exercise were issues linked to sexual equality and political emancipation.

In early twentieth-century Britain, advertisements for women's weight reduction multiplied. It was a time of growing social unrest, clamour for social change, and increasing fears about Britain's standing in the world. In the years before the First World War, journalists reported on the German 'cult of slimness'. Their affected amusement was mixed with unease at this further proof of German efficiency and economy. Germany's share of world manufacturing production had already outstripped Britain's; its share of world trade was also increasing, while Britain's was in decline. One reporter claimed that, in Berlin, 'the cult of thinness is universal. On the stage, on the picture postcard, the kinematograph, the advertisement, everywhere.'[57] In fact, this cultural change was more widespread: in the United States as in major European cities, the fashionable female shape was no longer curvaceous but typified by straight lines from armpits to knees.

Popular magazines routinely linked happiness and slimness. In 1914, the *Illustrated London News* published 'How to be Slender and Happy. A Word to the Modern Woman'.[58] The aim was no longer to preserve the constitution and balance the body as if it were a machine to be kept in good running order, but to reshape its outline instead by making a decisive intervention. Bulky women had to increase the body's powers of combustion and burn up stored energy from food by strenuous exercise. This active stance chimed with contemporary, socially progressive trends of thought which affirmed the power of humans to create, improve, and reshape their environment.

Hollywood stars had a huge influence on fans when it came to diet and exercise. Annette Kellerman, who made the first nude film scene, boasted perfect proportions: her measurements were nearly identical to the Venus de Milo and classical statues of the goddess Diana. As a child Kellerman wore iron braces for weak knees, but she perfected her adult physique through swimming, dancing, and fencing.[59] Health and beauty magazines explained that other female stars had taken to exercising with punch bags. Lillian Russell, a renowned beauty, was 'one of the most expert bag punchers of her sex'; Anna Held even had a punch bag fitted into her limousine so that she could exercise while travelling.[60] Readers were assured that 'bag punching is one of the best forms of exercise a woman could possibly engage in'; the Uppercut punch bag was available in Britain for a mere 12s 6d.[61] In 1926, First National Pictures added weight limit clauses to actors' contracts. If stars exceeded their contracted weight limit, they risked immediate dismissal. Magazines reported that as a result some lunched on just a slice of pineapple and two prunes, setting higher standards of abstinence for fans.[62] Intimate interviews with stars about their eating habits helped to authorise fad diets.

In the early twentieth century, weighing machines were too expensive for most households, but by the 1920s affluent women had incorporated bathroom scales into rituals of self-surveillance and weight loss. Their routines included using products like Clark's Thinning Bath Salts, said to dissolve superfluous fat through the pores of the skin to leave slim, girlish contours. The salts could be supplemented with Clark's Thinning Paste for restoring thick ankles to more graceful lines, 'a boon to dancers and persons moving in social circles', or with Clark's Fat-Corrective Pastilles, which claimed to alter 'the bodily habit of excess fat-formation'.[63] These products were also shipped to the British colonies, because slenderness was associated with social mobility and privilege.

Other products encouraged women who did have the use of a bathroom to view it as a slimming aid. Cyclax Violet Ray Reducing Salts promised to reduce weight through bathing, as Clark's salts did. The lower classes had to be content with La-Mar Reducing Soap, which claimed to wash away fat and years of age. Smoking soon became implicated in weight control. Advertisements for Clark's bath salts showed a slim woman in an elegant wrap, poised on the side of the bath with a cigarette in a holder.[64] By the end of the 1920s, smoking was openly promoted as an appetite suppressant. In one advert, women were advised to reject the temptation of a between-meal bite and smoke a Kensitas instead. This Kensitas campaign lasted just two years but embedded the link between smoking and weight management. Sadly, doctors had warned even in the eighteenth century that, although tobacco products could make people slim, they ruined digestion and introduced diseases.[65]

By the mid-1920s the pressure to be extremely slim had spawned an inventive range of quack products. They reflect the degree of competition that women experienced in the workplace and in life generally. There was the Vaco Reducing Cup for a protruding abdomen, no longer a matronly asset as in Victorian times; this suction cup guaranteed to loosen the congestion of fat and make it vanish. The Punkt Roller, if used daily for two hours, pledged to knead away unwanted fat while tuning muscles and nerves. There were several creams: Thinulene to cure the disfigurement of a double chin; Rodiod for thick necks or ankles; Espanol Solvent, which offered women the autonomy to reduce any part of their body by however much they wanted. The wealthy, figure-conscious woman could buy a portable electric Health Motor, which vibrated a wide belt around hips or thighs, allegedly sloughing off inches with no need for actual exercise. Sanatoriums offered mineral wax therapy, coating bodies with warm, liquid wax for health and weight loss. There was even electric shock treatment for those who failed to reduce by other means. Since none of these remedies worked, those with money for cosmetic surgery just had excess fat cut away, so that they could wear the androgenous styles in fashion. In the early twentieth century, French beauty magazines consistently ran advertisements for breast reduction as well as facelifts.[66]

By the 1930s, there was increasing concern about fad diets. Doctors reported early cases of models who starved themselves to extreme thinness to find work. Medical analysts noted that young women had not seen an improvement in the death rate from tuberculosis as most had, and that maternal mortality was high in this group. They hypothesised that both trends were due to malnourishment and dieting.[67] Social commentators speculated that restricted food intake was linked to depression and related to the lack of self-worth felt by 'surplus women' of the war generation.

In this context, new treatments explicitly offered weight reduction without dangerous dieting or harmful drugs. Marienbad Reducing Tea, taken first thing every morning, would keep women slim while allowing them to eat almost anything. A morning glass of Kutnow's Powder would also eliminate the need for fasting and dieting. Both were probably laxative. Other teas like Yerbama reduced the appetite. The beginnings of the diet food industry saw bread replacements such as Ryvita and Energen starch-reduced rolls. Both were advertised from 1925 as nourishing and beneficial to health. Energen products had formerly catered for the diabetic but would be marketed to weight watchers until the 1970s, offering to make dieting a pleasure: 'eat as much as you like and yet keep a fashionable, attractively slim figure'.[68] Arguably, from the 1920s, dieting was a means to keep the middle-class woman under surveillance, but otherwise free to enjoy life's pleasures.

A NEW PRISON

Weight control had long been linked to white women's reproductive health, especially among the middling and upper sort. These females were expected to play their part in revitalising white populations for the modern world.[69] In this context, the post-war athleticism of young German women was noted with disquiet and envy in Britain. In 1928, the *Illustrated London News* reported that German women were devoted to weekends of open-air exercise. Female telephonists in Berlin's Post Office had physical exercises programmed into their working day, while the fastidious could sample 'decalorised food' through a glass tube at the city's Kaloridorado Café, the first scientifically equipped eatery to supply a modern nutrient that would not lead to weight gain.[70] English women were now told they needed 'a natural "corset" of muscle'; after all, fitness experts had recommended breathing exercises to harden the abdominal muscles against 'ballooning' since the beginning of the century.[71]

Britain soon had its own mass fitness movement. In 1930, Mary Bagot Stack set up the Women's League of Health and Beauty. She herself had overcome serious illness through rigorous exercise. Across

Britain, women embraced the new movement, which cost just 2s 6d to join. The League's ethos reflected the class, racial, and imperial prejudices of the period. In the minds of its supporters, weight control and fitness were closely linked to women's reproductive health and class. In the British colonies, such eugenic ideas were inseparable from issues of race; branches of the League rapidly spread to Canada and Australia. But the League did offer a supportive context in which thousands of women learned the value of exercise, and many reported that they felt happier as well as healthier. Much of the attraction was the fun of doing synchronised routines to the latest hit tunes. The League marketed exercise to music, using the latest gramophone technology, although this had already been pioneered by W. K. Kellogg, inventor of the breakfast cereal and health guru. The League raised interest by staging a display of synchronised exercise at the Royal Albert Hall in 1931, but it was their 1939 televised performance at Wembley, involving 5,000 women, that really put the movement on the map.

Since at least the late eighteenth century, when news reached Britain that in Paris revolutionaries were giving meat rations to pregnant women as well as to the sick, pundits in Britain had turned a spotlight on women's health in times of crisis. They talked up the national importance of women's childbearing role and, increasingly, their productivity as workers. On the eve of the First World War, an enquiry found that low-paid female clerical workers were trapped in a vicious circle: they did not earn enough to eat well, became less productive because undernourished, and then their low productivity was used as an excuse to pay them less than men.[72] In 1938, experts claimed that nearly half the British population faced malnutrition, either through poverty or through poor understanding of cooking methods and food values.[73] They noted developments such as communal feeding in Soviet Russia, allegedly offering scientifically balanced diets, and the Women's Labour Service in Nazi Germany, which took women from different levels of society to camps for months at a time, giving them physical fitness regimes and training them to become good mothers and housewives.

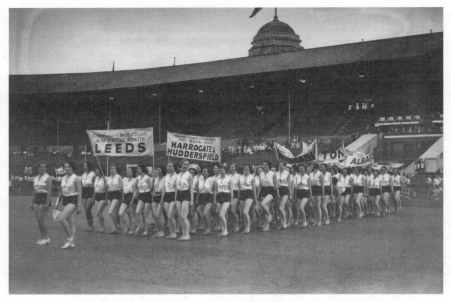

6. A demonstration by the Women's League of Health and Beauty at Wembley, 1935.

As with the Women's League of Health and Beauty, the implication was that girls should develop fit, healthy bodies for the good of the nation.

During the Second World War, rationing made diets redundant but also led to a better understanding of food values and a growing awareness that it was possible to be fat but undernourished. All the same, when war ended, advertisements for diet therapies took on a more sinister, coercive tone. 'How will you look when he returns?' demanded one, as British forces were about to be demobilised. 'If you have a spare tyre, pinch and pummel it mercilessly.'[74] The bikini craze swept French beaches in 1947, giving women more reason to buy products for a youthful figure.

The 1950s saw overtly manipulative marketing techniques that played on women's guilt. 'Can't be Jones's Wife', a man declared in one advertisement for abdominal exercise belts; 'She used to be such a slim, pretty woman! Another case for a daily 5 minutes with the Rallie Health

Belt.'[75] 'Too fat for fashion?' questioned another advertisement for the Health Belt. It featured a chance meeting between a dowdy, middle-aged woman and her svelte acquaintance. Their conversation about the belt ended with the larger woman saying, 'I'd do anything to get rid of this awful fat and it sounds so easy. Do tell me how I can get one.'[76] Social pressure to 'age well' was already established.

Scientific advances helped to validate a controlled food intake. In the 1950s, research into calories and the workings of the metabolism exposed common food fallacies: lemons are not slimming; toast is just as fattening as bread, Ryvita not less so. There was disheartening news about exercise: nutritionists worked out that dieters would need to run forty-three miles to work off a pound of excess fat.[77] Calorie-controlled diets already existed: an American doctor, Lulu Hunt Peters, had published *Diet & Health: With Key to the Calories* in 1918, the first diet book to become a bestseller. She herself had suffered problems with body image, growing up in a period when the ideal female shape morphed from a full, rounded figure to a flat, boyish one. In her book she simplified calorie counting for a mass audience – and handed women the shackles with which to imprison themselves. By the end of the 1950s, the Swedish Milk Diet, just vitamin and mineral powder stirred into milk, encouraged women to live on a mere 650 calories a day. Dieting became normalised and a lucrative slimming industry took off.

The evil of sugar was newly exposed. In 1963, Pepsi introduced Diet Cola and Coke launched sugar-free Tab, just days apart from each other. Schweppes followed with its slimline range (although in the 1920s the company had been recommending three glasses of their cider daily for glowing health and slimness). London restaurants began to offer diet lunches, and counting calories became another burden for the successful housewife. One cookery writer insisted, 'The clever hostess, however, will remember that most guests want to stay slim. She should be able to serve a superb meal with an enviably low calorie count.'[78] The modern girl weighed herself every day; personal scales, now reduced in price, were pitched as essential aids to beauty not just health. The jogging craze took off in cities. Television and mass advertising broadcast images of Twiggy and other super-thin role models so that, by 1969, girls as young as eleven were skipping breakfast to remain slim. Teenage girls were especially vulnerable to the stigma of being larger bodied; in 1971, the Inner London Education Authority ran a summer programme to slim down the 'fat' ones.[79]

Underwear manufacturers noted and helped to publicise changes in women's vital statistics. In Britain, a 1979 study even compared regional variations in women's weight and body measurements at different stages in life. It found that women in eastern counties were consistently larger and heavier. More plentiful food had resulted in a thicker female body; the hourglass figure was a thing of the past. The development was trumpeted as a threat to masculinity: in bold type a newspaper warned that women were 'growing more like men'.[80] The latest female silhouette produced other responses. Appearance has always influenced the judgement of character, but female body shape increasingly became an indicator of class; in some circles it became socially unacceptable to be fat. Slenderness and fitness became widespread indicators of moral worth.

All these pressures accelerated the diet industry. Audrey Eyton was a founder member of the influential *Slimming Magazine*, which appeared in 1970. Just when slimmers were enjoying chocolate-laced meal replacement bars, she published her ground-breaking F-Plan Diet; in 1982–3, her book was on the *Sunday Times* bestseller list for over a year. It showed readers how to cut calories and at the same time increase their intake of dietary fibre from unrefined cereal foods, fruits, and vegetables. It was followed, in 1985, by Miriam Stoppard's High-Fibre Diet, which had the attraction of assuring dieters that they would always feel full. By now the concept of losing weight was all-pervasive. Researchers found that girls as young as nine were unhappy with their body shape, and ironically blamed the 1980s health boom for this situation.[81] Young girls were dieting and paving the way for a damaging relationship with food that could last a lifetime. Yet Black girls were more satisfied with their bodies; they valued self-assurance and attitude more than zero-sized contours.[82]

Despite the concern of educationalists and some parents, all media perpetuated the notion that beautiful women had to be extremely thin. Commercialised fad diets like the cabbage soup diet or the grapefruit diet filled column inches, an ascetic counterpart to society's increasing appetite for highly processed foods. Such obvious fads were punctuated by regimes able to attract a mass following. The high-protein/low-carbohydrate Atkins Diet, which first appeared in 1972, moved main-stream during 2002–4, boosting the sale of high-protein energy bars. As with Banting's diet, its high meat content appealed to men, but a version with salad was marketed to women. By now the diet industry had completely usurped the calendar year, with predictable pre-Christmas, New Year, and summer beach diets.

As early as the 1980s, disillusioned weight watchers were exposing the paradox that dieting makes you fat. Doctors and scientists readily denounced the unbalanced Atkins Diet as a massive health risk, but dieting had become so normalised that the insidious impact on the metabolism of restricting food intake long-term had only intermittent publicity. Those who slowed their metabolism by prolonged dieting regained lost pounds, and sometimes more, on reverting to normal meals. Next time they dieted they found it harder to reduce weight. After nearly a century of faddish regimes for weight loss, dieters were faced with one choice: the lifestyle that the Victorian New Woman had espoused. Only strict dietary control and regular exercise, built into a daily routine, would keep the pounds at bay.

Women's relationships with food cultures are complex; their food choices can be inflected by social hardships and discrimination. In the United States, some Black women face additional dietary challenges that are partly due to systemic racism. Traditional African American soul food is high in carbohydrates and fat; low-calorie alternatives seem bland and alien. Women of African heritage can feel caught between conflicting aesthetics: the slim, white standard of beauty, and curvier Black ideals with the extra weight in all the right places. The anti-racist writer Vena Moore complains: 'Dieting while Black can be a huge headache when you either don't have access to healthy food, have to figure out how to navigate two widely different sets of beauty standards and/or don't wish to eat foods that are considered "white people food" . . . Essentially, we start to associate healthy eating with whiteness.'[83]

In Britain, female migrants from Black and brown ethnic groups have been found to have larger body sizes, a trend which increases with the length of time since migration.[84] The reasons are complex but the adoption of Western fast foods and low levels of physical activity are certainly implicated. The Fitness2Flash group is one of several prompting South Asian women worldwide to 'put themselves and their well-being before anything else' and maintain a healthy lifestyle.[85] Black Britons have a long tradition of exercising to feel fit rather than to change their body shape, and the goal of better health remains a powerful incentive for all individuals to lose weight.[86]

All the same, despite what amounts to a cult of slimness and health, populations are getting fatter. Researchers have found that dieting and binge eating are linked; the concerted pressure of the diet and fast-food industries have contributed to an 'obesity epidemic' bringing poor health. Since the 1990s, obesity rates have risen steeply. That said, the definition of obesity is problematic. The optimum weight range is based on a calculation of body mass index (BMI), an assessment of weight against height and bone structure, which does not allow for the differing weights of muscle and fat. Women of colour point out that the ratios widely used to define obesity are based on studies of white people and do not allow for different ethnic norms.

The BMI screening tool for obesity is low-cost and easy to use. Yet it may be helping to institutionalise long-standing prejudices against women of non-Western heritage and heavier build. After all, slenderness has long been used to signify racial as well as social superiority.[87] There is no easy solution to defining or addressing obesity; weight-loss surgery and injections that suppress the appetite bring risks and side effects with no guarantee that results can be sustained long-term without a change in lifestyle.

In earlier Western societies, it was the self-indulgent rich who were more likely to be fat. Today that position is reversed: it is the poor who are more likely to be larger bodied, their poverty serviced by an increasingly unhealthy takeaway culture. As George Orwell remarked in the 1930s, the less money you have, the less inclined you feel to spend it on wholesome food. The rich 'may enjoy breakfasting off orange juice and Ryvita biscuits', he wrote, the poor do not: 'When you are unemployed, which is to say when you are underfed, harassed, bored, and miserable, you don't want to eat dull wholesome food. You want something a little bit "tasty".'[88] Wherever home cooking facilities are limited, or when adults are depressed or working unsociable hours, takeaway meals are an easy option. And low-income families can live in 'food deserts' where shops simply do not stock fresh fruit and vegetables. Political systems do little to curb a food industry intent on profit from selling unhealthy snacks.

We cannot know how bodies were experienced in the past but certainly today, when weight loss is a commonplace goal, many women say they feel trapped in a cycle of failure and guilt. The diet industry sells dreams. Just starting a diet gives a temporary boost to self-esteem. The gym industry promotes wellbeing but partly depends on a supply of unfit people who need to lose weight. The food industry slips unhealthy ingredients into ready-made foods to increase sales and perhaps to lengthen shelf life. Fitbit technology helps people to keep to health regimes but easily inspires guilt when goals are missed. Even the body positivity movement, which encourages people to be happy with the shape they have, has become commercialised. It has increased diversity in the beauty and fashion industries and encouraged the diet industry to focus on health and wellbeing, but entrenched attitudes to body shape mean that women who differ from perceived norms are rarely at ease.

Every culture has a favourite body shape, however much that preference is exposed and contested, so individuals will always be judged on their silhouette. Sympathetic commentators may attribute fatness to poverty and mental health issues, but it remains strongly linked to a lack of self-discipline. Many women, afraid of censure, walk a tightrope between eating well and eating the minimum to slim down, between doing physical activity for wellbeing and extreme exercise to shed pounds. And as *Bridget Jones's Diary* memorably portrayed in the 1990s, women often battle issues of weight and self-image alone, despite the fake intimacy of slimming advertisements. The enticing possibilities of creating a new identity by changing body shape only make failure harder to bear. Ideals of slenderness and fitness, seeming to promise autonomy, can lead to new servitude.

₰3₰

SKIN

In 1714, the surgeon and physician Daniel Turner published the first book in English on skin disease. The case histories he described reveal the suffering caused by quite common skin conditions and the inability of contemporary medicine to do much about it.

In one case, Turner examined a young woman with a scattering of crusty blisters on her face. Every morning she picked the scab off the most conspicuous sore, only to find the next day it had grown a new crust. He suspected impetigo and explained, 'I desir'd she would show me her Elbows, and (if she pleas'd) her Knees.'[1] The woman readily showed him the sores on her elbows and modestly confirmed that the tops of her knees were rather worse. Turner prescribed ointment laced with mercury, which in time gave her both colic and mouth sores, and caused her to retch. Her gums swelled until they covered the tops of her teeth but still the doctor could not bring her to the plentiful salivation he hoped would cure her. After three weeks he tried sweating and purging. He put his patient on a restricted diet for a month, washed her sores in an alkali lotion as corrosive as she could bear, and sent her to try the spa waters at Bath. She returned after two months with the pustules still evident. Finally, he resorted to dabbing her sores with a solution of sulphuric acid. The woman bore this long and painful treatment with great courage, fearing the disease would further blemish her face. But at length, Turner had to admit that he was foiled. His therapies were good for nothing; the patient would have to live with the condition.

This story also shows the pressure that skincare placed upon women. Men as well as women suffered from skin diseases, but a blemished skin was much more likely to affect a woman's life chances. Her face might literally be her fortune if it enabled her to marry well. After marriage, a woman's beauty remained a social asset, so her husband would also wish to see it preserved. Samuel Pepys, for example, was so agitated about a swelling on his wife's cheek that he sent for a surgeon, lest it 'spoil her face, if not timely cured'.[2] The visible surface of a person's skin was in any case bound to be scrutinised because it was believed to give clues about their inner condition. Yet what could be seen and what was hidden? While all kinds of disorders might be going on inside the body, external signs would be unnoticed on those parts that were kept clothed. The face and hands were therefore of paramount importance as key locations where medical, moral, and social meanings converged. And the face got most attention.

Skin has always evoked a spectrum of associations. In the eighteenth century, victims of robbery were often described as having been stripped to the skin, which conveyed poverty, ill-treatment, and vulnerability all at once. Great value was placed just on keeping the skin whole because disfigurement and injury were common. One reason why inoculation for smallpox met with resistance in that century was that it required deep incisions (as well as the introduction of foreign matter into the body). Before the invention of synthetic materials, there was good reason for taking a utilitarian view of skin; so many items were made of different leathers. There were breeches of doe or buck skin; waistcoats of swan skin; memorandum books of asses skin, which could be written on in pencil, rubbed clean, and reused; cases covered in dog skin; overcoats of bear skin; muffs and trimmings of rabbit skin; and sword hilts that came wrapped in dried fish skin for a good grip. The process of cleaning, restoring, and preserving leather goods was familiar, and was echoed in advertisements for creams to cleanse, restore, and preserve the face, neck, and hands. Animal skin was a valued commodity but in women fine skin was a commodity overlaid with added meaning. It signified class, worth on the marriage market, and the possession of a healthy constitution. Invariably, the ideal complexion Westerners had in mind was Eurocentric and white.

Individuals have always been prepared to choose and arrange the messages conveyed by their skin. They might wear makeup, as we shall see in a later chapter. They might get tattoos or take steps to modify their skin colour. But, before the twentieth century, acceptable treatments for the complexion were mostly precautionary or remedial, so the ability to manage skin disease was vital. This chapter looks at advances in the scientific knowledge of skin and its medical care. It then explores beauty therapies and the work of transnational pharmaceutical and cosmetics corporations which dominate the skincare market today. What is at stake when women seek products and processes to treat their skin? Has the value of a fair complexion changed over the centuries? Are attitudes to skin tone evolving still?

Skin, the largest human organ, accounts for up to 20 per cent of body weight. Its biological functions were only slowly discovered, although doctors have known since classical times that skin consists of two main layers: a renewable outer layer, or epidermis, and a deeper layer covering subcutaneous fat. In the seventeenth and eighteenth centuries, human skin was commonly considered more of a mesh than a barrier; as microscopes improved, more investigations were carried out on its pores, which obviously allowed humans to sweat. The prevailing humoral theory of medicine encouraged a belief that diseases caused by disorders in the blood could be treated by drawing out impurities through the pores. As doctors noted that some people were prone to skin breakouts during spring and autumn, they also advised keeping the pores open and encouraging a healthy perspiration. Even today there are fad treatments for sweating out toxins, though the amount of matter that can be released from the body in this way is minuscule.

Before twentieth-century advances in medicine and hygiene, the complexion was much more likely to be affected by disease. This was doubly unfortunate since the skin's condition was thought to indicate lifestyle as well as health. A sallow, dull, mottled, or waxy complexion could signal some underlying illness, poor hygiene, or even moral decay because skin disease was so often implicated in venereal complaints. In the eighteenth century, newspapers helped to normalise a strongly negative response to skin disorders. One correspondent wrote, 'When there are any uncommon Eruptions or Appearances on the Skin, we justly conclude something unsound in the Constitution of the Body to be the Occasion of it.'[3] And even minor blemishes might denote flaws of character. Victorians took this further, claiming that, for women, a fair and bright complexion was a sure indication of a rightly directed mind.[4] In contrast, livid red skin rashes such as erysipelas were associated with violent passions. Such views reinforced the value placed on an alabaster complexion.

The causes of skin disease baffled doctors. Did patients suffer from humoral imbalance? Had they eaten improper food? Been infested by insects? Touched irritating substances? Often doctors were at odds with each other. By the early nineteenth century, most assumed that sailors on long voyages caught scurvy because they lacked fresh vegetables. But others still thought that the bleeding sores and tender gums of scurvy victims were due to poor ventilation on ships, filth on board, or too much alcohol. Medical diagnosis of skin disease was hampered because, in folk speech, people meant different things when they named their symptoms. The 'rheums', 'tetters', 'scalds', 'itches', and 'manges' they complained about could include syphilis, eczema, or disorders caused by parasites.

Many doctors could not even distinguish syphilitic eruptions from other conditions, although admittedly syphilis, or the pox, was a rampant health problem. It accounted for between a fifth and a quarter of all hospital patients in early modern London, and many more suffered at home.[5] Since syphilis was mainly expressed on the skin, the study of that disease and of skin itself progressed together. A range of disorders were attributed to the pox, and the shame and secrecy surrounding the disease meant that it was often deliberately confused with scurvy. That said, all kinds of spots and rashes on the face were wrongly labelled scorbutic, even though by the early decades of the nineteenth century scurvy was increasingly rare, not least because potatoes had become a staple food.

The side effects of treatments for syphilis were as well known and stigmatised as the bodily signs of the illness itself. The standard cure was salivation, induced by the local application or ingestion of mercury. Doctors advised early treatment, before the disease became entrenched or could be passed to unborn children. In this respect, prostitutes had an advantage because they were more alert to symptoms than unsuspecting wives who caught the pox from errant husbands. Men often renounced society while they endured mercury treatment, but women were less able to find privacy if their workplace was the home. When face patches were in fashion, women used them to conceal syphilitic sores, but there was no disguising the ultimate sign of syphilis: the collapsed nose.

Women also feared smallpox, because even those who survived were mostly disfigured. Fanny Kemble, who caught the disease in 1825, reported that 'besides marking my face very perceptibly, it rendered my complexion thick and muddy and my features heavy and coarse'.[6] Some female sufferers covered their pocks with poultices and powders, hoping to prevent pitting, but doctors thought these precautions made scars worse and sometimes helped to kill patients.

Other skin conditions, triggered by malnutrition or scant washing facilities, were a common and distressing sight; the poor had little chance of beautiful skin. Testimonials used to advertise patent medicines offer graphic descriptions of human suffering: Maredant's Antiscorbutic Drops, heavily marketed in Britain and North America from the 1770s, allegedly cured one young woman of 'white, scabby eruptions' which spread over parts of her body to form 'one dry hard scale'.[7] Bacterial and parasitic skin infections were close to endemic among children; many sported the tell-tale circular patch of bumpy skin that indicated ringworm, a fungal infestation. Scabies, or 'the Itch', was also both highly contagious and common. Caused by mites burrowing into the skin, it visibly disfigured the hands if not the face.

The Itch was a stigma because people knew it was linked to dirt and poverty. Sufferers mostly sought remedies that would not further reveal their condition by staining their linen. Nothing seemed to work, not even the ashes of soles of old shoes which some tried, until Parisian doctors introduced sulphur baths in the early nineteenth century. Meanwhile, doctors marvelled that skin diseases were not confined to the squalid poor but even afflicted young ladies of scrupulous cleanliness; if the Itch entered clean households, it spread rapidly through all family members.

The prevalence of skin disease meant that, before the mid-nineteenth century, many turned to doctors for creams to improve the complexion, or ointments to smooth the neck and hands. Superstitions lingered. Even in 1714, Daniel Turner came across women who believed that skin infections around a fingernail could be cured by thrusting the finger into the ear of a black cat, or that shingles could be healed by anointing the rash with blood from a black cat's tail. Turner was merely sceptical about the first notion but adamant that cat's blood aggravated shingles. Fallacies long persisted in the treatment of warts or skin growths. These had once been a means of identifying witches, since the 'familiars' or demonic animals associated with witches were thought to feed on their blood by sucking on these 'teats'. Even in the late nineteenth century, women still wore charms if they wanted to remove warts.[8]

Most traditional remedies for skin disease, carefully preserved in early household manuals, were harmless if futile. A fragrant poultice of wheat steeped in wine and mixed with frankincense was recommended for the Itch.[9] Spa waters were drunk to purify the blood. Essence of water dock was used on scorbutic rashes and even sold in the eighteenth century as a commercial product. Advertisements claimed, 'it removes gradually these external and unsightly Blemishes; gives a clean Skin . . . and prevents other illnesses arising from a Want of Perspiration'.[10] Everyday ingredients found in home remedies, such as rosemary, lemon juice, bitter almonds, and tar, continued to be used on the skin into the nineteenth century.

Other medical treatments for skin conditions were positively harmful. The overuse of mercury, today known to be toxic, badly damaged health. Doctors also prescribed arsenic drops and dabbed patches of discoloured skin with diluted acids. They used irritants to blister patients, drawing blood to relieve local inflammation. Charlotte Brontë was so worried about the blister treatment inflicted on her life-long friend Ellen Nussey that she begged her to visit, writing, 'when you come here we will give up Medical prescriptions and try what exercise and fresh air will do'.[11] Jane Welsh Carlyle wore a mustard blister for a pain in her side much too long. She applied it for four whole days until forced to visit a surgeon, 'to show him the pretty state into which I had reduced my skin with the mustard!' He snorted at her zealous application and recommended patience, which if pursued to comparable excess would have no ill effect.[12] In short, before the middle of the nineteenth century, clinical medicine had almost no beneficial effect on the management of skin disease and may have done more harm than good.

IMPROVEMENTS IN DERMATOLOGY

There were signs of hope. In Paris, the Hôpital St-Louis specialised in dermatology from 1801; in London, the first hospital for diseases of the skin was set up in 1841. Other European nations followed, creating dermatological departments in universities or hospitals. Such institutions also helped to promote public knowledge of skin disease. Resident doctors collaborated with artists to make wax models or *moulages* of patients' diseased body parts, the pus and rashes accurately coloured, so that medical students could practise their diagnostic skills. Horrific medical waxes might then be included in public wax model displays of celebrities, as in Spitzner's travelling wax museum which toured Europe in the nineteenth century. Medical models were usually grouped in a special section, possibly intended to dissuade visitors, mostly male, from using brothels. Similar wax collections toured the US in spectacular freak shows or circus sideshows.

Wax was thought to be an ideal medium to capture the smoothness and transparency of human skin, and particularly white women's skin. Touring wax exhibitions often included lifelike Venuses that could be taken apart, or cutaway models of women showing internal organs and the stages of pregnancy. In the West, popular wax anatomical displays

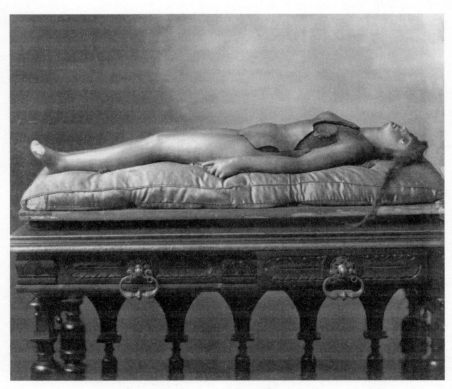

7. *An anatomical model by renowned anatomist and wax modeller Anna Manzolini (1714–74). She taught at the University of Bologna.*

helped to normalise and idealise the smoothness and pallor of female skin, whiteness as an ideal of beauty, and roundness of the female figure.

In the decades leading up to the mid-nineteenth century, new medical theories emerged about the nature and properties of the skin. The humoral theory of ascribing skin disease to impurities in the blood that somehow had to be drawn out was discredited. Instead, doctors gave meticulous attention to individual blotches and sought topical applications to relieve what they now thought were local skin problems. Unfortunately, their remedies still included the toxic mercurial ointments and assorted concentrations of sulphuric acid used when the humoral theory of medicine held sway.

Medical works also began to emphasise that the skin is semi-permeable, able to regulate body temperature through perspiration and to absorb substances through the pores. The notion of the skin as a wrapper, marking a border between the individual and the external world, became old-fashioned. Instead, skin was held to be a sensitive, communicative membrane protecting a unique self.

New findings brought about other changes in emphasis. Evidently, the skin could convey emotions by touch; fresh discoveries about the nervous system heightened awareness that humans are responsive individuals, communicating with the world through sensitive tissue. By the end of the nineteenth century, it was this view of the skin that family doctors propounded to women:

> Our skin . . . is not merely a secure covering which shuts in all the complex machinery about which we know so little. It is, of course, a most satisfactory covering, but it is something more. By means of the nerve fibres which have their terminations in the skin . . . every other portion of our body conveys sensations of pleasure or otherwise by the aid of the sense of touch.[13]

Since the skin interacted with every part of the nervous system, some pundits warned that 'The slightest disturbance, whether physical or mental, is certain to affect the skin, and may seriously deteriorate its beauty.'[14] The sensitive individual was likely to be susceptible to allergies and stress, both linked to blotchy skin, while persistent rashes were ascribed to forms of depression, when the skin condition might be implicated in both cause and effect.

Women, already credited with fine nerves and delicate skin, were thought to be prone to skin problems. In 1900, a prominent physiognomist, Professor Boyd Laynard, ascribed skin disease to strong mental emotions. In a book widely sold for just ninepence, he also claimed that a woman's habitual thoughts could make or mar a complexion, giving a new twist to the link between beauty, character, and personal responsibility.[15] Even so, many women had little choice about the condition of their skin, which might be damaged by their occupation, not by character or lifestyle. Factory workers, deprived of air and sunlight, acquired a dingy pallor; laundresses exposed to harsh soaps got 'washerwoman's itch'. In the mid-nineteenth century, artificial flower makers handling arsenical greens suffered painful running sores. Other toxic substances were equally dangerous and disfiguring: matchgirls exposed to white phosphorus contracted phossy jaw; women in munitions factories during the First World War found that the TNT turned their hair and skin yellow – they were dubbed 'Canary Girls'.

The physical and mental suffering of those tormented by skin disease in an age when there was little relief is now hard to imagine. Mary Josselyn, a New York skin specialist, claimed in 1879 that she had seen desperate patients tear at their itchy flesh until the blood flowed, and some who vowed they could cut the flesh from their limbs, so great was their agony. She knew women so badly disfigured that they shunned society, mistakenly dosing themselves with ever larger quantities of arsenic and mercury in the hope of improving their appearance. In her medical practice she had trialled new Cuticura products, developed by a drug company in Boston from 1878, and was happy to promote them. Cuticura products were being sold in Britain by 1880 and in British India, where American pharmacists promoted Western medicine as something practised in civilised countries.[16] Josselyn may have exaggerated the benefits of Cuticura soap but is unlikely to have overstated the shortcomings in contemporary medical knowledge. She wrote, 'It is no unjust reflection upon the medical profession to say that its efforts in the cure of skin diseases have been a failure.'[17] No wonder that newspapers and magazines carried so many advertisements for skincare products. Doctors' failings boosted that trade, although many commercial preparations were fraudulent.

FIXING THE COMPLEXION

For centuries, women in the West, and in Britain especially, set great store by a clear, milky complexion. Smooth, white hands, face, and neck signalled health and status, setting refined women apart from those who toiled in the wind and sun. Lady Mary Wortley Montagu, her face disfigured by smallpox, remarked bitterly that 'if 'twas the fashion to go naked the face would be hardly observed'.[18] Yet the whiteness and smoothness of the visible parts of a woman's body remained crucially important, and genteel women aimed to use the quality of their skin to social advantage.

Since so many English women chose to cultivate a pale, opal-like complexion, this delicate pallor became a mark of English nationality. Consensus about the nature of English beauty was a way to promote national unity while avoiding party politics. Foreign travel accentuated the trend: English women noted, for instance, how the sun roasted Spanish complexions. The concept of 'whiteness' depended on comparisons with other nations, as well as with the weather-worn appearance of Britain's labouring poor. In the imperial era, white skin was complacently associated with progress and civilisation. For example, an advertisement for Rowland's Kalydor, a lotion sold from the 1820s to remove sunburn, pimples, and freckles, claimed that it was in general use 'over the civilised parts of the world'.[19] By the mid-nineteenth century even the medical press in Britain patriotically upheld the excellence of British skin tones. One contributor noted that English women exposed their upper chest and neck more than other nationalities, adding, 'the custom probably arises from the superior development and colour of the bust in the Englishwoman. The French have always expressed their admiration of it.'[20] Such comments show how firmly skin colour had been racialised.

Since a perfect skin was hard to achieve and maintain without some artificial help, women early resorted to washes and potions that would disguise blemishes and improve their appearance. Bathing the face in May dew, for instance, was long thought to be an innocent and effective way to obtain a beautiful complexion. Pepys records his wife getting up before dawn on several occasions to collect spring dew from the fields. May dew was a key ingredient in eighteenth-century lotions for suntanned skin, including one to make the neck, shoulders, and breasts 'as white as Alabaster, though before of a dusky tann'd, or swarthy Colour'.[21]

Homemade recipes were popular, but in Britain, mainland Europe, and the North American colonies the need for a smooth, untanned complexion meant that skin lotions were early commercial products. In 1707, one perfumer advertised 'the only famous Beautifying Water for clearing and making the Face fair, tho of the brownish Complexion', claiming it would also 'take off all Pimples and Redness'.[22] It cost as much as five shillings a bottle, so was clearly aimed at the well-to-do. Overt makeup or 'paint' was associated with prostitutes, although trendsetting aristocrats brazenly wore it. Consequently, eighteenth-century manufacturers anxiously drew a line between skincare products and blatant cosmetics. An advertisement for 'The Princely Lotion' insisted that 'it is not Paint to put a false and unnatural Gloss on the Skin, but a true Remedy, that by its Use really adds a Lustre to the most beautiful, by shewing the fine Features of the Face'; another wash for the complexion was said to be so pure that it could be drunk as a cordial, even though it gave a luminous pearl colour to the skin.[23] And innocent spring dew continued to be associated with commercial face washes until at least the early 1800s.

In the eighteenth century, women could buy tinctures and lotions for the complexion from a variety of outlets: taverns and coffee houses, perfume shops, snuff shops, china shops, book shops, and 'toyshops' which sold novelties and luxury goods. Some premises, run by women, advertised that they dealt only in the toiletry needs of women and children, which indicates that the market was large enough to support specialist shops. Such women sometimes used their trade as a cover for other services, possibly including abortion. One retailer assured customers that she gave medical advice 'to her own Sex, who thro' Modesty cannot relate their Disorders to a Male Physician'.[24]

Skincare products for women, and the raw materials needed to make them, became important items of international trade, even though practices varied with different cultures. Britain imported several iconic products from Europe and the demand was so great that staple preparations circulated even between countries at war. In the eighteenth century, herbal Arquebusade Water for problem skin was sourced in France and Switzerland. The best kind of Hungary Water, infused with rosemary, came from Montpellier in southern France. Hungary Water was said to be good for aches and pains, but women also used it as a cleanser, diluting it with more water or milk and using it as a facewash to prevent spots. It was also supposed to preserve youthful beauty. High-quality lavender water came from France too, although it could be made in Britain. Holland Water, sometimes called Utrecht Water, was used to lessen wrinkles and smallpox scars. Retailers claimed that its action preserved the skin from harsh weather, 'by insinuating itself into the Skin, and nourishing it, as Grease insinuates itself into Leather, nourishes, and renders it more durable'.[25] The innocent-sounding Eau de Fleurs de Venice, or Venetian Bloom Water, was supposed to whiten the skin and remove pimples, while refined liquid soap from Florence blanched and polished the skin.[26]

Other standard items were proudly marketed in Britain as home-produced. The Royal Chemical Wash Ball was a favourite soap throughout the eighteenth century. Makers claimed that it smoothed and whitened the skin while being so safe it could be eaten. Milk of Roses, manufactured from home-grown flowers, was also popular. Other products traded on their alleged 'oriental', imperial, or classical associations, an advertising ploy that would be refined in later centuries. Women of means could smooth their skin with the 'genuine fat' of the mountain or forest bear, as used by Egyptians, Greeks, Arabs, and even ancient Britons; they could buy the kind of almond soap apparently favoured by the Queen of Palmyra, recently rediscovered by a caravan of pilgrims travelling to Jerusalem, and stolen from them by a troop of Arabians who, not given to washing, exchanged it for opium at Aleppo; or they could purchase Imperial Powder, which softened and whitened in all climates.[27] Here was further evidence that European skin-whitening products were spreading to tropical colonies. Equally, building on international trade and colonialism, European consumers now routinely expected to have access to ingredients from across the world; huge profits were to be made in satisfying this demand.

Despite assurances from retailers, many early treatments for a fine, lustrous skin carried hidden dangers. On her travels in Turkey, Lady Mary Wortley Montagu was given a small quantity of the valuable Balm of Mecca, a resinous juice used as an exfoliant to soften the skin. She expected a wonderful improvement to the beauty of her face; instead, it 'swelled to a very extraordinary size' and remained inflamed for three days. When the swelling subsided, she detected no visible change for the better and declared, 'I never intend to endure the pain of it again; let my Complexion take its natural course, and decay in its own due time.'[28] Mercury was routinely used in eighteenth-century skincare lotions and absorbed through the skin. As we have seen already, white women also danced with death by eating arsenic which, being poisonous, encouraged the paleness and transparency they so desired. Skin damage by these means was so commonplace that specific washes were developed to whiten and heal complexions that had been yellowed and corroded by mercury or arsenic. By the end of the eighteenth century, as women grew alert to these dangers, there was a specific market for creams guaranteed to be free of toxins.

Even so, mild caustics continued to be used to bleach out age spots and freckles. Early domestic recipes had directed women to strong animal ingredients: one called for goat's gall thickened with flour; another involved washing the face 'with the distilled water of the gut of an ox mixed with a small quantity of salt'.[29] Alum was commonly added to face washes to add lustre to the skin, although it was known to be damaging over time. In 1760, one doctor warned, 'It is true such water makes the skin shine: but it will certainly at length cause wrinkles; for allum [sic] is a very powerful astringent.'[30] But as late as 1868, *Harper's Bazaar* still recommended washing with alum to disguise wrinkles.[31]

It is remarkable how many beauty tips for the skin endured in some form over generations. Directions for making washes and scented pomatums, carefully transcribed into household manuals in the seventeenth century, were printed in pocket-books for women in the eighteenth century. And just as seventeenth-century housewives were urged to boil veal then wash their face in the water, so in the nineteenth century women were told that the secret to a velvety complexion was to sleep with a piece of raw veal on each cheek, strapped in place with linen bandages.[32] In the 1890s, Parisian fashion magazines still explained how to make age-old lotions for softening and whitening the skin from rose petals and other common ingredients. Girls' magazines of the time also gave instructions for making unprocessed face washes at home and recommended natural oils.[33]

Cold cream, an emulsion of water and fats, usually including beeswax and mixed with scenting agents, had been used to soften the skin since at least classical times. Shop-bought versions could still be suspect: one eighteenth-century cream was implausibly advertised as good for chapped lips, piles, chaffing caused by walking or riding, removing pimples, and preventing smallpox scars.[34] Until lanolin began to be widely used in skincare products from the 1880s, cold creams had a fatty base, commonly bear or pig fat, which turned rancid. These greasy preparations suited only dry skins, and some were even suspected of encouraging facial hair growth. Yet they may have worked when liberally spread into gloves worn overnight to improve hands and arms. In the eighteenth century, women could whiten their hands by wearing expensive French 'Chicken Gloves'; these were impregnated with almond oil and spermaceti, a waxy substance found in the head of the sperm whale. Cheaper gloves were treated with a mixture of lime, alum, and salt. Fawn-skin socks dressed in fine oil from venison were sold to smooth and soften the feet.

Victorians were adamant that a fine skin, as well as a small waist, were key beauty factors. At the time, a third of British women lived a single life, but even publications by women insisted that it was every female's duty to maintain her beauty and influence. Typical of such advice is the statement in a manual by a 'professional beauty' that a woman 'should endeavour by every means in her power to make herself pleasant to look at'.[35] Thanks to developments in print technology, periodicals now carried more persuasive illustrations and reached a wider market; standards of beauty became harder to ignore.

COMPLEXION AND MORAL FAILURE

Predictably, Victorians were convinced that good digestion was essential to a clear complexion. Nineteenth-century doctors had already traced a sympathy between the skin and the alimentary canal: 'When the digestion is deranged, the skin is dry, wrinkled and discoloured', one specialist wrote.[36] Because skin was known to be porous, one quack salesman even claimed that a poultice strapped over the liver would cure indigestion.[37] The link between indigestion and skin trouble became axiomatic; anxious mothers dosed their children weekly with brimstone and treacle to keep their bowels open and their skin nice. Eno's Fruit Salts were credited with fixing a pasty complexion as well as sluggish organs.

Poor skin became another reason to upbraid women and dictate their lifestyles. One self-proclaimed beauty specialist wrote of the complexion, 'Most of the elementary disorders may usually be traced to late hours, want of cleanliness, over-indulgence at the table, etc. (this with married women especially), and tight-lacing.'[38] Skin trouble was now all about personal will, choice, and moral responsibility. To what extent should doctors take women's skin problems seriously when they were judged to be a matter of personal failure?

From the 1840s, active management of the skin was an essential aspect of women's personal routine. In part, this was due to the latest discoveries about the functioning of the skin's pores and glands. Erasmus Wilson, a British dermatologist, counted 3,528 pores in a square inch of skin and estimated that the length of the tubular perspiratory system of the whole human body must be nearly twenty-eight miles.[39] These astounding statistics were much repeated, reinforcing the belief that the skin had to be kept scrupulously clean so that its excretory functions could proceed uninterrupted. Blackheads, once thought to be grubs or worms, were identified as clogged ducts. Now that the function of the skin in removing waste from the body was better understood, blackheads were a sign of poor hygiene.

The growing acceptance towards the end of the nineteenth century that skin had to 'breathe' added weight to criticism of tight corsets. And some columnists advised that the best way to avoid summer freckles was to let the skin perspire naturally and gently 'simmer', rather than clog the pores with chalk or powder. Victorians now applied themselves to the business of toning the pores. Since the early 1700s, a few physicians had recommended cold bathing for medicinal purposes, arguing that 'cold water concentrates the spirits, and strengthens the nerves and musculous fibres by bracing them'.[40] In the late Victorian period, such views no longer seemed eccentric. Doctors advised women to get used to a chilly bath on rising because 'the cold bracing shock of immersion in cold water each morning preserves the tone of the skin'.[41] They also thought this routine would leave women less susceptible to cold weather. Belief in the benefits of exposure to icy water or cold air proved long-lasting. In the 1930s, mothers were still being told to expose their babies naked at an open window, once bathed, to keep their skin active.[42]

White Victorian women were also obsessed with polishing the skin with scented oil to achieve a captivating sheen. In this respect, the Turkish letters of Lady Mary Wortley Montagu had lasting influence. She had vividly described the beauty of the ladies she had seen at the hot baths in Turkey, 'all of them perfectly smooth and polished by the frequent use of bathing'.[43] A version of the Turkish bath was revived in Britain from the 1850s and, in contrast to those women boldly taking a cold dip first thing in the morning, some privileged women followed the Turkish custom and polished the skin after a hot bath.[44]

Unfortunately, the restricted lives of Victorian middle-class women presented daily perils for the skin. White women were told that they could get an 'irregular brown spot or freckle' simply by sitting too close to the fire.[45] Those consigned to mourning clothes were dismayed when their skin became stained with black dye. In frosty weather, particularly if dark clothes were worn, hands soon became soiled and needed frequent washing. These trivial circumstances were felt to be hardships because standards of self-presentation were so high. For example, women were advised that, if their arms were not 'well formed and white', it was imperative to wear long gloves at balls and dinners.[46]

From the early eighteenth century and the first newspaper advertisements for skin creams, white women had been encouraged to consider the impression their complexion made on observers. In 1716, one cream guaranteed 'transcendently Fair, Plump, Smooth, and delicately Beautiful' skin 'tho' before it was never so Foul, discolour'd, wither'd and wrinkled', promising a complexion that 'causes admiration to the Beholders'.[47] Over time, an insidious link developed between health care and attention to the impact a woman's appearance had on others. By the 1890s, even a family doctor writing about constipation reinforced his arguments with, 'A good complexion makes a plain woman look handsome, and an otherwise handsome face most striking.'[48]

Once the biological properties of skin became better known, mothers with daughters to bring up and marry off were encouraged to learn some anatomy. Lydia Huntley Sigourney, an American educator and poet, wrote, 'Mothers, if you would do your duty . . . At least, acquaint your-self with the physiology of the skin, the lungs, the circulation of the blood, and the digestive organs.'[49] She insisted that the skin excreted more than twenty ounces of waste matter every twenty-four hours, and that, if this process were hindered by clogged pores, a girl's other excre-tory organs would be overtaxed. Neglected skin might even encourage pulmonary disease, a cause of early death in so many women of the time.

By the 1880s, college girls in the United States had weekly lectures on physiology, 'on the heart, blood, lungs, muscles, and skin', accompa-nied by warnings against tight-lacing their corsets, now routine.[50] In Britain, women were bombarded with magazine articles and even public lectures on the functions of the skin. Yet ill-informed practices continued. In 1889, the author of *Beauty and How to Keep It* claimed that English women owed their dazzlingly fair complexions to the extreme care of their mothers, who not only saw that their daughters always wore gauze veils, but also fed them a diet 'of white meats with an abundant use of milk'.[51]

Victorian elegance manuals encouraged the notion that care of the complexion was a proper subject for the female mind. This was not just intellectually limiting but anxiety-inducing. Women were told that they must avoid wind, sun, sea air, and hot rooms. A veil and a layer of face cream should be worn outdoors, the cream to be washed off on return. This meant that wealthy women travelled with baskets of washes and creams even on short journeys, as if venturing into a danger zone. Victorians favoured Rowlands' Kalydor milk for the face and Walton's Kaloderma to combat any change in temperature. The latter was adver-tised as 'delightfully cooling, healing, soothing, and refreshing after the ride, promenade, or drive, heat of ball-room, exposure to the scorching sun, sea air, and saline vapour'.[52] This same advertisement underscored the supposed danger of such mundane activities because it also recom-mended Kaloderma for inflamed wounds.

In the seventeenth century, some European women had resorted to full face masks to preserve their complexions. By the nineteenth century, masks were firmly out of fashion for daytime wear on both sides of the Atlantic, but 'toilet masks or face gloves' were worn at night to bleach and lubricate the face.[53] Madam Rowley's mask, patented in 1875, was made of flexible rubber and had to be worn three times a week. Other models were made of chamois leather or flannel, lined with a sticky preparation that included white wax mixed with honey and almond paste. The masks were unsightly but had some followers, being fairly cheap and long-lasting. Today, overnight 'face masks' still offer women the hope of waking up with clear, glowing skin, but most are just heavy creams.

The stigma once attached to skin disease, and the cultural value in the West of a pale, camellia-like complexion, restricted women's behaviour. Whether self-imposed or encouraged by others, this constraint on activity was a form of social control, at least for the middle classes, and might even involve sensory deprivation. A Norwegian who emigrated to

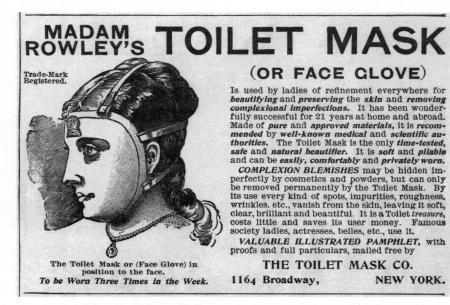

8. *Made of flexible India rubber, this mask was popular in the 1890s and was meant to be worn overnight.*

Iowa in 1853 was amazed to find that in the American Midwest she could get sunburnt in the shade, writing, 'I have never had such an experience. I found it so pleasant to have the wind blowing on me.'[54] All the same, she did wonder how her husband would react to her tanned skin. Some women rebelled. Fanny Kemble reported from New England: 'The women here, who are careful, above all things, of their appearance, marvel extremely at my exposing myself to the horrors of tanning . . . but . . . I prefer burning my skin to suffocating under silk handkerchiefs, sun-bonnets, and two or three gauze veils, and sitting, as the ladies here do, in the dark till the sun has declined.'[55] Kemble's neglect of her complexion elicited further disapproval when she returned to England. After one stage performance Henry Greville, an officer in the royal household, criticised her deportment and appearance, offering to lend her his personal hairdresser, 'to whitewash me after the approved French method, *i.e.*, to anoint my skin with cold cream, and then cover it with pearl powder; and this, not only my face, but my arms, neck, and shoulders'.[56] Kemble refused to submit to what she termed 'manipulation'.

All the same, an ivory sheen seems to have been admired by most women. When Queen Victoria was crowned, the author Maria Edgeworth found fault with the length of her drapery and her figure, 'short enough already', but admitted that the royal neck and arms were beautifully fair, so 'the better half of her looked perfectly ladylike and Queenlike'.[57] In her view, an alabaster skin could compensate for physical defects because she appreciated the great effort needed to achieve it. Before appearing in full evening dress, some women patiently sat for hours under an old piece of linen, their neck and shoulders covered in a paste of egg white and alum.[58]

HAZARDS AND ENTREPRENEURS

Late Victorian manuals on beauty and hygiene repeatedly warned readers to use only traditional preparations known to be safe. One of the reasons why magazines for women and girls included recipes for homemade cosmetics was because shop-bought, chemical preparations were still dangerous. Just like cosmetic surgery in Britain today, the Victorian beauty industry was largely unregulated and even well-advertised brands could be harmful. Older white women, finding pearl powder dusted over the face and shoulders too evanescent in strong light, resorted to enamelling with a preparation called liquid white. It dried to a hard, enamel-like finish that was difficult to wash off. Although it lasted longer, it damaged the skin, as did depilatories made of caustic lime or sulphide of arsenic, and treatments for acne containing mercuric chloride, a virulent poison.[59]

Nineteenth-century innovations posed fresh hazards. Synthetic aniline dyes, by-products of coal tar, were discovered in the 1850s. They yielded clear, bright mauves, and other colours followed, more intense than any available from natural dyes. But Victorians soon had cause to be wary of striped socks and coloured undergarments, so eye-catching in shop windows. The cheaper aniline dyes caused pain, swelling, and skin eruptions. Flannel underclothes, dyed in the scarlet shades popularly thought to guard against rheumatism, triggered dermatitis when the colours, modified by perspiration, stained the skin. Women's feet were even damaged by the red lining of their boots as toxins from the dye seeped through their stockings.

The upper classes spurned bright colours when the dangers became evident, preferring instead tastefully coordinated pastels. But the poor, used to drab clothing, were attracted to vibrant shades that once only the rich could afford. Contemporary warnings issued by dermatologists, and their descriptions of dye-related injuries, paint a picture of poverty, sweat, dirt, misdiagnosis, misery, exploitation, and a lack of industrial regulation. Yet even today allergic reactions to dyed textiles are not unknown.

The harm caused by cheap aniline dyes may have dented faith in progress, but in the later nineteenth century women were being swiftly drawn into a consumer culture offering enticing ranges of branded skin products. Skincare companies increasingly emphasised the need to preserve youth as well as a clear complexion. Women had always looked for treatments that would smooth wrinkles and plump cheeks, but home remedies had been laborious and sometimes hazardous. One dangerous eighteenth-century idea was to heat myrrh powder on a fire shovel until red hot, fill the mouth with white wine, spit the wine onto the shovel, and inhale the fumes from under a napkin.[60] No wonder women looked for over-the-counter products that would target problem areas with less fuss.

In Britain, ranges of skincare products were developed from the 1890s by Mayfair beauty salons. The Cyclax range came from Mrs Hemming's salon, founded in 1896; Mrs Pomeroy, who moved her salon to Mayfair from Chancery Lane in 1896, developed another range of treatments; and Mrs Adair, an army wife who claimed she had learned her beauty secrets during a posting to India, opened her Bond Street salon in 1900. All three women used an alias, since operating a beauty business, even for high-end clients, was not entirely respectable; clients themselves often visited incognito. Yardley was an existing brand (the company had been established in 1770), but it specialised in soaps and perfumes, developing toiletries only in the twentieth century when the soap market became crowded. The three female salon owners went on to open premises in other major cities on the Continent and in the United States. Their skincare ranges were soon even available in parts of the British Empire, through established routes for supplying British goods to colonial households. Some salon owners also offered the latest electrolysis technique for hair removal and treatment of discoloured skin. The procedure had been invented in the 1870s but machines for commercial use were not sold until the early 1900s. Eleanor Adair used stick electrodes, the ends filled with cotton wool soaked in skin tonic, to stimulate facial nerves, shrink enlarged pores, and allegedly whiten the skin.

These self-made beauty experts were immensely entrepreneurial. They built up international businesses, exploiting a growing female consumer base in capital cities, where mass public transport and new department stores lured women into centres to lunch and shop. As beauticians, they often recycled earlier therapies, but as businesswomen they marketed their creations using the latest visual techniques and graphic design. Their products seemed to reflect the essence of modernity. They understood the pressure that women were under to retain flawless complexions and youthful looks, turning this to commercial advantage. Other entrepreneurs followed. Elizabeth Arden (another alias) got her start in the business by working at Adair's salon in New York. One of Arden's employees went on to open her own salon with its brand of products, using the name Dorothy Gray. Meanwhile, Helena Rubinstein, who already had a beauty salon in Melbourne, opened another in London in 1908, then extended her business to Paris and New York. All these entrepreneurs had great marketing flair and a natural talent for selling product. Several became lifelong rivals.

Women's magazines and newspapers offered these businesswomen far-reaching platforms for advertising skincare products. Mass-circulation magazines became more general after 1900, and by the 1920s some titles had over a million subscribers. This reach was vital, since many cosmetics were sold through mail order. By 1927, women in North America were buying 52,000 tons of cleansing cream, 26,500 tons of skin lotion, and 17,500 tons of nourishing cream a year.[61] Beauty gurus aimed to get women hooked on their products early, warning young girls about dry skin and untimely wrinkles; simultaneously, they offered mature women the dream of regaining lost bloom. Elizabeth Arden cannily targeted white women who had spent their lives in the torrid outposts of empire, 'who sometimes lose heart regarding their complexions, rather dreading the time when they will go home'.[62] Wealthy older women were an important market for her skincare products, which were not cheap.

Arden, copying Adair, insisted on a three-step beauty routine which helped to sell a suite of branded products. Rubinstein would also claim, 'Give me 10 minutes a day – I'll add 10 years youth to your skin . . . How is it done? By *faithfully* following these three indispensable rules of beauty . . . *cleanse* . . . *nourish* . . . *tone*.'[63] She was adept at using pseudo-scientific language to make her skincare goods sound both cutting edge and trustworthy. For instance, her Skin Life Turgosmon treatment to plump out ageing skin combined the words 'turgor' and 'osmos', which she claimed were the proper terms to describe the balance of fluids within cells. Yet when Rubinstein wanted to persuade users that a product applied daily would benefit all women, she reverted to the simplest of descriptions like 'Skin Dew'. Beauty houses energetically introduced new products for each season to maximise sales. Some claimed to have made a study of the needs of 'winter' skin, and by springtime they would be ready to persuade customers that they needed a different lotion to counteract the damaging rays of the sun.[64]

Skin products offered some women the hope that presumed defects would fade, freeing them to become their true selves. Beauty entrepreneurs promoted a classification for skin according to its nature and needs, defining types as normal, oily, or dry. Rubinstein, who specialised in skin problems, later added combination skin to this list. The categories had been implicit in Victorian beauty books but were particularly useful to the skincare industry, helping to sell whole product ranges. Heavy promotion invited users to identify with a particular skin type, so that a woman's sense of self was, to some extent, bound up with her skincare management.

At the same time, targeted products, which ostensibly met individual needs, were marketed as liberating. In 1979, for example, women were told that 'Estee Lauder brings a fabulous new freedom to skincare'; the company offered a free, personalised skin analysis so that women could pinpoint the right product for their needs and get the quickest results.[65] Skin analysis and focused treatment soon became popular relaxation packages at spa retreats. Spas encouraged women to take time out, address their personal wellbeing, and consider the impact of their lifestyle on the skin. Body oils, once used to polish the skin, were reconceptualised as relaxation and healing aids.

Some skincare innovations became true forces for good; Germolene, developed in Britain in the early 1920s for pimples, became a trusted antiseptic. Other innovations to improve skin health contained hidden dangers. In the late 1920s, scientists finally identified vitamin D and showed that it was essential to prevent rickets. They discovered that humans needed sunlight to make vitamin D in the skin, so developed equipment to produce ultraviolet light for patients lacking the vitamin. Soon people were encouraged to buy ultraviolet units or 'sunlight baths' for home use. Advertisements promised that there was no chance of an overdose of UV radiation, but enthusiastic purchasers who used the equipment without supervision risked major health problems.

The latest skin treatments offer a varied picture. Retinol-based products are popular these days and may reduce the appearance of fine wrinkles but they irritate sensitive skin. Many face creams are laced with vitamins. They possibly have a cosmetic effect on the surface of the skin, but few such nutrients, if any, penetrate the skin's outer layers. In the absence of controlled, clinical trials, the value of such products remains controversial. Costly anti-ageing creams containing hormones prompt similar debate. Hollywood, where beauty is big business, sets the standard for cosmetic skin procedures. The choices today include laser treatments, skin retexturing, collagen and vitamin injections, antioxidant serums, liposuction, fat replacement, and Botox injections. Many celebrities owe their youthful appearance to ongoing anti-ageing treatment from a discreet surgeon or dermatologist. But these procedures are generally expensive, short-term, and, in the hands of unskilled practitioners, potentially catastrophic.

In parallel, there has been a movement towards natural skincare. For example, traditional African products like shea and cocoa butter, displayed as novelties in the Great Exhibition of 1851, have become mainstream. The Windrush generation and their descendants have helped to make these creams familiar in Britain. The Body Shop further popularised them from 1976, and now heavily processed versions can be bought in any chemist, although shops run by those of African heritage usually stock the full-strength kind.

SKIN COLOUR

Before the 1920s, European women did all they could to avoid tanning, which was associated with low-class manual labour and ugly, wrinkled skin. Betsey Freemantle, married to a naval officer, lamented in 1797 that she had burnt her face 'shockingly' in Gibraltar, and it being a novel experience she remarked how unpleasant and painful it felt.[66] Times changed. Mata Hari, a Dutchwoman who reinvented herself as an erotic dancer in the early twentieth century, happily dyed her skin to look Eastern. And in 1925, *Country Life* reported a sudden vogue for sun tans – not natural but obtained by iodine baths or ochre powder. It described the effect as innocuous and becoming, unlike genuine sunburn which only coarsened the complexion.[67]

The fashion designer Coco Chanel seems to have started the trend. She had returned from vacation with an accidental tan, and it became a craze in North America and Europe. By 1930, the film star Loretta Young assured fans that 'the complexion that any woman envies and men admire is an even, healthy tan'.[68] It was hard to achieve. Allegedly, during the Second World War, women resorted to gravy browning and, second choice, cold cocoa to disguise their pallor. As the post-war market for foreign holidays grew, tanned skin became a coveted mark of affluence, only lessening in appeal when the damaging effects of overexposure to the sun's rays were publicised in the 1980s. Today's fake tans send conflicted signals about wealth and class, demonstrating our ability to draw complex meanings from subtle grades of facial evidence.

Before the vogue for tanning complicated matters, white women regularly lightened their skin to obtain the economic and cultural benefits of a creamy skin tone. When they first encountered peoples with Black and brown skins, many praised the beauty and sheen of darker skin. But the cultural investment that Europeans had made in smooth, fair complexions was too deep-rooted to be soon displaced. And when Black skins were appreciated, it was often as a foil to pale complexions, the aesthetic effect reinforcing the apparent rightness of enslaving and silencing other peoples. In plantation societies, because the bodies of African women were valued as a commodity, they were less likely to be appreciated for their beauty. Artistic representations of colonial landscapes might erase Black bodies and the labour they performed altogether.[69] In colonial societies, a socially constructed, ideological whiteness was used to reinforce structures of power. Skin colour became a distinguishing marker between ruler and ruled, and beauty ideals reinforced the imperial system.[70] By the nineteenth century, people of European heritage readily took 'white' skin to be a badge of civilisation: not only a sign of gentility and class privilege, but also of racial privilege.

In Caribbean island colonies, light brown skin became a symbol of the middle classes because some residents with this skin colour, the descendants of slave owners, were emancipated before their darker-skinned neighbours. They then benefited socially and economically in the post-emancipation period. The white elite perceived light brown skin as a respectable form of Blackness with which it could align. It relied on the often light-skinned middle class to help maintain colonial order, and this class was privileged under the legal system.[71] In addition, light brown skin was fetishised by men who wanted a glamorous sexual partner but only wished to 'flirt' with Blackness. Many women therefore sought to lighten their complexions not because they wanted to appear whiter, but to gain social advantage.

The privileging of white, or lighter, skin is still prevalent in many parts of the world. It is an affront that has proved hard to dislodge, despite the Black is Beautiful movement of the 1960s. This movement was aligned with the Black Power movement, which had notable links to fashion and writing, but arguably the Black is Beautiful movement continued to centralise whiteness, using it as a benchmark and positioning 'authentic' Black beauty as its opposite, demanding natural hairstyles and dark skin.[72] In a reversal of earlier customs, white women today often strive to be tanned, while women with darker skin might aim to bleach and lighten it. Just as European women once preserved a pale complexion to gain status, respectability, and the opportunity to marry well, so across the world women with darker skins apply lighteners for similar reasons, not repudiating their skin colour but pursuing success and recognition. Many begin to use lightening creams before marriage: in North America and the West Indies, successful Black men have tended to choose lighter-skinned wives to help secure social mobility.[73] The prominence of light-skinned celebrities like Beyoncé or Bollywood film stars like Aishwarya Rai Bachchan, endorsed by Oprah Winfrey in 2005 as the most beautiful woman in the world, encourages other women of colour to emulate their appearance.

White women who tan to the extent of transforming their skin colour can be viewed as toying with a specific form of Blackness. The notion that skin colour is a marker of 'race' is evidently unstable. That said, skin colour is always read in relation to other features such as nose shape and hair texture, which help to determine how 'Black' someone is perceived to be. Similar assessments are made for other 'races' – for example, when determining how 'white' someone is observed to be.

The use of skin-lightening products has mushroomed internationally, and their manufacture is now a multibillion-dollar industry. In the United States, skin lighteners have been used by women of African heritage since the nineteenth century, although historically the largest market for them in North America was among women of European descent striving for a milky complexion. In Japan, where light skin in women has long been prized, everyday beauty products often include ingredients designed to make skin appear paler; the same is true in other Asian countries such as Korea and China, where light skin indicates someone who does not have to labour in the sun. In India, the Philippines, and Africa (notably in Nigeria, Ghana, and Zimbabwe), skin bleaching can be viewed with extreme ambivalence, as a legacy of colonialism, although some point to pre-colonial influences, such as the caste system in India, which may have encouraged a preference for lighter skin tones. Critics of skin lighteners argue that those who use them have internalised racism. Certainly, the penetration of Western consumer culture across continents has helped to make skin bleaching popular.

Tremendous economic forces are at work in making, advertising, and selling skin lighteners worldwide, impeding the positive acceptance of diverse types of beauty. Persuasive advertisements for skin lighteners, which promise happiness and social success once the user has achieved paler skin, may accentuate prejudice. Research has shown that colour bias negatively affects the health and prospects of darker-skinned African Americans, and their experience is replicated on other continents.[74] Giant, multinational skincare companies unwaveringly associate lighter skin with beauty, progress, joy, confidence, and achievement. Their seductive advertising aims to make skin lightening seem normal, and suggests that the modern, upwardly mobile, cosmopolitan woman in Africa or Asia routinely 'tones' her skin to realise her potential.

Even so, in some countries there is a degree of shame in applying skin lighteners, and women are reluctant to admit that they use them. This secrecy can have serious health consequences because the cheaper creams that companies offload in disadvantaged, less-regulated communities often contain toxic mercury or chemicals that cause skin damage. Even the use of trusted, safer brands can uncomfortably restrict women's lifestyles in hot climates, discouraging users from outdoor sports or swimming in the sun.

Skincare companies argue that they are responding to demand not creating it, and that their lightening creams are aimed at all skin tones. The claim has some truth since their products can also treat age-related skin pigmentation in fair skins. But advertisements for skin lighteners work to reinforce a colour bias that needs no encouragement. Critics of the practice in India explain that 'It starts when children are young: the moment a child is born, relatives start comparing siblings' skin colour. It starts in your own family – but people don't want to talk about it openly.'[75] There is little sign of the market for skin lighteners diminishing because they are so strongly associated with social mobility, liberalisation, and success. Some may find that lightening the skin empowers them, but the practice does nothing to eliminate discrimination on the basis of skin tone. It promotes idealised whiteness as a beauty standard, while obscuring the beauty of people of colour and the cultural benefits of diversity.

White skin is still associated with social and racial privilege, and definitions of female beauty are still mostly centred on white stereotypes. That said, aesthetic views about skin colour are shifting as Western societies become more multicultural and as activists, including people of colour, demand change. This is important for social well-being, not least because the children of mixed heritage can have different hues, and face prejudice from both Black and white communities. They may have to come to terms both with strong views about who can claim Black identity and with the belief, stemming from the colonial era, that it is better to be white. The work of notable women of colour in public life encourages people to re-examine prejudices about skin tone and to see that they are increasingly outdated as well as unjust.[76] The media, especially the persuasive film and music industries which once put a premium on light-coloured skin tones, is changing fast to reflect diverse audiences.

TATTOOS AND PIERCINGS

One sign of changing attitudes to skin is that more women have chosen to get tattooed in recent decades. Tattoos have been worn across the world for millennia but the modern practice of tattooing in the West mostly derives from contact between eighteenth-century sailors and Polynesians. Whereas in the colonial world, the tattooing of Europeans was a mark of cross-cultural engagement, elsewhere it was popular only with seafarers and marginalised groups such as criminals. Despite this, or even because of it, tattoos suddenly became fashionable among the British elite in the early twentieth century. Members of the royal family had them, and county sportsmen liked to decorate their skin with hunting scenes. Magazines noted that, once people had been tattooed, they were often keen to add more designs.[77] The electric tattoo machine, invented around 1890, had already made tattooing quicker, less painful, and more precise. A few socialite women braved the needle: Winston Churchill's mother had a coiled snake tattooed around her left wrist. It was a daring statement, since the first Western women to be tattooed did it for commercial gain: circus performers in nineteenth-century North America revealed colourful body decoration in shows that were perilously close to striptease acts.

The revival of tattooing from the 1960s, and its ongoing popularity, suggests that it satisfies a range of desires. Do tattoos increase self-esteem? Enhance a woman's sexual attractiveness? Indicate a refusal to accept feminine passivity and go against expectations that women should aim for flawless skin? Much of the attraction of tattooing is its mystique. Skin decorations are linked to individual identity and control of the body. They often have personal significance but can also signify compliance with group expectations. In some cases, they can be a mark of belonging to a subculture. Across different cultures, tattooing is a recognised form of communication, yet designs are intriguingly capable of more than one meaning.

The practice has moved from dingy port-town back streets to tattoo parlours in town centres, and is now common in many parts of the world where, since antiquity at least, there has been no culture of tattooing. There is an increased acceptance of body art in wider society. Visible body inscription has almost become a fashion accessory, with social media allowing people to share and get reactions to even those tattoos that might generally be hidden by clothes.[78]

Piercing and body jewellery also allow people to adapt the skin to communicate something about themselves. Body piercing for both sexes is an ancient practice and ear piercing remained common among Western nations into the twentieth century. But it was only from the 1970s that piercing other parts of the body became popular, not least because it was embraced by the anti-establishment punk movement.

Among women, body piercing appeals most to the under twenty-fives. Some younger teenagers get a piercing to make people think they are more interesting than they feel, but motivations vary. These include celebrating a milestone in life, signalling rebellion, or just for pleasure and aesthetic reasons. Piercings are no longer so controversial; some treat them like any piece of jewellery. The most common piercings for women, apart from in the ear lobe, are in the navel, nose, other ear parts, tongue, and nipple. Genital piercings are far less popular but estimated to rise. Unlike a tattoo, piercings are easily undone. And for those worried about complications, which are reported in about a third of cases, there are always fake piercings.

If tattooing and piercing allow women to assert their individuality and exert control over their bodies, the international use of skin lighteners indicates the continuing pressure on women to conform to social expectations for economic benefit. At the heart of this tension are vital issues of power and influence. The global skincare market is set to rise to $185.5 billion by 2027, its steady growth largely due to the demand for anti-ageing and sun protection products.[79] That said, young women now think nothing of sharing images of their latest face blemishes on social media. And when an advertisement appeared on Twitter for a flawless colour-correction cream, allegedly able to cover wrinkles, old tattoos, age marks, flecks, and acne, the immediate response was 'Why do we need to be flawless?'[80] The body confidence movement encourages women to disregard blemishes and champion such genetic conditions as vitiligo and albinism. The beauty industry increasingly embraces these skin conditions, as in the Dove Real Beauty campaign which seeks to reassure young women who face social media pressures and who might be prone to low body confidence. Today, a woman's skin can be a site of both protest and repression.

MAKEUP

I n January 1943, Marta Gorick, an American nurse, spent a terrifying
night in a lifeboat in the north Atlantic Ocean; a German U-boat had
torpedoed the transport ship carrying her nursing corps from England
to North Africa. After seven and a half hours, the sun rose, and a British
destroyer came into view. Afterwards she wrote, 'I put on my rouge,
lipstick, and powder before being picked up, thinking I might look at
least a little bit glamourous, although worn-looking.'[1] Perhaps she
wanted to mask her fear. Perhaps she wanted to signal her patriotism –
after all, women were encouraged to wear lipstick to boost morale in
wartime. Whatever the motive, makeup was among the essential posses-
sions she grabbed when abandoning ship.

Some feminists have argued that, by wearing makeup, women conform
to standards of beauty imposed by a patriarchal society, and acquiesce in
a ritual that limits their freedom. Others take the view that those who
object to makeup are fetishising 'natural' feminine beauty or seizing an
opportunity to moralise about women's artifice. But as Marta Gorick's
story affirms, makeup can be empowering; queer and trans women can
feel hugely emboldened and affirmed by makeup. Many types of performance art depend upon it. And criticism of makeup today is often bound
up with negative views of the cosmetics industry more broadly.

Historically, women fought to wear makeup; they themselves set up iconic cosmetic businesses. And when cosmetic production became a multi-billion-pound industry, many found ways to negotiate its marketing pressures. In the twenty-first century, women have mocked the slick advertising of cosmetics, using it as material for satire and social comedy. So why do women wear makeup? And how has its use changed over centuries? This chapter takes in practical information such as what makeup was made of, how it was applied, and whether it was safe to use. It also explores the layers of meaning attached to painting the face, which has long been associated with moral ambivalence, power, and performance.

Cosmetic use is hardly a modern phenomenon. Ancient Egyptians used red pigments on their cheeks and lips more than five thousand years ago. They wore green eye paint and lined their eyes with kohl, which they made chiefly from galena (a grey lead compound). Kohl protected them from the sun's glare and from the eye infections to which they were prone, thanks to Nile bacteria, insects, and dust storms. The effect of their makeup was aesthetic but also infused with spiritual meaning.

The use of cosmetics continued into classical times and never entirely died out, although opposition from the Church grew strident in the Middle Ages. Contemporary conduct books advised women to be modest and submissive. That said, Italian women started to use juice from the dark berries of deadly nightshade to dilate their pupils and flush their cheeks, giving rise to another name for the plant: belladonna, or beautiful lady. Some painted their faces to achieve a smooth, pale complexion, often using white lead makeup (ceruse). Elizabeth I is said to have routinely applied ceruse after contracting smallpox in 1562. As queen she relied on face paint to achieve her iconic mask-like image. White women also used red dyes on cheeks and lips, mimicking the balance of colours in a delicately flushed complexion. This was thought to indicate a healthy balance of humours in the body, with blood considered to be the most positive of the four humours.

In 1650, England's government tried to outlaw face paint. Puritans complained that it was against biblical teaching, that it would lead men and women into vice, that it was inherently deceitful (a failing associated with women), and that it meddled with God's creation. This government bill did not make it into law but gained some popular support. John Bulwer, a London physician, carped, 'Our English ladies who seem to have borrowed some of their cosmetical conceits from barbarous nations are seldom known to be contented with a face of God's making, for they are either adding, detracting, or altering continually.'[2] The diarist John Evelyn was shocked when he noticed that more females were painting their faces, 'formerly a most ignominious thing & used only by prostitutes'.[3] Respectable women were expected to mind spiritual matters, not waste time on vanity.

Evelyn was behind the times. In England the puritan restraints of Oliver Cromwell's rule were on the wane. The aspiring cleric and writer John Gauden certainly sensed the way popular opinion was flowing; in an influential book on 'artificial beauty' he argued that what women called 'little private *helps* to their looks' harmed no one, if discreetly used.[4] His turn of phrase may deliberately blur the boundary between cosmetics and skin treatments, but household manuals were full of recipes that show an overlap between culinary, medical, and beautifying advice. Women could claim they used beauty products for health reasons or to repair damage, not out of vanity. The practice holds true today, given that makeup is routinely blended with sunscreen; women are still assured that they can 'protect and perfect' at the same time.

Gauden's book also reveals a link between cosmetics, nationality, and class. He pointed out that in other European nations face paint was openly used among the cultured elite. Only the vulgar and ill-informed objected. In 1660, when Charles II returned from exile, he helped to make Continental fashions popular in London. Yet references to face paint were still used negatively against Catholic Spain and France, and against Charles's own lax court, as in this satire:

Give the Devil his due.
Whoring and *Painting* flourish now so well,
We hardly know where *Honest Women* dwell:
Virtue is out of Fashion; she's a Saint
That can with Art and Skill, *Sing, Whore,* and *Paint.*[5]

By the end of the century, calmer voices prevailed. Commentators pointed out that attitudes to makeup should depend on context and intent: 'The Harlot dresses herself up to allure and ensnare the Unwary into her Embraces, the virtuous Lady for Decency and the Credit of her Family.'[6] The old argument had been upended: when women from good families beautified themselves it was a sign of respectability. Painted faces just had to be decoded.

Women were already sending out social and political signals by wearing face patches. Made of gummed silk, velvet, or paper, these were variously shaped into moons, stars, birds, or beasts. Tory and Whig supporters patched on different sides of the face. The position of a patch could have other meanings: near the lips, for instance, it was termed 'the coquette' and invited flirtation. Patches were the height of fashion until about 1700; the French called them *mouches* (flies) and kept them in attractive *boites à mouches*. The most coveted boxes were made of ivory, mother-of-pearl, or gold, with perhaps a mirror inside. To possess such trinkets, to know how to name and use each patch, was a sign of fashionable sophistication. But observers had to be wary: patches covered smallpox scars but could also mask rampant syphilis.

As the vogue for patching extended down the social ranks, critics from the middling sort labelled it 'barbarous' and compared patches to the face decoration of native peoples that sailors encountered on voyages of exploration. Contemporary illustrations show a Black woman and a white woman side by side, the Black face adorned with white patches; such images seem to mock both women equally.[7] Patches fell out of fashion completely towards the end of the eighteenth century, not least because a vaccine had been discovered for smallpox.

At the same time, cosmetic use became more acceptable among the white English elite in the eighteenth century; posthumous editions of Gauden's book in 1692 and 1701 explicitly urged women to apply makeup to make the most of their charms. In Britain, as on the Continent, women began to buy manufactured cosmetics, although home production continued, and some endures in the present.

COSMETIC MATERIALS AND TECHNIQUES

Ceruse was a popular cosmetic ingredient. This was lead carbonate, dense and opaque, which clung to the skin so could be applied quite thinly. Ceruse was also used by painters. Due to high demand, it was manufactured on a large scale in England from the seventeenth century, by exposing lead to acetic acid in the presence of water and carbon dioxide. In London, there was a substantial white lead factory in Islington by 1786, with a windmill for grinding the pigment to powder. By the nineteenth century, the factory had steam-powered mills and a workforce of about fifty. Two-thirds of the workers were women because most thought they could better tolerate the pollution.

While some women continued to favour ceruse in the eighteenth century, white makeup was also made from bismuth compounds or aluminium sulphate (alum), finely powdered and then blended with oils. Safer alternatives included starch, burnt bones, and ground alabaster. For a slight sheen, women applied pearl powder. The most expensive sort was made from seed pearls dissolved in lemon juice or vinegar before being dried to a powder, but there were inferior mixtures, often including bismuth. Women could also buy a lead-based 'liquid pearl' which promised a soft, genteel glow. Lead and bismuth were known to be corrosive, and sometimes so-called pearl products gave a faintly blue shine. By the 1780s, retailers were offering a safe French alternative made from the scales of small ablet, fished from the River Loire. Such light-reflecting cosmetics evened out skin tone and were mostly intended for evening wear.

Rouge was available in various tints and at different prices depending on quality. Carmine, a crimson pigment, was made from the cochineal insect, still used for red colouring today. Cochineal was enormously expensive, so vermilion was often substituted. This orange-red pigment came from grinding natural cinnabar or mercury sulphate, but it had also been manufactured in Europe since the Middle Ages by melting and subliming mercury and sulphur. Cheaper red lead, or lead oxide, was sometimes passed off as vermilion. The lower classes might only have been able to afford inferior rouge made from red ochre, a clay containing iron oxide. But vegetable dyes were also used, made from red alkanet root, safflowers, saffron, gum benzoin (wood resin), brazil-wood, or sandalwood.

Women applied the colour to their cheeks in several ways. Spanish wool, a hair pad soaked in red pigment and then dried, was popular for a while. Spanish papers – strips of paper thickened with carmine – were more easily stored. Red leathers were also used. Women rubbed these materials on the cheeks to transfer the dye to the skin. Others preferred powdered rouge, which was put on with a rabbit's foot; face cream would make the rouge stick if women chose to omit the white base layer. Some used liquid rouge, applied with a brush of camel's hair. From the mid-eighteenth century, the French moved to an oil-based rouge and British women soon followed suit. A small rouge pot survives in London's Foundling Hospital, among the objects left with children, should mothers wish to identify and reclaim them.

Tinted lip salves could be made from any red dye. Elizabeth I favoured cochineal mixed with gum arabic, egg whites, and fig milk. A popular eighteenth-century guide contained recipes for making lip cream from alkanet and white wax, or roses and hog's lard, a distinct improvement on seventeenth-century advice to blend the dye with sweat from behind the ears.[8] Other recipes fixed organic dyes for the lips in wine or brandy.

Eye makeup was adopted more slowly in western Europe, although early travellers remarked that the Turks used kohl to set off the white of their eyes. When Lady Mary Wortley Montagu was in Turkey in 1717, she admired the lustre that kohl gave the eyes in candlelight.[9] A beauty manual of 1760 advised English women to darken their eyebrows with a paint made from the soot of burnt ivory or cherry stones mixed with oil of amber.[10] With less trouble, eyebrows could be dyed black with a lead comb or rubbed with burnt cork. Bushy eyebrows might be thinned first with depilatory cream.

There are few reliable sources for the total effect of eighteenth-century makeup comprising such vibrant ingredients. Contemporary portraits flatter the sitter and have anyway faded over time. Paintings from the later eighteenth century showing white skin and pink cheeks may simply depict an ideal of female beauty. But writers often satirised the use of cosmetics, and older women were an easy target. In William Congreve's play *The Way of the World*, staged in 1700, Lady Wishfort calls upon her woman, Foible, to repair her makeup so that she can live up to the portrait sent to her suitor:

FOIBLE: Your ladyship has frowned a little too rashly, indeed, madam. There are some cracks discernible in the white varnish.
LADY WISHFORT: Let me see the glass. – Cracks, say'st thou? Why, I am arrantly flayed: I look like an old peeled wall. Thou must repair me, Foible, before Sir Rowland comes, or I shall never keep up to my picture.[11]

As this extract shows, the link between painting the face and portraiture was a familiar one. Not only were the same pigments often used but painterly skill was needed to apply makeup.

ELITE MAKEUP AND NATIONAL DIFFERENCES

Why would women use such bold cosmetics? Doubtless they wished to look their best and feel confident. But in applying white and red pigments, elite women were also asserting their status. This was evidently the case in

France during the reign of Louis XV. Rouge was even implicated in court politics: on the cheeks of Madame de Pompadour, the king's mistress, it was a sign of social success, royal favour, and her fidelity to the Crown. The king's pious wife from Poland, Queen Marie, did not favour rouge.

By the eighteenth century, France was already the centre of production for perfumes and cosmetics; British perfumers often advertised their cosmetic goods as the latest imports from Paris. Yet the style of makeup varied in the two countries. Among the French elite, the fashion was to rouge heavily; in London, this would be considered poor taste. Lady Mary Wortley Montagu thought women in the French court 'Nauseous' and labelled them 'grotesque Dawbers': 'So monstrously unnatural in their paint! . . . on their cheeks to their Chins, unmercifully laid on, a shineing red japan, that glistens in a most flameing manner, that they seem to have no resemblance to Human faces.'[12] Some ladies painted blue veins at their temples and on the neck, which further racialised standards of beauty because veins, visible through the skin, emphasised whiteness as well as delicacy.

French dressing tables showed how much aristocratic French women valued makeup as a badge of rank. The tables were designed with more ingenuity and decorated more expensively than any furniture women owned for washing the skin. The French were in any case dubious about washing; to the end of the century, their physicians feared that water would enter the body through open pores and damage vital organs. Women spent long hours at the dressing table so made the best use of their time: once preliminary work was complete, they applied the finishing touches before a favoured, select company. Their toilette was a performance of status and an opportunity to catch up on gossip. British men larded fictional accounts of the French toilette with salacious innuendo. One character boasted, 'I have handed many a Marchioness out of Bed with only her Under-Petticoat on, and a loose Bed-Gown; sat afterwards by her at her Toilet while she dress'd her Head and painted her Face.'[13] In fact, the dressing table ritual was essentially a sociable activity not a sexual one.

Clearly, French women made no secret of painting. In any case, by the mid-eighteenth century the Parisian elite wore elaborately curled and white-powdered hairstyles; the effect was simply too ghostly without some red tint. The middling sort were more sparing with the rouge but still clamoured to wear this mark of status. British writers underscored distinguishing national traits in Paris and London. One commented, 'A Woman there *without* much Paint, is as ridiculous as a Woman *with* much here.'[14] Another mused that, if he thought an opera box of French ladies resembled a bed of full-blown peonies, a Frenchman might compare English beauties to a bed of lilies, or a border of light-coloured pinks.[15] By the 1780s, all but the very poor in France wore makeup; it was claimed that French women got through two million pots of rouge a year.[16] After the French Revolution, a less dramatic, liquid rouge gained ground; a light sweep with a wet rag took away the tell-tale colour from soft facial hair, leaving it just on the cheek.

As is still often the case, women had to conform to customary standards of appearance. Aristocratic women were notably on display and, like artworks, subject to aesthetic appreciation or pretended connoisseurship. Even so, eighteenth-century moralists insisted that beauty had to be accompanied by virtue: 'No Woman is capable of being Beautiful, who is not incapable of being False. . . . How much nobler is the Contemplation of Beauty heightened by Virtue.'[17] The ideal woman had to look beautiful, sexually appealing, and virtuous at the same time. This helps to explain why, in Britain, rouge was a particular target for criticism; men worried that rouge would obscure a woman's true emotions. Since blushing denoted modesty, a mask of makeup gave room for false delicacy, and plentiful rouge was associated with shameless women. What is more, men who aspired to possess a beautiful wife did not want to find her beauty owed more to art than to nature. Consequently, aristocratic women who painted, and the middling sort who aped them, drew censure, while the supposedly unadorned virtue of the simple country girl attracted praise: 'No Midnight-Masquerade her Beauty wears, / And Health, not Paint, the fading Bloom repairs.'[18]

But, although the British elite disapproved of makeup in theory, it was still normal to wear a little rouge in society.[19]

Advertisements indicate that painted women in Britain aimed at a natural look. For example, the innocent-sounding white makeup 'Balm of Lillies' promised 'a very beautiful and natural bloom, which cannot be distinguished from real nature'; nor would it come off 'by wiping or perspiration'.[20] In his novel *Roxana*, Daniel Defoe plays with these ideas. Roxana, who traded her virtue for money, assures her French aristocratic admirer that her fine complexion owes nothing to art: 'I have not deceived you with false Colours.' She washes her face before him in warm water to prove her point. Afterwards, 'he kiss'd my Cheeks and Breasts a thousand times, with Expressions of the greatest Surprize imaginable'.[21] Here Defoe takes aim at the stylish French, swayed after all by natural British beauty. But there is a twist: Roxana may be deceitful at bottom, given the advertised qualities of contemporary face paint.

Natural-looking or not, cosmetics helped to produce a socially created stereotype of beauty linked to wealth and luxury. In Britain, as in France, cosmetic use spread from the aristocracy until face paint was worn by all who could afford it. The middling sort were expected to be more virtuous than the elite but, since face paint was potentially an aid to social mobility, white women of this class wore it to emulate their superiors. One author described how society in Edinburgh had changed by the 1780s: 'The daughters even of tradesmen consume the mornings at the toilet, (to which *rouge* is now an appendage).'[22] Inevitably, the trend spread to the British North American colonies: Martha Washington had her own recipe for alkanet-tinted lip salve.[23]

ANXIETIES AND COMMERCIAL BENEFITS

Many cosmetics were dangerous with prolonged use. Belladonna caused blurred vision and even blindness. Ceruse prompted the typical effects of lead poisoning: abdominal pain, muscle weakness, tingling in the hands and feet, and memory problems. It could damage and blacken the skin, and make hair fall out. Mercury-based red pigments resulted in tooth loss and stinking breath. A 1724 Act forbidding apothecaries from selling poison did safeguard Londoners to some extent, but even recipes for homemade beauty potions sometimes called for toxic metallic compounds.[24]

Medical writers in England had cautioned against using corrosive ingredients in cosmetics from the beginning of the seventeenth century. John Bulwer complained that mercury washes stripped women's skin and made them look like 'peeld Ewes'.[25] There were also high-profile deaths from the effects of face paint. The beautiful Maria Gunning hooked an aristocratic husband in 1752 to become Countess of Coventry. She died aged just twenty-eight in 1760 from tuberculosis, exacerbated by poison from her lead-based makeup. The artist and letter-writer Mary Delany remarked:

> What a wretched end Lady Coventry makes after her short-lived reign of beauty! Not contented with the *extraordinary share* Providence had bestowed on her, she presumptuously and vainly thought to mend it, and by that means they say has destroyed her life . . . the white she made use of for her face and neck was rank poison; I wish it may be a warning to her imitators.[26]

Some twenty years later, Fanny Burney recorded the fate of two 'unnaturally white' sisters, suspected of using face paint. One had died already; the other looked 'upon the point of death'.[27] In the 1780s and 1790s, advertisements for vegetable rouge and other innocent cosmetics multiplied, but women whose social status depended on their beauty, or who were just determined to have their own way, seemingly ignored warnings about toxic makeup.

Increased cosmetic use in western Europe prompted anxieties: some feared it signalled that the lower orders were attempting to climb the social ladder. Face paint also retained its association with prostitution. Women were aware that makeup elicited a complex response. In 1720,

Lady Lansdowne sent a present of rouge from Paris to her friend the Countess of Suffolk, confident that it would be appreciated, but wrote tactfully, 'not that you have any occasion to use it'.[28] Some women could not quite explain their visceral reaction to makeup. In the 1780s, the playwright Elizabeth Berkeley visited Vienna and was shocked to find that 'Every lower class of women paint white – and even girls of ten years old going of errands in the street are painted', adding, 'What their reason for so doing is I cannot guess; for the Germans are generally fair.'[29] Berkeley, who came from an aristocratic family, perhaps resented lower-class pretensions, but she also seems troubled by face paint on young girls, which hinted at premature sexuality.

Negative reactions to face paint were fanned by the outrageous public performances of women who used makeup to bolster their celebrity, or just to have fun. The actor and writer Mary Robinson was a chameleon-like icon in the late 1770s. One commentator gushed, 'Yesterday she perhaps had been the dressed belle of Hyde Park, trimmed, powdered, patched, painted to the utmost power of rouge and white lead; to-morrow she would be the cravated Amazon of the riding house; but, be she what she might, the hats of the fashionable promenaders swept the ground as she passed.'[30] Robinson was the first public mistress of the future George IV. Her fame coincided with a visible increase in the use of cosmetics, which seemed to help bold women make their fortune. Scandalous displays like hers prompted attempts to assert social stability and conservative values by denouncing makeup. Painted aristocrats drew sharp criticism. In the 1780s, when the radical intellectual Mary Wollstonecraft was a governess in the household of Lord and Lady Kingsborough, she wrote home to share her outrage at the time her mistress and other ladies of her circle spent dressing; she found great fault with their use of rouge.[31]

But there were commercial forces at work helping to promote the use of face paint. Perfumes and dyestuffs had been traded across the world for centuries; by the mid-eighteenth century, cosmetics, too, were having a significant impact on international trade and on the economies of major European cities. The British cosmetics market centred on London. The most prized perfumes, powders, white cosmetics, and rouge were imported from France and Italy. Some vermilion came from Holland. The ingredients for other commercial and homemade cosmetics came from all over the globe, including red sandalwood from southern India, brazilwood from Brazil, and the finest otto or oil of roses from Bulgaria. The poet Alexander Pope expressed his fascination at the global aspect of a rich woman's dressing table: 'This Casket *India*'s glowing Gems unlocks, / And all *Arabia* breathes from yonder Box.'[32]

Merchants based in Marseille imported a wide range of products from the Levant for the European cosmetic trade. These included perfumes, incense, benzoin, and other resins like frankincense, some of which reached Turkish markets from East and Southeast Asia. From the Ottoman Empire, Marseille's merchants also imported alum, used to fix colours in the dying trades, as well as for cosmetics. They re-exported cochineal and indigo. Cochineal, which gave the colour carmine, came from crushed insects found in Spanish America and was almost as valuable as gold or silver. Much of the cochineal harvest was shipped to Spain before being traded to the rest of Europe, then further afield. France, with dynastic links to Spain, obtained cochineal at a good price, which was fortunate as rouge was in such demand there. French merchants also imported from Spain the expensive Cyprus Powder, a cosmetic made from the starchy root of the plant commonly known as lords-and-ladies.

The costly and obscure imports needed for cosmetics had drawn censure in Elizabethan England. But merchants quickly saw the potential for lucrative trade and so encouraged early travellers to record where ingredients for possible cosmetic use could be found. Handbooks for novice merchants and dictionaries of trade and commerce listed imports of cosmetic value, including vermilion, benzoin, borax, and bismuth. Their worth might otherwise be overlooked. The manuals explained how to recognise the genuine article and how to distinguish the purest grades from inferior products.

In the mid-eighteenth century, the British apothecary and chemist Robert Dossie noted that the demand for rouge had greatly increased imports of carmine from France.[33] The market for cosmetics became so large and the trade so profitable that in 1786 Prime Minister William Pitt decided to tax perfumes, cosmetics, and hair powder, anticipating significant revenue for the state. Britain was at war with France from 1793 to 1815, but illegal trade with the enemy persisted. During these years, British merchant ships gratefully loaded whatever cochineal they could get direct from Cádiz.[34] Yet in France, after revolution broke out in 1789, the populace turned against the heavily rouged look of the aristocracy. Physicians stepped up their warnings about the toxins in face paint. Critics blamed female deceit for a range of social evils and emphasised that mask-like cosmetics blurred social status and veiled a woman's true character. In 1790s Paris, stark white makeup and brilliant red rouge gave way to a look seemingly free from artifice. Women coveted a natural flush that would complement the vogue for Grecian fashions. They turned to beauty manuals which were often based on doctors' advice and seemed to offer permissible recipes to improve their looks.

In Britain, garish face paint remained strongly associated with Paris. War with France therefore bolstered the preference for a more natural look in Britain too, although women may also have feared the tax on imported cosmetics. In the popular mind on both sides of the Channel, social upheaval was linked to aristocratic debauchery and alleged female sexual deceit at all levels – another reason for women to avoid heavy makeup. But the natural look was contrived; the cosmetic trade flourished still, even if women were drawn to innocent-sounding, plant-based preparations. Since there was now less dependence on toxic ingredients, the consumer base for cosmetics even widened. In Britain, although political unrest in France led some to think that women needed careful supervision, even Quaker women could paint. Elizabeth Fry, a Quaker and later a famous prison reformer, visited London in 1798 before her marriage. She wrote in her diary that she had been given makeup to wear before an evening concert, 'I was painted a little, I had my hair dressed, and did look pretty for me.'[35]

Crucially, British women of the period were expected to show a lively sensibility, which was virtually impossible if they had painted on an artificial complexion. As the author of one beauty manual exclaimed in 1811, no one can look on a face 'bedaubed with white paint, pearl powder, or enamel, and be deceived for a minute into a belief that so inanimate a "whited wall" is the human skin'. A little vegetable rouge might be excusable; wartime anxieties caused many to lose rosy cheeks. But on no account should women copy the French use of rouge: 'Frenchwomen in general, and those who imitate them, daub it on from the bottom of the side of the face up to the very eye, even till it meets the lower eye-lash, and creeps all over the temples. This is a hideous practice.' Likewise, pencilling or darkening the eyebrows were 'clumsy tricks of attempted deception'.[36] As war with France dragged on, British women's use of cosmetics was more than ever contrasted with a caricatured view of French practice.

British women were encouraged to revert to making lip salves, pastes, and health-giving skin washes at home. Even Caroline, Princess of Wales, made her own concoctions. Her peevish lady-in-waiting thought it absurd: 'I was called by Her Royal Highness into her secret chamber, where there was a fire, though the thermometer was at eighty; but she makes cosmetics and dirt pies, and there were various pots and pans boiling. What a droll amusement!'[37] Even so, European standards of restrained makeup were increasingly contrasted with fashions in non-Christian countries. White British female travellers censured women in Gujerat for overtly using cosmetics to increase their beauty; they scorned the painted faces of lower-class Turkish women.[38] Makeup use helped to cement a sense of Western superiority.

VICTORIAN TRENDS

In the nineteenth century, British women did seem to support the view that painting the face was deplorable. Queen Victoria set the tone: she disapproved of cosmetics and praised soap and water. In 1843, Jane

Welsh Carlyle gave a typically damning description of a woman who used makeup. The American poet Lydia Huntley Sigourney came to a social event 'beplastered with rouge and pomatum – barenecked at an age which had left *certainty* far behind – with long ringlets that never grew where they hung – smelling marvellously of camphor or hartshorn and oil'.[39] Carlyle's disapproval was probably heightened because Sigourney made eyes at her husband all evening, trying to get the famous social commentator to take centre stage. But early Victorian women did mostly aim to maintain their looks by rigorous skincare.

As in the early eighteenth century, popular literature insisted that women had to cultivate goodness and modesty, which would shine through the skin as loveliness. In 1853, *The Family Treasury*, a journal for women, gave clear expression to typical Victorian values:

> It is not the smiles of a pretty face, not the tint of her complexion, nor the beauty and symmetry of her person . . . that compose a woman's loveliness . . . It is her pleasing deportment, her chaste conversation, the sensibility and purity of her thoughts, her affable and open disposition, her sympathy with those in adversity, her comforting and relieving the afflicted in distress, and, above all, the humbleness of her soul, that constitute true loveliness.[40]

True beauty came from within, and a woman's outer appearance ought to reflect inner purity. Given this mindset, rouge was a badge of sin, an affront to the increasingly powerful middle classes who valued morality, propriety, and restraint. Men were credited with superior reasoning powers, whereas women had to fight for intellectual stature. The very language of advice books reminded women that their brains would be judged from their appearance. 'Paint should never be resorted to', insisted one; 'It is a senseless piece of hypocrisy, betraying a mean and degraded mind.'[41]

Victorian beauty culture therefore posed real difficulty for plain women and those who were no longer young. Magazines offered scant comfort: one declared that 'A plain woman, who has a cultivated brain and good taste, will always be able to hold her ground against pretty women', while 'a homely face' would look good-humoured in old age.[42] If some readers were reassured, others acted. The dangers of metal-based cosmetics were still routinely publicised, so middle-class white women, largely confined to the home, became skilled at make-do cosmetics. Some applied brightening makeup under the guise of using a gentle cream to preserve the complexion. Household recipe books featured innocent-sounding preparations like 'Mamma's lip salve', which contained red alkanet dye fixed in alcohol.[43] Some women reddened their cheeks by rubbing them with geranium petals.

In the 1830s, the novelist Fanny Trollope noticed that women sweltering in a New York summer powdered heavily with 'pulverised starch'. 'The effect', she wrote, 'is indescribably disagreeable by daylight, and not very favourable at any time.'[44] But soon more British women used powder, which was prevalent by the 1860s. For an even complexion, they primed their skin with cold cream. The technique was a hundred years old, but now the powder, whether of rice, maize, or orris root, was often tinted. The recent vogue for 'baking' the face – setting foundation with a generous layer of loose powder – is similar.

Luckily, a new substance was found on the steel rods of oil pumps which helped to meet the demand for cold cream. In 1872, Robert Chesebrough, a chemist from New York, patented a way to purify this petroleum jelly, which he branded Vaseline. Soon he was selling thousands of jars of Vaseline each year. Unlike animal fat, it never turned rancid. It proved a cheap, effective base for various products, from cold cream and hair tonic to axle grease. Doctors warned that face powder might clog the skin but did allow that, with a cream barrier, starch was less likely to ferment in the pores and face cream might also protect against dangerous substances.

Skilful Victorian women rarely betrayed any trace of commercial makeup. They incorporated it into their performance of femininity, but observers were never meant to notice it. By this time, better cosmetics were available. Women could buy little pocket-books of rose-infused blush sheets; the colour was lifted off with a moistened fingertip and applied to the cheeks. Eyebrows were darkened with kohl. The British regularly accused French women of touching up and correcting their faces but did the same thing in the privacy of their own homes.

POISONS AND PROSTITUTES

Victorian cosmetics still had shortcomings. At balls, women had to be careful not to sweat and spoil the effect of cream and powder. In the theatre or at church, any escape of gas from the lighting could turn a powdered pink and white complexion to green and yellow, because sulphur vapours reacted with bismuth. Sitting too near a coal fire could have the same effect. And health dangers remained. Face powders were sometimes tinted with cheap toxins, not least because the secrecy surrounding makeup made it easier for manufacturers to use them.

In the 1860s there were high-profile cases of lead poisoning among Parisian actresses who used liquid pearl as a foundation; there were also injuries among women whose depilatories contained quicklime. In the United States, many assumed that bismuth had wholly replaced white lead in skin creams, but the American Medical Association published details in 1869 of three cases of lead poisoning in young white women who had used Laird's Bloom of Youth. One woman, who had used the product for about two and a half years, had almost completely lost the use of her arms and hands: 'she was unable to feed herself, comb her hair, pick up a pin, hook or button her dress, or in fact make any movements whatever with her hands, except the very slightest flexion of her fingers'.[45] Yet the lotion was still being advertised in *Harper's Bazaar* in the 1880s; federal laws regulating food and drugs in the United States did not cover preparations sold as cosmetics.

Before the twentieth century, fear of being poisoned remained perhaps the greatest barrier to everyday cosmetic use. The consequence of making the wrong choice about some commercial product could be nervous debility or even insanity. In 1896, some twenty years after American doctors exposed Laird's Bloom of Youth, Britain's local press was still reporting cases of 'Cosmetic Paralysis' caused by mercury poisoning:

> A woman feels a queer sensation in her arms, accompanied by shooting pains and numbness. She usually supposes she has rheumatism or something of that nature, and it will pass away in a few days. Instead or getting better it grows gradually worse, and she finds her feet becoming uncomfortable. They feel as if needles and pins were being run into them. In fact, her whole nervous system appears to be going to pieces.[46]

Carefully phrased advertisements ought to have raised suspicion: lip and face rouge was 'indelible', pearl powder made users 'glow and bloom'. Cosmetic ingredients were rarely stated on the packaging.[47] A batch of innocent-sounding 'Violet Powder' – usually just starch scented with orris root for brightening yellow tones in the skin – was found to be 38 per cent arsenic.[48] Astute retailers claimed that their products were free from all injurious substances, sometimes falsely, and even described home tests that would alert users to poison in other cosmetics.[49] Ultra-cautious white women applied only damp chalk to the face; it was safe but rarely looked good.

Another curb to makeup use was its enduring link with prostitution. As in earlier centuries, much of the pressure on women to avoid 'paint' was to ensure a visible difference between 'virtuous' females and sex workers. Class anxiety was a contributing factor. Some feared that prostitutes, whose deceit was legendary, and actresses, often assumed to be women of easy virtue, would use cosmetics to disguise their social background and trick men into disastrous liaisons. In the nineteenth century, an apparent increase in prostitution caused huge concern. To preserve their social status, men often postponed marriage until they could afford all the trappings of a middle-class family lifestyle. Meanwhile, they resorted to brothels. In the 1830s, the number of prostitutes in New York, Paris, and London was anxiously compared. Accurate statistics were impossible, but New York, with a population of almost half a million, was estimated to have 10,000; Paris, with about 900,000 inhabitants, was thought to have 18,000; and London, a city of over two million, was reckoned to have up to 10,000 prostitutes, although a charitable society for the protection of young women judged that it had as many as 80,000, with a substantial number being under fifteen years of age.[50]

The widespread fear that society would be morally contaminated by prostitution was probably more important than bald statistics. William Acton, a gynaecologist, wrote that prostitutes did not die early 'in hospitals, workhouses, or obscure degradation', as many assumed, but merged with the population over time.[51] How was a man to recognise a woman of the town? There were clues: a veil, or lack of it, and bright clothes, but above all makeup. Even so, respectable women complained of being accosted in the streets because men found it hard to distinguish prostitutes by appearance alone; any woman could innocently give glimpses of ankle as they lifted skirts over dirty pavements.

In Britain, the Contagious Diseases Acts passed between 1864 and 1869 meant that women redoubled their efforts to avoid being taken for prostitutes. These Acts aimed to reduce venereal disease in the armed services but had an increasing impact on women in the general population, not just in military towns. Females could be arrested on the mere suspicion of being sex workers, subjected to humiliating examination, and, if found to be infected, held in a lock hospital for twelve months. The Acts, a blatant instance of Victorian double standards, were suspended only in 1883 and repealed in 1886. The number of innocent women who were detained is unknown, but fear of arrest certainly impacted on how women dressed and behaved. Opposition to these Acts also helped to unify women in a cause and strengthen their growing agitation for equal rights. Wives thought it particularly unjust that, if they experimented with makeup to enhance their looks and keep husbands faithful, they risked sexual harassment on the streets and perhaps arrest.

Despite all these dangers, the late Victorian period was one of increasing cosmetic use among fashionable women. Heavily veiled ladies left their carriages a hundred yards down the street and slipped furtively into salons for treatments and products. Society became more tolerant of older women wearing lip rouge, not least because an ideal of feminine beauty persisted and was a matter of national pride. The middle classes remained averse to makeup, especially to rouge, which they still associated with immorality. But women who said they paid no attention to their beauty were open to accusations of false modesty. The middle classes were therefore ready to be seduced by floral cosmetic brands that seemed related to cleanliness. Since a woman's reputation was affected by the skill with which she could apply makeup, beauty manuals were popular. Authors seemed to write from personal experience and often gave inexpensive tips. One writer advised young girls to dab beetroot juice on the cheeks and rub it well in with chamois leather.[52]

The nineteenth century also saw a growing appreciation of eye liner, partly due to the publicity surrounding archaeological digs in Egypt from the 1860s. Finds included eye makeup containers. As more evidence of ancient Egyptian cosmetics emerged, one beauty specialist enthused, 'Egyptian women are famous for the art of arranging the eyelids and eyebrows', and gave details of how to emulate their skill.[53] Archaeology did help to legitimise eye makeup, but beauticians had been recommending kohl from the mid-nineteenth century, dismissing charcoal and burnt cork as fit only for amateur dramatics.[54]

Eugène Rimmel is credited with inventing the first commercial non-toxic mascara. The son of a French scent manufacturer, he opened his own shop for beauty products in the Strand in 1857 and was selling Egyptian kohl by the 1860s. Early eye makeup was termed 'eye-black' and associated with theatricals. Romantic pulp fiction helped to promote its use more widely. One story featured a young woman who attracted a rich admirer by acting in an amateur play. Afterwards, 'All her rouge and eye-black washed off, she was once more to most people a sallow, uninteresting girl. But he could not forget those deep, earnest eyes, the intense fervour of her voice, the passionate emotion expressed in her gesture.'[55] The key point is that eye-black could help to attract a man, and that this attraction would continue even when the makeup was removed. But beauty manuals insisted that eye makeup had to be subtle. Coconut oil was praised as less easily detected than eyebrow pencil; lampblack was recommended to darken lashes for evenings; kohl had to be applied with a light hand; cologne on a sugar lump would add secret sparkle to the eyes.[56]

Visible makeup was tolerated earlier in North America than in Britain. But a distinction was drawn between the western states, where wives were deemed too busy with chores to consult a mirror, and eastern states, where fashionable women devoted hours to their toilette. Even so, by 1870, magazines reported that, mostly, 'The time has gone by when it was a matter of church discipline if a woman painted her face or wore powder.'[57] Canny salesmen inverted the adage that face paint insulted God's creation: they explained that women who neglected their toilette were failing to honour God's handiwork, going against God-given instincts, and disregarding nature's first law: self-preservation.[58] In New York, shops selling cosmetics stayed open on Saturdays until 10 p.m. to cater for women with jobs, and a mail order service supplied households across the United States. Illustrated sales catalogues opened women's eyes to the range of beauty aids available. These were mostly aimed at white women, but 'olive tinted' powders were available for 'ladies of dark complexion'.[59] Mail order was doubly useful because customers did not have to risk being spotted buying makeup.

Despite known hazards, commercial products became increasingly popular as women sought to save the time it took to make cosmetics at home. By the 1880s, the consensus was that no woman past thirty should be ashamed of using makeup; the extremes of the North American climate and life under gaslight meant that older women with good skin were rarities.[60] Some women fiercely demanded the right to wear powder and rouge: 'Is not beauty in many instances a woman's fortune, and has she not a right to make herself as attractive as she can? . . . Is the use of powder to be made a sin, and the application of rouge a crime?'[61] What mattered was the power of individual choice.

INFLUENCERS AND ENTREPRENEURS

On both sides of the Atlantic, some white women were even drawing blue veins on their bosoms once more, although beauty culturists advised it should only be attempted by the practised hand. Apart from following beauty manuals, how were women to learn makeup skills? Photographic studios had clients from all levels of society and sometimes used face paint to improve their looks. But middle- and upper-class Victorians and Edwardians seized opportunities to wear makeup in amateur theatricals. These included plays and tableaux vivants (the latter quite distinct from professional versions, when scantily clad performers arranged themselves in erotic poses). Heavy makeup was perfectly acceptable for home theatre; magazines at first advised women to copy actors who seemed to have learned how to apply cosmetics for the stage without skin damage. Some dancers and public singers had visibly coarsened their complexions by using bismuth powder, but safe theatrical greasepaint (lead-free powders mixed with lard) could be bought from the 1870s in handy stick form. Some women were even tempted to make light use of greasepaint for evening wear.

The term 'makeup' comes from nineteenth-century theatre slang for the process of making up before a show. It hints at invention and deceit, long associated with cosmetics, and at the idea of compensating for defects. By the 1820s, 'makeup' could also refer to a person's hardwiring, which helped to confuse notions of outer appearance and inner character. Home theatricals grew in popularity and, by the late nineteenth century, magazines carried detailed articles explaining how to apply stage makeup. *Harper's Bazaar* assured readers that with practice they would be able to apply it almost by touch alone, implying regular use.

When the magazine listed essential cosmetics for 'any young woman about to embark on the rather serious pastime of play-acting', several could be put to discrete daily use.[62] Leading ladies like Sarah Bernhardt shared cosmetic 'tricks' in magazine and newspaper articles, although most insisted that they never wore makeup offstage. Star performers, with an appeal that crossed classes, were increasingly accepted as social influencers rather than relegated to the fringes of respectable society. In short, magazines and readers colluded in a pretence that makeup advice merely helped amateur performers to emulate professional actors, when it also encouraged routine cosmetic use.

In the 1880s, fashionable women carried tiny kits, often disguised as watch cases, which allowed them to touch up their makeup during social engagements, but beauty writers still advised secrecy, explaining that men did not like to see how it was done.[63] Wives could buy lockable bathroom wall cabinets in which to hide their beauty secrets. These were glass-fronted, but there was room for an embroidered hanging or panel on the inside of the glass for privacy. Women also purchased toilet boxes for the dressing table, which were useful when travelling. Most of these boxes had locks; some had secret compartments. But in any case, patent cosmetics could easily be decanted into ordinary bottles and hidden in toilet boxes alongside acceptable beauty aids and medicines. The most expensive toilet boxes were crafted in fine woods and lined with velvet, but cheap metal versions were also available.

Light has always been key when applying makeup. Lead-based white proved a seductive product because it was luminous in candlelight. When Lady Mary Wortley Montagu saw Turkish women using kohl, she noted how it added to the blackness of the eyes at a distance, or by candlelight. English ladies, she thought, would be glad to know the secret but kohl was 'too Visible by day'.[64] In the nineteenth century, white women adapted their cosmetics to gaslight: powders included blue and lavender tints, so that complexions appeared pale even in the yellow aura of candlelight or brighter gas. Magazines advised that theatrical makeup was best applied by gaslight to achieve the right colour balance, and that evening makeup was also best applied by gaslight.

When electric lighting came in at the end of the nineteenth century, women had to adjust again. Clear electric light minimised colour distortions. It could help women make up in glamorous detail but gave some cheek colours a blue tinge, so face powder with mauve and pale green tints was introduced for evening wear. Dressing tables were designed with an electric lamp either side of the mirror to help women achieve a flattering effect. In contrast, daytime makeup applied by electric light could easily be overdone; specialists advised placing dressing tables where they could best catch natural light. Today, the cool, bluish light of LED lighting can lend an unwelcome sharpness to some makeup colours. Beauticians advise never buying foundation creams tested under shop lights alone; a sample must be viewed in natural daylight.

The burgeoning cosmetics trade offered welcome opportunities for female entrepreneurs. After all, there was a long tradition of female involvement in the beauty trade. In eighteenth-century France, most small rouge-sellers were women, kept out of other professions; unsurprisingly the wives of French perfumers who emigrated to London often specialised in making rouge.[65] In the 1790s, an 'inventress' who claimed to have studied under the ablest chemists in Europe advertised that she could improve British complexions with a year-long programme of care.[66] She set a precedent for the scandalous Madame Rachel, whose spurious cosmetic treatments in the 1860s were accompanied by fraud on a wider scale.

Beauty specialists were well placed to win clients' trust by promising secrecy; many were also innately skilled at business and marketing. Harriet Hubbard Ayer founded the first cosmetics business in North America, setting up her Recamier Manufacturing Company in New York in 1886. A former socialite, she was struggling to support herself and her daughters after a messy divorce but was able to trade on her former status to sell a range of preparations. She persuaded unscrupulous chemists to guarantee that her formulations were safe, and paid celebrities to endorse them. She did so well that she planned to open a manufacturing branch in England for the British and European markets. But the men in her life schemed to take over her business. They had Ayer institutionalised for insanity in 1893, and by the time she was freed she had lost control of her company. Undaunted, she found a job writing the women's pages of the *New York World*, still working to extend the cosmetics market. By the time of her death in 1903, doctors and chemists had exposed the fact that costly Recamier products were made of cheap ingredients, including mercury compounds. But the brand name Harriet Hubbard Ayer was sold on and profitably applied to cosmetics for the next forty years.

Another American, Anna Ruppert, extended her beauty business from New York to London in the 1890s, using 'Mrs' not 'Madame', to avoid comparisons with Madame Rachel. She set up a salon in Regent Street and lectured on natural beauty to large audiences. Sensitive to public opinion, she insisted that beauty came from within, but still sold a range of products that were effectively cosmetics. When her rejuvenating skin lotion was found to contain mercury, she was prosecuted; her salon never recovered. But the medical men who exposed quacks gave good advice, and improved safety also helped to make cosmetics respectable.

Not all self-styled beauty experts were charlatans. In the early twentieth century, Madam C. J. Walker, an African American, made a fortune by developing and marketing skin and hair preparations for Black women. At its height, her business provided jobs for some 100,000 people. Her door-to-door sales technique allowed her to explain how products should be used and, at the same time, to get an understanding of customer needs. This was essential to her success. Later cosmetic companies, notably Avon, copied her technique in the 1950s and early 1960s, when women were still mostly found at home. Walker is also remembered because she devoted so much of her business income to philanthropy and activism, determined to improve the lives of fellow African Americans.

MASS MARKETS

In the United States, the number of manufacturers of cosmetics and perfumes quadrupled in the twenty years from 1879, at a time when the population only increased by just over half.[67] By the early twentieth century, cosmetic firms in North America had the assurance to claim that their products improved a woman's character as well as her appearance.[68] Women were insisting on their freedom to wear makeup, and their attitude became associated with the suffragette movement. When women marched through New York to demand the vote in 1912, they wore red lipstick as an act of defiance and to demonstrate their power. The story that Elizabeth Arden joined the marchers, joyfully handing out lipstick, is often repeated but not true. She saw a marketing opportunity and inserted herself later into the narrative of women's rights, when lipstick was already a badge of independence.

Early Hollywood movies helped to develop a mass market for cosmetics. Heavily eye-blacked stars made a great impact, especially after the First World War, when the cinema was no longer viewed as entertainment for the poor. But if movies helped to normalise visible makeup, among the working classes rouge was still frowned upon. One Londoner recalled, 'My father would say, what have you got on your face? If I see any make-up on your bedroom dressing table it'll go through your window and you after it.'[69] Such girls resorted to makeshifts such as strawberry juice, or the dye from soaking red ribbons in water. Artificial flower workers stole the red ones and rouged their cheeks with them.

North America led the way in the use of lipstick. Early department stores in London and Paris did not dare place such controversial goods on prominent display, but B. Altman & Company in New York launched its makeup counter in 1867, allowing women to browse a full range. In Britain, Harry Gordon Selfridge, who opened his Oxford Street store in 1909, is credited with being the first retailer to display makeup on open counters near a front entrance. Makeup use accelerated as women entered the workforce in great numbers during the First World War. Men returning from the battlefields noticed the difference. One recalled that, before the war, if a woman entered a public house with lipstick on, 'well they were put down as prostitutes, you see, and people wouldna speak to them, and that was that', but by 1918 factory girls in Britain wore lipstick openly.[70] And women wore makeup to please themselves rather than to attract men. In London's Holloway prison, women used shoe polish for mascara and glossed their hair with margarine; in North America, too, female prisoners found the means to paint their faces despite being forbidden makeup.[71] Increasingly, the girl who wore no makeup at all seemed not just behind the times but also lacking in self-respect.

Packaging added much to the allure of makeup and helped to make its use seem the height of modernity. Pretty boxes and showy glass bottles had always been in demand by those who could afford them, enabling women to show off their wealth and good taste. Now the market offered attractive powder compacts and petite rouge cases with mirrors. Lipsticks came in a push-up metal tube from 1915, which was both practical and attractive, especially after the swivel case was invented in 1923. In the 1920s, a North American firm even sold a makeup kit disguised as a pocket pistol, with powder and rouge in the handle and lipstick in the barrel: it was the ultimate symbol of the power of makeup.

Cosmetics, always performative, allowed women to construct themselves as cosmopolitan and modern. Some used makeup to transcend social class, just as they had in earlier centuries. Applied with skill and judgement, it could be part of a process of reinvention as well as an aid to attracting a partner. Increasingly, women touched up their faces in public, although the conservative middle classes still preferred not to. Some cosmetics gained ground because they were carefully advertised as enhancing a woman's existing beauty. By 1925, a magazine columnist could claim that women in Britain and North America had won the 'battle' to wear cosmetics and would never relinquish their 'victory'.[72]

But women were slowly caught in a growing web of commodification. By the 1930s, manufacturers were pushing to capture new markets, and targeting defined groups. In North America, some pursued students leaving home for the first time, proclaiming that no college packing was complete without a cosmetic kit. Here, a marked change took place in public opinion: applying lipstick became a rite of passage, signifying that a young woman was reaching maturity. Cosmetics were among the first branded goods to have such emotional value.

Photographs, now more common in promotional material than line drawings, lent authenticity. Advertisements helped to standardise a type of beauty that relied on cosmetics and suggested that, with the right products, beauty was within every woman's grasp. *Harper's Bazaar* even assured readers that being beautiful was as much a social obligation as being clean or using a knife and fork properly. Women who were not beautiful must act as if they were: 'If you make believe long enough, and hard enough, you can will it to come true'; yet the magazine also implied that makeup was a great leveller: 'the sublime lady who believes that she doesn't need cosmetics overestimates herself'.[73] Advertising claims for makeup had extended beyond the enhancement of natural beauty towards transformation; in an ironic reversal, the absence of makeup now denoted vanity.

PREJUDICE AND LARGE-SCALE MANUFACTURING

Technical advances in makeup helped to extend the market. As products improved it was easier for women to adapt their style to bright sunlight or dinner-table candles; the vamp look of earlier Hollywood stars faded. In 1935, an important new cosmetic followed the release of the first Technicolor feature film. Technicolor had to be filmed under hot, bright lights. In these conditions, theatrical makeup was too reflective to look natural, and when actors perspired it streaked and produced odd colour effects. Max Factor, who had worked with the film industry for over two decades, solved the problem by inventing Pan-Cake Make-Up, which was matt but transparent. A lighter version for daily wear went on sale to the public in 1939 and soon became a cult classic. It can still be bought online.

By the 1930s, women routinely darkened their lashes. Waterproof eye-black was invented just in time for the wearing of gas masks in the Second World War. Ordinary eye-black melted inside the mask due to the heat. Eyes began to smart and eyelids to spasm, and women were tempted to rip off the mask, 'with dangerous results if gas is present'.[74] Even so, waterproof mascara cannot have been all that common: in North America, one cinema introduced three-minute mascara breaks after tear-jerking movies so that women could repair the damage in privacy before lights were raised.[75]

Although more women were wearing makeup, some remained conflicted about it, African American women in particular. Makeup was still associated with prostitution. Given that the ethnic stereotypes developed to justify the shameful practices of plantation slavery had included the Black woman as innately promiscuous, the last thing many wanted to do was to draw attention to their sexuality.[76]

During the Second World War, metals and glycerine were needed for explosives, so makeup was in short supply. Even so, British women were strongly encouraged to wear it in order to support the cosmetic industry. Cosmetic exports were vital, not only for foreign exchange, 'but to win and hold new markets and avoid unemployment after the war'.[77] In contrast, Nazi Germany promoted a clean, no-makeup look for women that would help to emphasise national purity. All the same, most German women aspired to be fashionable, and the wives of high-ranking Nazi party members eagerly embraced French fashions and makeup. German magazines for women continued to advertise the latest international trends, perpetuating a normality that helped to cloak the totalitarian regime.

Refugees who fled to the United States from Nazi Europe noticed that American women wore more makeup, and from a younger age.

They marvelled that, here, 'a woman is never properly dressed if she doesn't use lipstick'; by 1948, about 90 per cent of women in North America wore lipstick and rouge.[78] Europe followed. After two world wars, old proprieties were on the wane and the market for cosmetics mushroomed. It was fed by television advertising and Hollywood films. In the 1950s, when the ideal woman was expected to be ultra-feminine, there was even a Daimler model 'designed for the woman who has very definite ideas about the car she wants her husband to buy'; crucially, its luxury features included an 'elegant vanity case'.[79] By the end of that decade, the British cosmetics market was worth over £61 million. But large manufacturers and mass distributors were poised to mop up the profits of an industry in which the cost of production was notoriously far less than the retail price. In 1948, there had been 1,100 cosmetics firms in Britain. By 1960, through amalgamation or bankruptcy, this peak figure had shrunk to just 190 producers.[80]

Even so, the market for cosmetics kept growing, especially among teenagers, since young women were encouraged to experiment with a range of products. The only consumers whom large-scale manufacturers neglected were Black women and women of colour, who had to blend different foundation creams to get the tones they wanted. In Europe and North America, cosmetic companies made the default assumption that they produced makeup for white women. Companies created no mass-market lines for Black women until the mid-1970s, although Avon began to target Black consumers in the 1960s.[81] White privilege within the industry meant not only that women of colour were denied the pleasure of browsing a range of mainstream makeup created for them, but also that they were liable to make costly mistakes because some eyeshadows and lipsticks on the market had unexpected colour effects against darker skin tones. The first all-inclusive foundation range did not appear until 2017, when Rihanna launched her cosmetics brand, Fenty Beauty, which also accommodates albino complexions.

In the early 1960s, the Caribbean-born journalist and activist Claudia Jones seized the opportunity inherent in this situation to help raise the political awareness of Caribbean women recently arrived in London. She included a beauty column in the newspaper she edited, *West Indian Gazette*, effectively challenging racist beauty politics and the marginalisation of Black women.[82] She was also responsible for the first televised Black beauty pageant in Britain. The pageant was part of an indoor Caribbean Carnival which she and others founded, later to become the outdoor event in Notting Hill. Her beauty competition was broadcast live into people's homes, affirming that Caribbean women were proud of their beauty and identity, and demonstrating how beauty culture could be used as a tool against oppression. *Flamingo*, a pan-Caribbean lifestyle magazine published in Britain from 1961 to 1965, included articles on skincare, hairstyling, and makeup. A piece in the first issue, 'Dark Beauty', advised women never to apply fair foundations or powders but to heighten their natural skin colour with bright lipsticks and neutral powder bases. Yet later issues also carried advertisements for skin bleaching creams, available by mail order. The most popular brands were those already fashionable in the United States.[83]

In the United States, progress in getting white-owned cosmetics companies to cater for women of colour came at the expense of companies owned by African Americans. For a while this went unnoticed; by the 1930s, African Americans had largely ceased to purchase cosmetics from Black sales agents and instead bought from stores. They were largely unaware of which companies manufactured the cosmetics. Yet in 1986, when Revlon suggested that Black manufacturers made inferior products anyway, the Reverend Jesse Jackson successfully organised a boycott of Revlon's products, and the company was forced to backtrack.

In the period of post-war expansion, the beauty business had been quick to introduce products for mainstream markets: over thirty styles of false eyelashes were available by 1968. Aspects of the industry were flexible enough to respond to fashionable consumer concerns: a Beauty Without Cruelty cosmetics range, not tested on animals and free of animal derivatives, was launched in 1963. Not surprisingly, although female entrepreneurs had been central to developing the industry in its early days, consumers began to feel manipulated rather than in control. Even when feminists rejected makeup in the early 1970s, the beauty business cashed in and introduced translucent ranges that catered for the unmade-up look. Companies understood that most people's skin is in poor condition (due to a lack of sleep, too little exercise, a diet of junk food, and filthy city air), and that a natural look can be hard to achieve without grooming aids.

The industry adapted with equal ease to the grunge culture of the late 1980s and early 1990s, bringing out lipsticks in dark browny red and even black, and adjusted to the rave scene of the 1990s, producing unusual colours like blazing orange or bright yellow as well as neon hues. Even old-time 'favourites' were recycled as classic luxury. Shoppers found themselves on a roller-coaster of rapid variation, as manufacturers reworked the finish and texture of makeup, from matt to glossy or pearlescent; changed ingredients, from flower and fruit to mineral-based; and altered the overall facial 'look', whether minimalist or extravagant. Is it ever possible to stop the ride? The author of a thrift book for women with no money advised buying a single cosmetic. An expensive look is mainly a matter of good skin, she decided, so just dab illuminating cream on the cheekbones to look 'quite shiny', because 'Matt looks poor rather than luxey.'[84]

When mass-market companies eventually began to cater for darker skin, they tended to be the producers of expensive brands, often only stocked in central stores. And the names given to foundations and lipsticks for women of colour were less positive compared to those for light skin tones. They referenced foodstuffs, for example, rather than valuable goods like ivory or coral, although a neutral numbering system, marking a light to dark gradient, would always have been an option. Some brands did follow a neutral route but, in the main, a complacent cosmetics industry slid into practices that subtly reinforced discrimination based on skin tone. Their advertising was not truly inclusive. And, in stores, makeup displays tended to centre on products for white skin, so women with darker skin found it harder to locate what they wanted. In cosmopolitan cities this is changing. After all, mainstream marketing always aims to maximise profit, and Black women spend more on cosmetics than white women, experimenting with many products to find shades that suit them best.[85]

Beauty culture is still a site for activism. And the web of communication around makeup is increasingly multi-layered as consumers become wise to marketing claims pitched at identities and lifestyles. Can the new product be applied in the back of a swerving cab? The scenario has already been parodied in the British sketch show *Smack the Pony*, which ridiculed the notion that career women can apply faultless makeup on the move.[86] Cosmetic advice on social media is often playful and sophisticated, drawing on the rich history of makeup. Some vloggers ironically reference feminist opinions about cosmetics in videos that uphold feminist arguments when appreciated as parodies. Whether or not such content strikes home depends heavily on the skill with which vloggers manage codes of communication.

Some vloggers celebrate trends that started within the drag community, who in turn borrowed face-contouring and other techniques from theatrical tradition. Others target racist misconceptions or challenge gender norms in support of LGBTQ+ rights. Such platforms decentralise access to the media and allow different voices to speak. But makeup, although often mask or performance, is not always an adjunct to a fluid identity.

'You may not be able to change your face, but you *can* change the way it looks!' enthused Helena Rubinstein.[87] But is makeup really a means to creative self-invention? Or does it simply add to social pressures within a competitive culture? The debate is often simplified. The history of makeup shows that there is a subtler dynamic at work: women fought to wear overt makeup and so are more susceptible to the argument (often used in marketing) that makeup is a right, an essential product which allows them to create their own identity. Yet personal motives and makeup styles are bound to vary with the individual and social situation; there is always a balance of choice and constraint. Cosmetics may give confidence and help women to reveal their inner selves while concealing blemishes, but in ritual acts of purchasing and application, new users discover the makeup palettes that suit them; once a flattering look is found, most tend to stick with it. Sometimes the whole point of makeup is that it makes a perceptibly different impact to that of the wearer's true face, as when women perform as drag artists, or there would be no performance at all.

The open artifice of extravagant twenty-first-century makeup creations, featured online and in high-end magazines, might be compared to the painterly makeup of the eighteenth-century French court, which played with disapproval to create new meaning. Clearly, the face can be a canvas on which to express attitude and even rebellion, taking makeup style beyond the desire to look attractive. Across the world, cosmetic use is subject to different cultural practices and offers a platform for engaging with feminism, gender, and racial discrimination. In the West, where for centuries makeup was used to help construct a white identity, a marked change has taken place. Women of all skin tones freely use makeup to reflect their involvement in public life, their financial autonomy, their role in fashion, and their impact on the world economy.

ᛝ 5 ᛝ

HYGIENE

The author Maria Edgeworth stayed with friends in Hampstead during the severe winter of 1830. She was touched by their generous offer of keeping a constant fire in her bedroom, as well as in her sitting room. She refused the offer because she was never in the bedroom except when warm in bed or washing. And when washing, she explained, 'a body must be cold'.[1] Her stoic response is testament to the determination and fortitude a habit of cleanliness once demanded.

Hygiene is essential to health, and intimately connected to ideas of beauty: diseases can be disfiguring; filthy bodies are rarely attractive. Over the centuries, standards of hygiene in the West have altered substantially as medical understanding has advanced and housing conditions have improved. This chapter explores how changes in hygienic norms have affected women's lives and how they were used to bolster ideas of white supremacy.

Today, the word 'hygienic' is so often used to mean just 'clean' that we can forget it specifically relates to preventative medicine and defines behaviour that will help people avoid infection. With the take up of germ theory in the second half of the nineteenth century, people enthusiastically adopted the concept of hygiene, fearing that contagion would enter the body through damaged skin. From the 1880s, there was

151

growing pressure on women who managed households to boil laundry, ensure ventilation, and consider hygiene in all domestic purchases. Flexible corsets, braces for stooping shoulders, garters, perfumes, and even sewing machines were all advertised as 'hygienic'. In the case of sewing machines, retailers argued that without them needlewomen ruined their health by hunching over hand sewing, though they may have been anxious to counteract claims that the machine's rhythmic motion encouraged nymphomania.

Hygiene soon became firmly linked to a woman's responsibilities, both to herself (because fresh air, a healthy diet, and exercise for a fine figure were all labelled 'hygienic') and to her family (because it was her duty to instil sanitary habits and to ensure the wellbeing of children). Over time, mothers were more influential in changing attitudes to hygiene than even schools and hospitals.

HUMAN STINKS

In our deodorised cities with sewerage systems, litter may sometimes be a nuisance, but the potent stockpot of stinks and dirt that earlier ages endured is beyond our experience. We also manage personal hygiene in unprecedented privacy. Yet in the days of horse-drawn transport, the very streets would be excrement-sodden swamps in wet weather and reeking dustbowls in summer. Open sewers, middens, privies built over leaking cesspits, poor water supplies, and bad drainage added to the stench. The use of chamber pots polluted the air within doors and often caused embarrassment, as when Pepys surprised Lady Sandwich, the wife of his patron, on the pot in his dining room.[2] There were few public lavatories, particularly for women, who were not expected to venture far from home; as late as 1879, social reformers in Dundee complained about the heaps of human excrement on the common stairs in tenement buildings.[3]

Anyone entering a crowded public room would encounter a rich stew of body odours, a wall of foetid air only worsened by the reek of tobacco, tallow candles, and later gas lighting. In the seventeenth century, fastidious souls carried aromatic pomanders or nosegays; by 1700, they could also resort to smelling bottles. People in central Europe did manage to retain the public baths of classical times into the sixteenth century; the Church worried about immoral behaviour but sanctioned medical bathing. But by the eighteenth century, hot baths had come to be regarded as rather unsafe; French doctors thought that they weakened the constitution and, as already mentioned, that liquids might enter the body through open pores and damage internal organs. Even the rich seldom washed all over before the nineteenth century. Instead, they relied on clean linen, which became a mark of status, since a large supply was needed to last between laundry days.

The British were less prejudiced against washing. Famously, Elizabeth I is recorded as taking a monthly bath whether she needed to or not. Probably she bathed more often: she had a bath at Whitehall, a sweat bath at Richmond, and travelled with a hip bath.[4] Lower down the social scale, people also washed, if irregularly. In London, they could visit a bagnio or Turkish-style bathhouse. Some bagnios were places of assignation and seduction, but others were perfectly innocent, with separate bathing days for men and women. Elizabeth Pepys visited one in February 1665; afterwards she insisted that Pepys wash himself with warm water before bed as she meant to keep herself clean. Pepys washed his feet from time to time in warmer months, though he once complained that it gave him a cold. Labourers bathed in rivers and canals. Women had fewer opportunities for complete immersion, especially since bathhouses never wholly lost their taint of the brothel and slowly went out of business in the eighteenth century. The respectable were mostly content to display clean hands, face, and linen.

Elite bathing habits are thrown into relief by Elizabeth Montagu's experience in 1741. She fell ill when staying with her friend the Duchess of Portland, and the doctor prescribed a warm bath. Already a practised author of witty letters, she sent an amusing account to her mother. First, there was a delay because the wooden bathing tubs on the ducal estate were found to be in such a state of disrepair that they would not hold water. Then, as she had packed no bathing costume, she was forced to get into the tub in her chemise and skirt. To bathe naked, even in her own chamber, was unthinkable. No wonder perfume was a staple item in the household budget of the well-to-do.

Misogynistic satire of the time criticised women for rarely washing their private parts. A lady could be 'very fine and very filthy'.[5] Diaries and letters offer some supporting evidence. In 1777, Fanny Burney was told to expect a visit from David Garrick, an actor she deeply admired. The extent of her best hygiene seems limited today: on four mornings, she got up at 7 o'clock, and was 'at the trouble and fatigue of washing face and hands quite clean, putting on clean linnen, a tidy gown, and smug [clean, neat] cap'.[6] Sadly, Garrick never came at all. Bathing continued to be rare in France, too, where piped water was scarcer than in Britain until at least the end of the nineteenth century. And modesty still required rich provincial women taking their monthly summer bath to soap themselves through their bath shirts.[7]

Personal hygiene was even more of a challenge for the poor, especially in cities polluted with coal smoke. They followed the clean linen standard as best they could but might only have one change of clothes; in winter they tended to wear all they had for warmth, with dirt providing an extra layer. They rarely washed, whether from a distrust of water (some considered dirt a protective barrier) or because they lacked the means. In France, clean water was so expensive that the poor had no option but to be dirty. The evangelist John Wesley famously promoted the view that cleanliness is next to godliness, in a sermon he gave 'On Dress' around 1791, but the idea took a long time to become established. When Queen Victoria moved into Buckingham Palace, in 1837, it had no bathroom.

As most people emitted strong body odours, constant exposure bred acceptance. That said, some individuals had sensitive noses. In the seventeenth century, Thomas Tryon, an author of self-help guides, denounced unhealthy domestic filth and chiefly railed against sweaty feather beds. Yet even he recognised that filthy housekeepers became inured to stale odours, 'the greatest Slut in the World does hardly smell her own House or Bed stink'.[8] Human reactions to smells are shaped by experience.

CHANGING ATTITUDES TO SMELL

From the mid-eighteenth century there was a dramatic change in people's sense of smell. The elite in many Western societies began to experience odours more keenly. Medical experts in Europe linked bad airs, termed miasmas, to disease, and reasoned that air corrupted with pestilential matter caused illness when inhaled. Clearly, not all stinks led to infection. But foul smells were thought to be implicated in health issues because they signalled dirt. Unfamiliar stenches were a matter of particular concern. In 1769, Lady Mary Coke, remembered for her letters and journal, was troubled by reeking garden drains in her house at Holland Park. A local workman botched the repair, which says much about contemporary expertise in drains and sewers. She remained so distressed that eventually she sent for the man who had lately remodelled the house.[9] City dwellers increasingly feared miasmas and nauseating steams from gutters and dunghills. Overflowing gutters might not only exude dirt likely to soil clothes but also spread disease. Chemists in France and England tried to find precise terms to calibrate these pestilential airs and studied the properties of aromatics that might counteract them. Their work heightened an awareness of smells among the upper classes.

Those in the vanguard of fashion now rejected heavy perfumes, suspecting that they masked poor hygiene, or worse. Animalistic perfumes, once popular, excited revulsion. In part this was due to their excremental nature: civet oil comes from the anal glands of civets, ambergris from the intestines of the sperm whale, and musk from a gland in the male musk deer left to putrefy after the deer is killed. This change in the sensibility of smell has been most closely studied in France but the same phenomenon occurred in Britain and elsewhere in Europe.[10] Lady

Mary Coke censured some Dutch women she encountered in Vienna in 1771: 'The Dutch Ladys have given great offence by their perfumes: everybody here is extremely delicate with regard to those things, & some are so little able to bear strong smells, that they can't remain in the room with anybody that uses musk.'[11] The Dutch women swore they did not have musk but, as they smelt of it, Coke did not believe them. She wondered how these foreigners could care so little about offending polite company. There is a whiff of prejudice here, as people often disparaged other nations as having a distinct odour. Yet clearly new forms of sociability, as well as medical opinion, were affecting perceptions of smell.

All the same, some English women were slow to give up their dependence on heavy scents. In 1785, the poet and classicist Elizabeth Carter complained that one of her routine headaches had been triggered by 'a fine fashionable lady from London, who poisons the atmosphere round her with highly perfumed powder', and continued, 'There is something to me very disgusting, as well as unpleasant, in people being perfumed; and I believe I am not singular in thinking there must be some secret reason for such artificial smells.'[12]

Of course, people were aware of the sexual attraction of body odours, which heavy perfumes may once have been intended to enhance as much as disguise. The sexual aspect of heavy perfumes may explain why single women like Carter took against them. But body odours were not attractive if they amounted to a stench, and some couples certainly appreciated good hygiene. The Sussex shopkeeper Thomas Turner chose his second wife in 1765 for her hygiene, not her looks: 'As to her person I know it's plain (so is my own), but she is cleanly in her person and dress (which I will say is something more than at first sight it may appear to be towards happiness).'[13] And when Charles Greville palmed off his mistress, Emma, onto Sir William Hamilton in 1785, he praised her as 'the only woman I ever slept with without having ever had any of my senses offended, & a cleanlier, sweeter bedfellow does not exist'.[14]

The lighter, floral perfumes which affluent women adopted towards the end of the eighteenth century defused natural body odour and distanced those strong smells linked to animal instinct. Women could signal their good hygiene while choosing fragrances to express a mood or personality. The new sensory experience proved so popular that the perfume industry centred on Paris and London expanded. It supported a myriad of smaller trades, including those who made stoppered and silver-mounted bottles, sprinkler tops, paste pots, corks, printed labels, and fancy boxes. London perfumers imported tons of fragrant substances annually, including citrous peels, oil of cloves, sandalwood, orris powder, and amber essence. Their needs helped to expand warehousing in the city's maritime districts, and supported firms specialising in packing and transporting delicate goods to the colonies.

IMPROVED CLEANLINESS

With this revolution in the sense of smell, and heightened sensitivity to putrid vapours that might carry disease, those with the leisure to worry about such things began to emphasise cleanliness to safeguard health. Yet, for most people, being clean still meant simply having clothes that were free from lice and odour. A bathroom was not yet an option. In 1782, a German traveller marvelled, 'the English are certainly distinguished for cleanliness', but only because he rarely saw a labourer without a shirt, and these shirts looked as if they had a history of being laundered.[15] Women could certainly buy washable corsets by the early nineteenth century, but equally they might choose to wear travelling corsets, advertised as never needing to be washed.

Doctors still did not understand just how skin pores functioned. Some thought a good sweat was purging and that obstructed perspiration was dangerous; they recommended fleecy hosiery and underwear to cure or prevent a string of ailments from deafness to gout.[16] Others worried that harmful vapours might enter the body through open pores, and still held that bathing might weaken a person's animal vigour. That said, from the end of the eighteenth century, the elite in France began to wash more often, using bidets as well as washstands. The British in

India noted that Indians took a daily strip wash with minimum fuss. Under both influences, the upper classes in Britain took to washing the body more often, although bathing the feet was still an operation to be managed with care. *The Ladies' Hand-Book of the Toilet* warned in 1843 that 'the evils connected with wet or damp feet are innumerable'.[17]

Even in the nineteenth century, some French doctors feared that excess bathing might make women infertile; they saw no need to make it a daily occurrence.[18] But others urged the well-to-do to wash all over at least once a week, which led to a modest uptake in the use of hip baths. These were more economical and practical than full-sized baths because they used less water. The bidet even became popular among the middle classes towards the end of the century. All the same, a witty comparison of the French and English around this time concluded that 'France and England may be ranked amongst the tolerably clean nations, England taking the lead; but real cleanliness is not general in either . . . The majority prefer a modest degree of dirtiness as being more conducive to their true comfort.'[19]

There are signs that in the 1860s personal hygiene was little better in the United States of America. A girl at boarding school described her morning routine to her mother: 'Well, I get up, put on my shoes and stockings first, then my underclothes, then my combing jacket, and wash myself, throw out the water into a tub that stands in the middle of the floor, wipe the bowl with a great towel and then comb my hair, put on my dress and by that time the bell rings for prayers.'[20] She clearly assumed that her mother would approve of this standard of grooming. Water rarely touched the whole head in the nineteenth century. In Britain, some working-class mothers feared that washing a child's scalp would give the child water on the brain.[21]

COLD BATHS AND CHOLERA

From the early eighteenth century, physicians and philosophers had occasionally recommended cold bathing to instil rigour and cure certain ills.

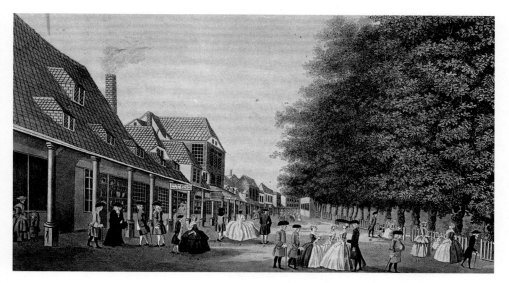

1. Spa towns attracted a variety of visitors. This view of Tunbridge Wells, 1748, includes Dr Johnson and his wife Elizabeth, David Garrick, Elizabeth Chudleigh, Samuel Richardson, and William Pitt the Elder. The diminutive fan painter, Thomas Loggon (left), produced such views of the town for sale to visitors.

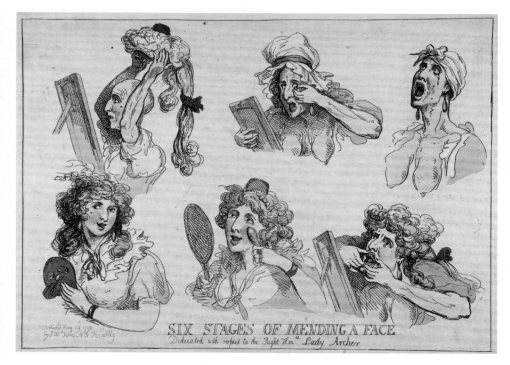

2. This satire of an ageing socialite trying to appear young is dedicated to Lady Sarah Archer, often mocked for her heavy makeup. Top right, she is an old woman in a night cap. With glass eye, wig, dentures, rouge, and mask in hand, she seems stylish and pretty.

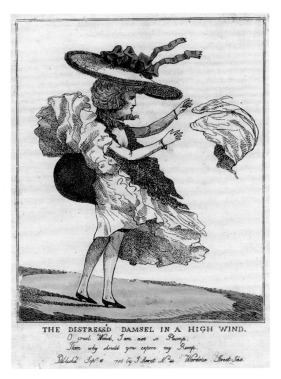

THE DISTRESS'D DAMSEL IN A HIGH WIND.

O cruel Wind, I am not so Plump,
Then why should you expose my Rump.

Published Sept. 8 1786 by I. Roach N. 44 Wardour Street Soho.

3. This hand-coloured etching shows the dangers of a blustery day to a fashionable lady. Her false bosom has flown off and her petticoats have been blown up to reveal a false rump apparently made of wickerwork.

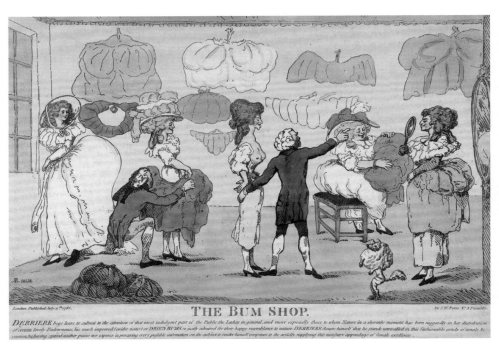

THE BUM SHOP.

DERRIERE begs leave to submit to the attention of that most indulgent part of the Public the Ladies in general, and more especially those to whom Nature in a slovenly moment has been niggardly in her distribution of certain lovely Endowments, his much improved (unlike nature) or DRIED BUMS, so justly admired for their happy resemblance to nature DERRIERE flatters himself that he stands unrivalled in this fashionable article of female decoration, he having spared neither pains nor expense in procuring every possible information on the subject to render himself competent to the artfully supplying this necessary appendage of female excellence.

4. Two salesmen supply ladies with false rumps which extend their dresses at the back. The shopkeeper facetiously claims his design will compensate those 'to whom Nature in a slovenly moment has been niggardly in her distribution of certain lovely Endowments'.

5. Albinia Hobart, satirised here, was targeted for her girth, gambling habit, and passion for home theatricals. The picture behind references the opera *Nina*; a small man kneels before a fat Nina, terrified, as she thinks him the ghost of her lover.

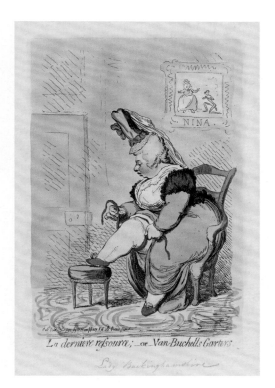

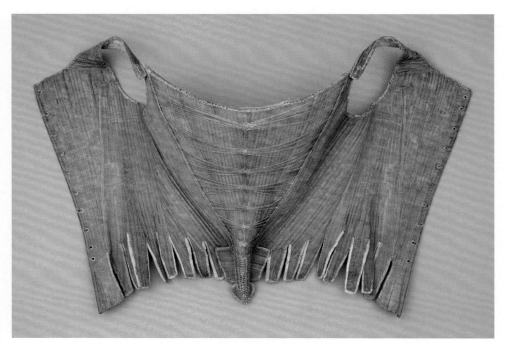

6. English stays from the 1730s–40s, made of stiffened silk moire, silk cording, and ribbons, with a linen lining. The lace holes are finished with thread. The centre back length is fifteen inches.

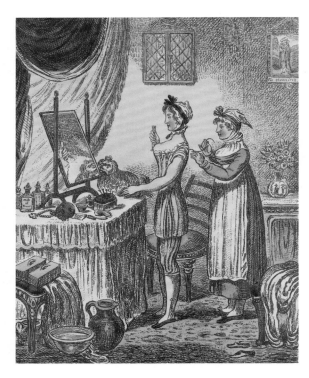

7. The first of three prints showing how women got dressed in 1810. A chambermaid laces her mistress in stays after a perfunctory wash. On the dressing table are pins, toiletries, including Milk of Roses, and rouge.

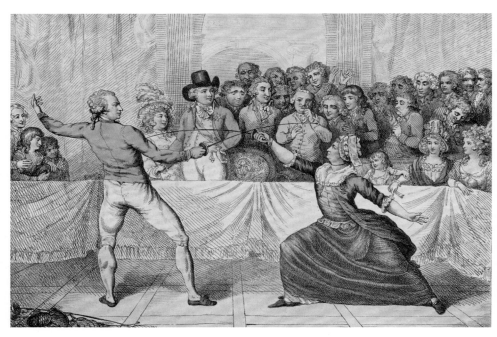

8. On the right, the Chevalier d'Éon, fencing in female attire. On the left, Joseph de Bologne de Saint-Georges, son of a plantation owner in the French West Indies and one of his African slaves, Nanon. The match took place in the presence of the Prince of Wales (centre).

9. A satire on women in control, this hand-coloured mezzotint shows a woman in quasi-military dress whipping her horses towards the military camp at Coxheath. By her side, a fat militia officer is fast asleep.

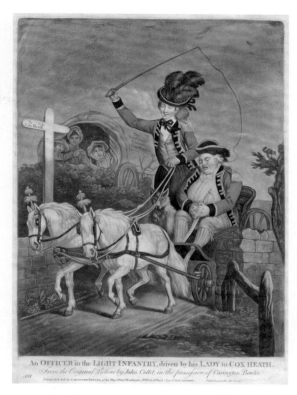

An OFFICER in the LIGHT INFANTRY, driven by his LADY to COX HEATH.
From the Original Picture by John Collet, in the possession of Carington Bowles.

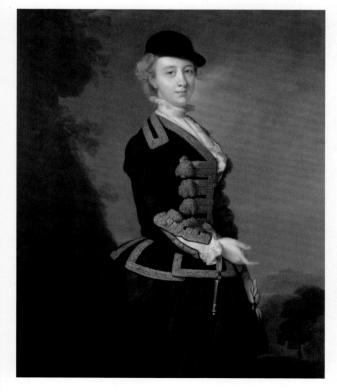

10. Princess Amelia, second daughter of George II, enjoyed riding and hunting. Here she is in her mid-thirties, in about 1745. She wears a cap and a close-fitting, dark blue riding habit with gold braid.

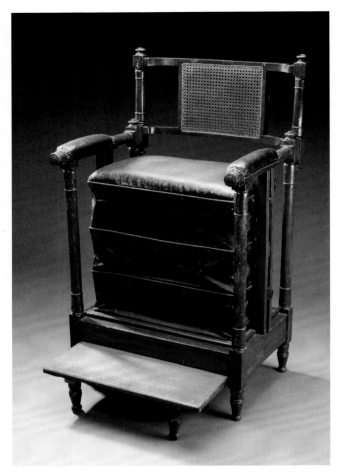

11. The chamber horse was invented in the mid-eighteenth century. It was said to offer the benefits of riding; the user bounced up and down as if trotting. This exercise chair is just over six and a half feet high and constructed of mahogany, concertina springs, and leather.

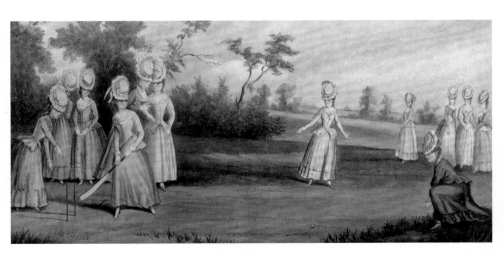

12. This watercolour shows the Countess of Derby and others playing cricket as a tasteful amusement at Knowsley Hall in 1779. There are regular press references to women's cricket matches from the mid-eighteenth century.

13. Archery was one of the few competitive sports that middle- and upper-class women could respectably enjoy. They wore special dresses with close upper sleeves that would not obstruct the bowstring.

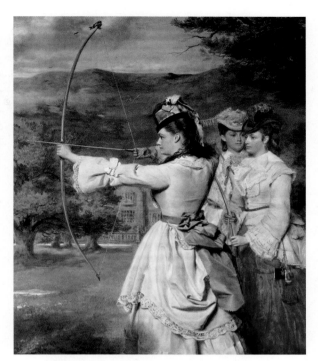

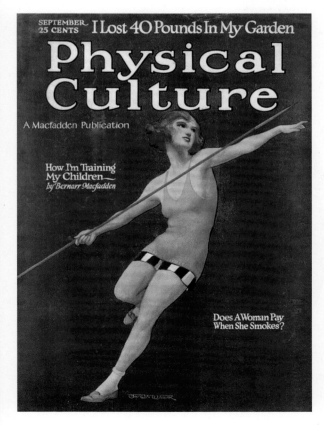

14. Macfadden's *Physical Culture* used inspiring photographs and appealed to a broad readership. Founded in 1899, it sprang from Bernarr Macfadden's tours in England during the 1890s when he sold home exercise equipment, charging for his lectures, and distributing a small pamphlet.

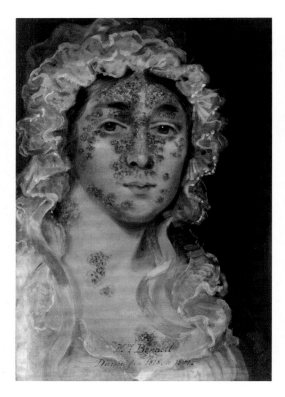

15. Mrs Bennett, in lace cap and nightgown, disfigured by a skin disease. The painting is paired with another showing her cured, in a series depicting gentlefolk of Leeds afflicted with serious illnesses.

16. Jeanne-Antoinette Poisson, Marquise de Pompadour, Louis XV's official mistress from 1745 to 1751. Cosmetics marked women as fashionable and aristocratic. After white face paint, Pompadour applies copious rouge with a brush, in the circular shape then fashionable in France.

17. This *boîte à mouches* (0.9 × 2.1 × 1.6 inches) is made of gold and agate. It has two lidded compartments – one for rouge, the other for black taffeta patches. The brush and mirror were kept in the larger, front compartment.

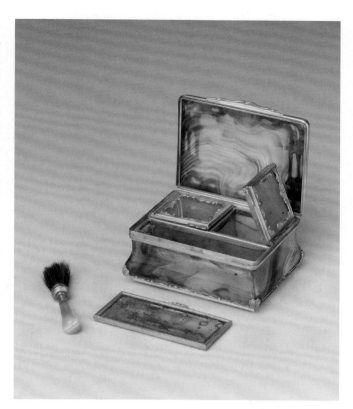

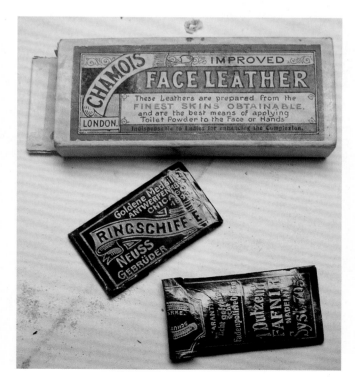

18. From the late nineteenth to the mid-twentieth century, women who wanted their makeup to look subtle might rub liquid face powder into the skin with chamois leather. This removed any excess and ensured the powder remained on longer.

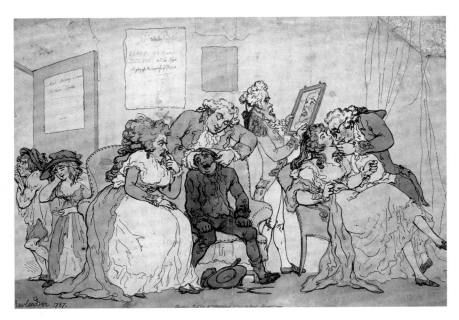

19. Here, fashionable dentists extract teeth from the poor to insert 'live teeth' into the mouths of wealthy patients. The lady centre left has endured an extraction and will receive a tooth from a chimney sweep. A boy and girl leave in pain, the girl looking at the coin in her hand.

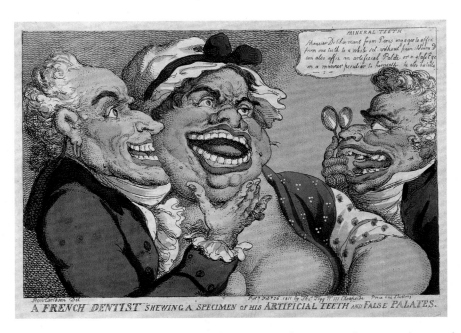

A FRENCH DENTIST SHEWING A SPECIMEN OF HIS ARTIFICIAL TEETH AND FALSE PALATES.

20. Dentist Nicolas DuBois de Chémant demonstrates his own, and a woman's, porcelain teeth to a customer, 1811. Alexis Duchateau invented 'mineral teeth' in 1744 but de Chémant overcame the problem of shrinkage in firing. His dentures did not look realistic and caused hilarity at the time.

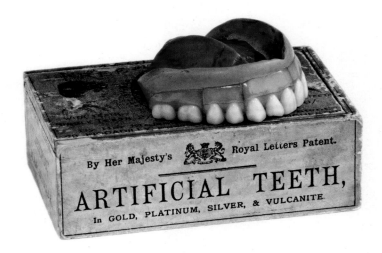

21. After the vulcanisation process was discovered in the 1840s, rubber became a viable material for dentures. The middle classes could now afford them. Anaesthesia had just been introduced, extractions were no longer painful, so people flocked to get false teeth.

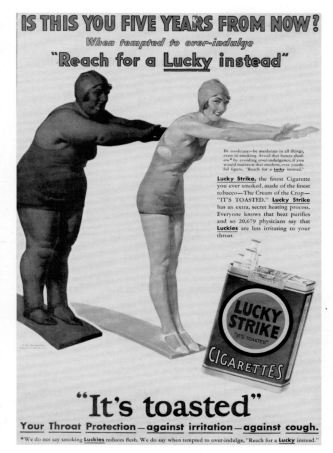

22. This advert from 1930 preaches moderation and advises women to smoke when tempted to overeat. But the small print carefully states, 'We do not say that smoking Luckies reduces flesh.'

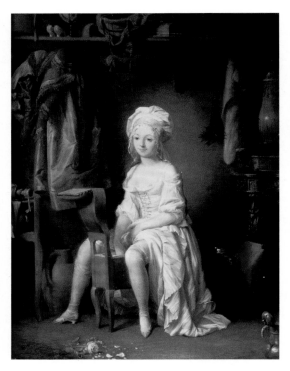

23. The bidet was introduced to the French court as a luxury item in the early eighteenth century. The seated washbasin was used for intimate hygiene, particularly by women. As this painting illustrates, the bidet became a focus of erotic interest.

24. The reverse of this advert for Lifebuoy Disinfectant Soap in about 1900 has testimonials from 'grateful mothers' who claim to have used it successfully to treat their children's eczema and ringworm.

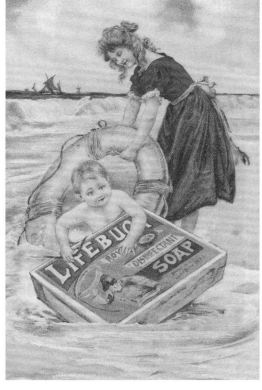

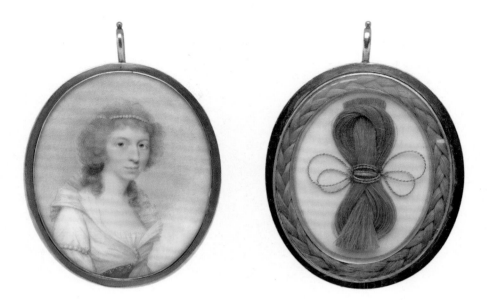

25. *(above)* The hair of a loved one, arranged artistically, has long featured in jewellery. This pendant depicts a woman on the front and contains her hair at the back. Hairwork in commemorative jewellery was particularly popular in Victorian times – memorialising the dead while stressing the fragility of life.

26. *(right)* A magazine insert from the 1890s directed at mothers. The British Medical Association, analysing patent medicines in 1909, found Edwards' 'Harlene' was mostly water, with about 6 per cent alcohol, 5 per cent borax, 4 per cent glycerine, 1 per cent ammonia, and traces of perfume and colouring.

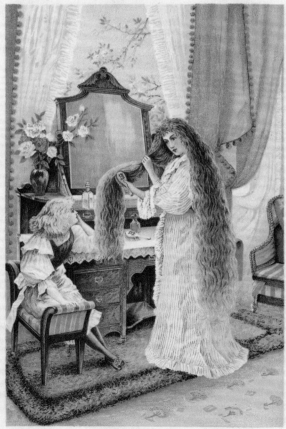

"Mama, shall I have beautiful long hair like you when I grow up?"
"Certainly, my dear, if you use **'Edwards' Harlene'**."

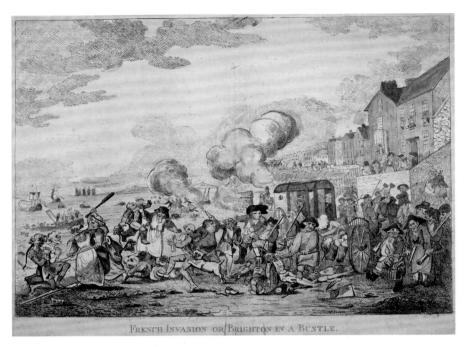

FRENCH INVASION OR BRIGHTON IN A BUSTLE.

27. Some Frenchmen have landed on Brighton beach and are being repelled by old women and yokels armed with pitchforks. A figure resembling Martha Gunn, the bathing-woman, holds at arm's length a kicking French soldier who has lost his wig.

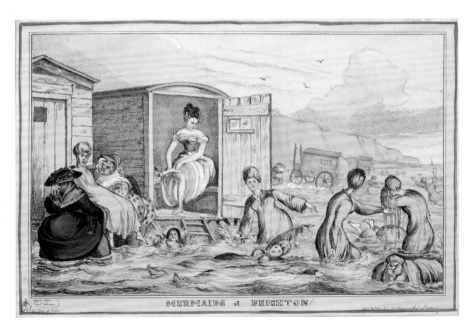

MERMAIDS at BRIGHTON

28. This hand-coloured etching, 1829, satirises women in flannel garments splashing or floating in the sea at Brighton. Two burly old women are about to dip a frightened bather. Another is undressing, or dressing, in a bathing machine.

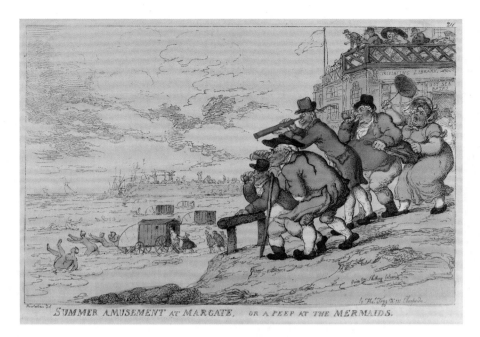

29. Men eagerly train their telescopes on naked women in the sea at Margate, 1813. The wife of one of them angrily pulls at his coattails. Nearby signs for hot sea baths and a circulating library point to more respectable amusements.

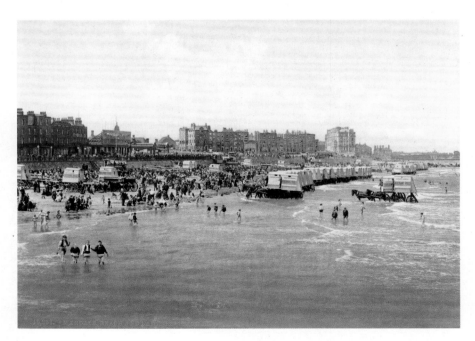

30. A photochrom print of the beach and ladies' bathing place at Margate around the end of the nineteenth century. Many women have simply rolled up their skirts to paddle but there is a line of bathing machines for hire.

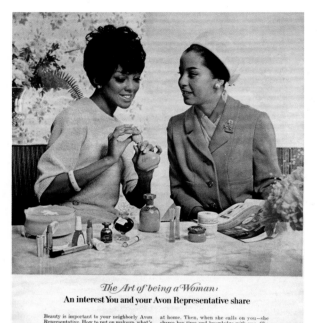

31. Avon expanded into the African American market in the 1960s. Its advertising campaign, 'Ding Dong! Avon Calling!', promoted its distinctive door-to-door sales service as well as attracting women to career opportunities in the company.

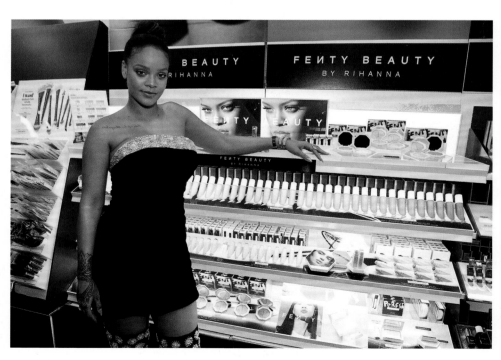

32. Rihanna at the launch of her inclusive cosmetics brand Fenty Beauty at Sephora in New York in 2017. The different shades of foundation are clearly seen in the background.

Some eighteenth-century landowners built cold plunge baths on their estates so that they could benefit from an icy dip. Caroline of Brunswick, estranged wife of the future George IV, added a plunge bath to the back of her house in Greenwich Park. It furthered the scandal surrounding her lifestyle, although it was probably intended as a health measure. The well-to-do condemned their children to daily immersion in a tub of cold water for perceived weaknesses, or used washing in cold water to harden children. Elizabeth Grant recalled winter mornings on her family's Highland estate around 1812: 'We were not allowed hot water, and really in the Highland winters, when the breath froze on the sheets, and the water in the jugs became cakes of ice, washing was a very cruel necessity.' She and her siblings began their piano and harp practice before fires were lit, and without candles since they could play their scales in the dark: 'How very near crying was the one whose turn set her at the harp I will not speak of; the strings cut the poor cold fingers.'[22] Washing in cold water meant discipline and stern effort; it helped to make cleanliness a physical virtue.

By 1800, the cold shower was a respectable treatment in a physician's armoury. It was reserved for certain disorders, including nervous afflictions, and was not to be attempted without a medical attendant. All the same, some households tentatively adopted the portable 'shower-bath'. Its great advantage was that it used far less water than a bath. In 1847, a public health reformer tried to encourage wider use of the shower, explaining how it worked: 'The shower-bath . . . consists in the fall of about a pail of water from a tin cistern pierced with holes, upon the head and body. Its great effect depends chiefly on the shock it gives to the skin, and consequently . . . to the whole system.'[23] Some models had pumps so that the water could be sent to the upper chamber again for a second dousing.

The mid-nineteenth-century fashion for hydrotherapy or water cures did much to encourage the British middle classes to wash all over. In the 1840s, Thomas and Jane Welsh Carlyle both submitted to a fashionable water cure: they were 'packed' or wrapped in wet sheets, then dry blankets, then put to bed for an hour. Thomas found it beneficial; Jane thought she would suffocate. But she did experiment with cold showers, regarding them as a great effort of virtue: 'Every morning I take the shower-bath – quite cold – and three pailfuls of it! The shock is indiscribable! and whether it strengthens or shatters me I have not yet made up my mind!'[24] The shower stimulated her appetite but also drove her to drink bottled porter. The Carlyles had no running hot water at home and seem to have washed all over two or three times a week in cold water, but when feeling unwell in 1854 Jane did go to the public baths for a warm soak on the advice of a friend. Doctors continued to uphold the virtue of cold baths. As we have seen, by the end of the century they routinely advised women to take such baths to bolster resistance to infection and to improve the tone of their skin.

If the middle classes followed the trend towards cleanliness, the poor had other priorities, although institutions like the workhouse did much to enforce the habit of washing and a regular change of linen. Upper-class women also inadvertently improved standards of hygiene in the general population. Any female servant hired was expected to be 'cleanly in her person'.[25] Fanny Kemble complained in New England in the 1840s that the only servants available were Irish people of the lowest order. The girl she engaged to help with her children 'had to be duly enlightened as to the toilet purposes of a wash-hand basin, a sponge, and a toothbrush, not one of which had she apparently been familiar with before'.[26] Men and women in the filthiest occupations were especially neglectful of their person and, from the early nineteenth century, reformers bombarded them with patronising advice. Campaigners told the poor never to sleep in the same shirt they wore for work; to change their linen not just on Sundays; to wash hands and face morning and evening; and to advance towards a daily all-over wash with a sponge or wet towel, standing on an oil cloth to avoid slops. The height of such 'personal purification' was a weekly bath, the consensus being that the English climate did not require more frequent immersion.[27]

Upper-class interest in the hygiene standards of the poor stemmed as much from self-preservation as altruism. The different social classes increasingly rubbed shoulders on public transport, and the well-to-do became uncomfortably aware that they could catch infestations from 'the great unwashed', as the politician Edward Bulwer-Lytton termed the London poor in 1830. Similar fears persist today. After a heatwave in 2018, pest controllers warned of hot spots on the London Tube network where passengers ran the greatest risk of catching bedbugs and bringing them home. In 2023, bedbugs made a resurgence in Paris, plaguing commuters and cinema-goers.

In the nineteenth century, cholera outbreaks brought sanitation and public health into sharp focus. Cholera, which originated in India, reached Sunderland in October 1831, despite quarantine measures. By February 1832, there were cases in London, and the disease continued to devastate other major cities. As with the plague, centuries earlier, poor people in overcrowded, unhealthy dwellings suffered most. Even before the pandemic, several northern industrial centres were at breaking point due to rapid population growth as migrants sought mill and factory work. Badly ventilated housing with no adequate sanitary provision, packed with undernourished families, created conditions for the rapid transmission of disease.

The upper classes, threatened with repeated outbreaks of cholera, were jolted into looking at the living conditions of the needy. It took decades for medical opinion to identify and then to accept that cholera was spread by contaminated water. Meanwhile, ineffective sewerage affected both rich and poor. But the plight of unfortunate labourers, living in filth, close to their own excrement, was taken up by social reformers who did not mince their words. They claimed that that the poor were well washed just twice in their lives – after birth and at the hour of their death.[28] Reformers saw much ignorance in working-class families: some were unaware of the health dangers of dirt; others thought there was no need to wash skin that was never exposed. The cholera epidemic showed that the wealth of the nation depended on public health, which in turn required individuals to adopt hygienic habits that would help to safeguard their neighbours. Reformers wanted a change of attitude and a new code of behaviour.

PUBLIC HEALTH

It is facile to argue that the unwashed masses were indifferent to dirt. Housewives habituated to buying clean water in pints and gallons found it hard to conceive of the amount needed for real cleanliness. For many, water came from a pump at the end of the street, and in 1840s London some 30,000 inhabitants lacked even that; in mid-century Paris, only a third of premises were supplied with water.[29] Much sanitary advice given to the poor was simply impractical. In 1840s Nottingham, there might be one privy for eight or nine houses; in one district of Manchester, upwards of 7,000 people were supplied by just thirty-three privies; women in the slums of Liverpool told one reformer how painful it was to be surrounded by filth and pollution that it was impossible for them to remove.[30] Mains drainage in British cities became an urgent health concern, not least because once experts published findings about the skin's own drainage system, helping to rid the body of impurities, people made an obvious analogy with the sewerage systems needed to cleanse major cities.

Medical men urged the British government to build public baths so that the lower orders could keep clean. Doctors had lobbied for baths in manufacturing towns from the early part of the century, but little action had been taken. A few public baths existed, including in London and at the Pier Head in Liverpool, but these were not aimed at the very poor. Cholera underscored the need for change, and the 1846 Baths and Washhouses Act empowered local authorities to provide facilities for the working classes. Even so, sanitary reform progressed quickest where it obviously supported local economic and business interests; employers looked to benefit from a healthy workforce, and authorities aimed to strengthen their position by reducing social unrest. Public baths were often architectural statements of civic pride and tools of social control, but they did also become community centres.

The baths were much used by the respectable poor. For one thing, workers found it easier to gain employment if they were clean. Women used them less, although the sexes were decently segregated. A private hot bath with soap and clean towels was a sensory pleasure; it could be had for just pennies, but women went without when money was tight. Young children might also keep women at home; and their long hair was a disincentive to bathing: some feared a chill if it got wet. Men's health was thought more important as they usually earned the main wage. Men also tended to have dirtier employments, although not exclusively. In South Wales, pit girls washed after work with male and female members of their family if employers provided no bath.

Women derived most benefit from the washhouses mostly attached to public baths. Laundry was hard physical work: clothes had to be trampled or beaten to remove dirt, then wrung or mangled to remove excess water. Well-off households often hired extra help on washdays; maids might be allowed an extra pint of beer. For many, laundry was not a weekly chore until the nineteenth century. Outer clothes – made of wool, leather, or felt – could not be washed, and dirty linen was amassed until the disruption of a wash day was worthwhile. Most families dreaded this chore. In the French countryside, it rarely occurred at all in the winter months. British taxes made soap expensive, so poor families often made their own from animal fat and lye, the latter prepared by leaching water through wood ashes. Homemade soap could irritate the skin; an alternative was to use stale urine. Boiling laundry made a house stink, and drying clothes afterwards was a major problem. A Monday wash made sense because, with food left over from Sunday, there was no need to shop, but the main point was that laundry would have all week to dry.

Liverpool opened a washhouse in Upper Frederick Street in 1842, inspired by the efforts of Kitty Wilkinson, who hired out her copper, or boiler, in the 1830s during cholera outbreaks so that neighbours could disinfect clothing. Their washing was hung to dry over her back yard on a network of ropes stretching from upper window ledges to the back of a house opposite. She is publicly honoured today in a rare memorial to a working-class woman. Although housing for the poor rarely made provision for doing laundry, at first strong objections were made to building public washhouses. Some thought it would be better to employ female workers to wash the clothes of the poor, others that it would be dangerous to encourage wives out of the home, neglecting their children and domestic duties. Critics warned that washhouses would encourage bad behaviour: gossiping, gin-drinking, and squabbles; laundries would become neighbourhood black spots, and places of assignation for the vicious. While none of these concerns proved valid, they did affect washhouse design – each woman had a washing cubicle, to prevent gossip.

In most washhouses, it cost a penny to use a trough and a copper for an hour. It cost threepence to wash, mangle, and use a heated drying closet and iron for a total of four hours. But after this time, women took clothes home almost ready to wear. No longer were they accused of driving husbands to beer-shops and keeping their dwelling-room 'in a state of steam and slop' all day when they were only doing essential laundry.[31]

Unfortunately, women now shouldered the burden of keeping up appearances through cleanliness. Authorities often made this explicit. After the George Street baths and washhouses opened near Euston Square, the founding committee produced a leaflet in 1848 informing the labouring classes of north-west London that they must practise sobriety, morality, and cleanliness. Only by these means could they rise to their proper place in the social scale. The new washhouse meant there could no longer be any excuse for dirty clothes. Meanwhile, the lower middling sort in Britain were also finding it difficult to wash and dry laundry, especially as there was no strong tradition, as in North America, of sending washing to commercial laundries. And in 1890s Paris, so few homes had safe piped water that clean clothes were a luxury even for the middle classes. Many endured niggling health problems caused by dirty linen.

A clean home was supposed to help keep husbands safely at the domestic hearth. Cleanliness, health, and the absence of strong personal

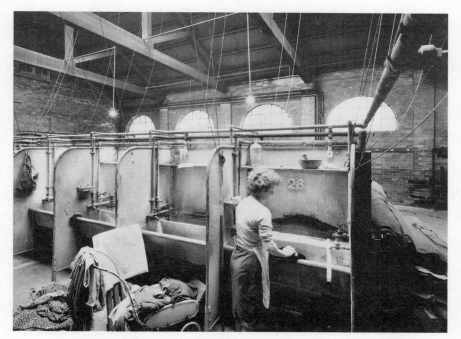

9. *The Boundary Estate, constructed in London's East End from 1890, had a public laundry still used in 1964.*

odour began to indicate moral as well as social superiority, and a certain snobbery became attached to household chores. At the same time, hard labour at the wash tub helped to keep women in their place. And hygiene became ever more demanding as better household lighting revealed latent dust and new technologies admitted higher standards. For instance, by the 1840s, even feather beds could be reconditioned and steam-cleaned to remove impurities.

Popular Victorian handbooks on health, beauty, and cleanliness were invariably aimed at female readers. By the 1860s, hygiene was routinely added to women's list of domestic tasks, alongside the care of children, overseeing the household and servants, nursing the sick, and food preparation. Harriet Martineau, who wrote about society and especially women's place in it, explained in her influential 1849 work, *Household Education*, that children should be brought up to think that a head-to-toe wash every day was as routine as having breakfast. It was understood that the reform of public health would largely begin with educating children, so reform was heavily dependent on mothers. Some now scrubbed their offspring in a disciplinary ritual; they felt ashamed if they had to send children to school in grubby clothes or without shoes.

Once the dangers to health of crowded dwellings and poor ventilation were better understood, wives were also expected to ensure a free circulation of air in the home. They were urged to keep houses clear of stale odours, to empty chamber pots daily, and to learn how to ventilate rooms without causing a draught. By the late nineteenth century, foul odours in decent working-class homes were unusual. But medical advice still reflected the patriarchal prejudices of the time. One expert wrote in 1896 that a wife would do well to let her husband smoke in whichever room he pleased, since tobacco was a useful form of disinfection.[32]

Hygienic norms did vary in different parts of Britain. In the countryside, washing all over was rare; in the industrial north, poor children might not change their clothes for months. But, by the early twentieth century, most respectable families had a weekly bath. If this was taken at home, a zinc bath would be filled with hot water from a copper and afterwards there would be clean clothes. In very cold winters, the bath might be omitted for two or three weeks, and in very hot summers it might be more frequent, but there was a firm expectation that it would be regular.

Attitudes had changed markedly. In the 1850s, one British commentator could breezily affirm, 'We are not a bathing people.'[33] A decade later, when the scandal of con artist Madame Rachel made headlines, the fact that clients undressed and took baths in her beauty salon added to the apparent seediness of her enterprise. But the United States helped to blaze a trail. When the American fashion magazine *Harper's Bazaar* was set up in 1867, one of its stated aims was to promote hygiene. In Europe, too, by the end of the century, it was accepted that a refined and cultured lady would be distinguished by the all-over cleanliness of her body. It had become a matter of personal responsibility to keep clean and ward off disease. A woman who had attained adulthood and not established a regime of personal hygiene was deemed 'an inferior being'.[34]

Nowhere, perhaps, were advances in hygiene and expectations of class differences in cleanliness more rigidly embodied than in the accommodation provided on ocean liners. The busiest liner routes were between Europe and North America, and steamships worked them from 1838. An Atlantic crossing took about two weeks, yet at first washing facilities on board ship were minimal. American women travelling to England on the SS *Great Western* in the 1840s were mightily relieved when they finally reached their hotel and could take a bath. After all, among the New England elite, domestic bathing had been routine since the early eighteenth century.

When the SS *Great Britain* entered service between Bristol and New York in 1845, it had baths for first-class passengers. They were sorely needed in coal-fired ships. As one woman exclaimed in 1861, 'You cannot think how dirty everything gets; hands, clothes, everything is black. The white in my dress is in a most disastrous state. I never saw such a dirty ship.'[35] In 1870, RMS *Oceanic* set a new standard by providing running water in almost all first-class cabins. Wealthy passengers had lavatories, not chamber pots, and bathrooms with water heated by steam. Third-class passengers, segregated by sex and marital status, had no such amenities. In steerage they were lucky to find space at a common sink to rinse faces and hands.

HYGIENE AND BEAUTY

Meanwhile, among the upper classes, cleanliness was becoming ever more firmly linked to concepts of beauty. The trend was especially notable from the late eighteenth century, when women began to favour light floral perfumes and aromatic vinegars to counteract stinks and foetid air. When in 1811 *The Lady's Magazine* printed rules for the preservation of beauty, these included cleanliness. Among the aristocracy and gentry in most of Europe, frequent, tepid baths were now the norm. Not so in Britain. Although some maintained that Britain's changeable climate abruptly altered the skin's secretions, making baths necessary to improve skin health, British ladies seemed 'ignorant of the use of any bath larger than a wash-hand basin'.[36] In North America, fashion writers began to think cleanliness essential for beauty. In 1868, *Harper's Bazaar* declared, 'the first great law of beauty, as of health, is cleanliness', and recommended a daily bath using rain or river water and soap.[37]

Much store was set on soft water. Conventional wisdom held that complexions could be ruined by hard water. The lower classes often collected rainwater in barrels, and some used lye to soften water and make their soap go further. But rainwater in cities could be sooty. By the 1870s, women were advised instead to stir products such as Maignen's Anti-Calcaire Powder into a jug of water and leave overnight. From the 1880s they could add the delightfully named Pasta Mack to their bathwater. These tablets were perfumed and contained carbonic acid so that they effervesced while softening water; advertisements claimed that they gave the skin a velvet-like texture. Some women adopted more rigorous bathing. One regime involved taking an ammonia bath before daily exercise, presumably because ammonia acted like smelling salts, increasing the breathing and heart rate. It was also a skin irritant. Another option was to use Bailey's rubber brush daily with soap and water for a healthy glow. The brush was flexible, with flat-ended, cylindrical teeth designed to open the pores and remove blemishes.

By the end of the nineteenth century, beauty advice on both sides of the Atlantic insisted, 'It is impossible to be beautiful without being thoroughly clean.'[38] In Britain, even popular girls' magazines recommended a daily bath. Aimed at young women entering new types of white-collar employment, these magazines implied that cleanliness would not only improve girls' looks but enhance their life chances, distinguishing them from lower classes who were not clean. Some medical authors encouraged this snobbery. One handbook for women claimed, 'Almost every lady's bedroom . . . has either a sitz [hip] or slipper bath stowed away in some corner.'[39]

Advice about the temperature of bathwater varied, but cold baths became part of a fashionable routine where before they had mostly been taken on medical advice. The self-discipline of a daily cold bath was touted for a healthy complexion; it also signalled moral worth. Middle-class girls were attracted to this new health and beauty movement, although probably many more advocated the regime than adhered to it. Working girls with limited access to piped water took early morning dips in London's parks; at Victoria Park, for instance, they were allowed to bathe until 10 a.m.

SOAP

Soaps were heavily marketed to women. Advertisements implied that it was a woman's business to thoroughly understand the properties of different soaps. In the eighteenth century, washballs made with vegetable oils were expensive and kept for cosmetic use to smooth and whiten face and hands. Other soaps were harsh and likely to chafe the skin, but what mattered was how well these soaps cleaned laundry. The French elite generally preferred savonette for washing face, neck, and hands. This was soap with powder and perfume which formed a thick paste in water. Savonette was also stocked by up-market retailers in London and Bath, where it was advertised, in French, to the upper classes, but really it was a whitening cosmetic. Not until the 1780s did British manufacturers begin to claim that their washballs cleansed as well as beautified users.

As the market for toilet soaps grew, women were cautioned against harmful ingredients. In 1800, one advertisement explained that the destructive effects of 'common Soap impregnated with strong Salt Ley' were easily seen from the red, chapped hands of servants; even soaps presented as refined and scented might be 'impregnated with the most pernicious and poisonous colourings, such as Red Vermillion, Powder Blue, &c.'[40] Expensive soaps could injure the skin even more than common soap.

Toilet soap remained a luxury until the reign of Queen Victoria, when the tax on soap was first lowered, then abolished in 1853. Soap was now produced on an industrial scale, and consumption rocketed as cleanliness was promoted to the masses. Soap advertising was mostly directed at female concerns: preserving the complexion or children's health. One of the most effective campaigns for cleanliness was the mass marketing from the 1860s of Pears' Transparent Soap. Pears was a family business. Andrew Pears, a barber by training, first produced soap commercially in 1789, having found that his Soho clients bought his powders and creams to cover up the damage caused by harsh soaps and beauty products. Pears' Soap hugely increased its market share in the 1880s after the stage star Lillie Langtry endorsed it. She was reputedly paid £132 for her statement that, since using Pears' Soap for the hands and complexion, she had discarded all others. The soap was also endorsed by Professor Sir Erasmus Wilson, Britain's highest medical authority on skin health.

French chemists soon discovered how different ingredients made better and cheaper soap. In Britain, where soap manufacturers were less dependent on animal fats or olive oil, soap became a product of empire. Manufacturers took advantage of copra from Ceylon, Trinidad, and the Pacific Islands, palm oil from West Africa and the East Indies, and cottonseed from Egypt and India. They exploited colonial labour and exhibited a level of blatant racism in their marketing campaigns that is shocking today. Jokey advertisements depicted Black children being soaped white, implying that the use of soap was a sign of civilisation. Advertisements for Palmolive, made with olive and palm oils, depicted seductive, eastern-looking women in evocative imperial settings. Promotions for most brands trod a careful line between suggesting that soap was a luxury product and presenting it as an essential purchase for grooming and hygiene.

Although toilet soap became safer, women were still advised to investigate the properties of different makes. The manufacturers of Pynozone warned women in 1906 that soap 'may look very nice, be gorgeously scented, and have a high-sounding name, but in spite of this it may be bad soap, which will work mischief to the skin'.[41] African Americans were targeted early, decades before the African market for toiletries expanded as African nations gained their independence from colonial rule after the Second World War. African American newspapers explained that 'even when a toilet soap is beyond reproach' it would not suit all skin types; readers should question retailers about a soap's purity and its effect on dry or oily skins.[42]

Women were also expected to know about the properties of antiseptic soaps, and their role in preventing disease. Yet, although women's purchasing power for both household and toilet soap put them at the centre of what was a global industry, soap advertisements remained condescending if not blatantly sexist. In the early twentieth century, Resinol was marketed as a soap to help the girl whose complexion made her a 'social failure'; in the 1930s, an advertisement for Palmolive bore the caption 'A wife can blame herself if she loses love by getting "middle-age" skin.'[43]

Campaigns for household soaps insisted that they saved labour, but still played on women's fears about status. A caption for Sunlight laundry soap claimed that 'Rubbing, scrubbing & steaming went out of woman's life when Sunlight Soap came into it.'[44] The cleansing powers of Pearline allowed 'weak women' to manage a large wash. The soap dislodged dirt so quickly that it was a boon to proud women who did not want neighbours to know they did their own washing; they would never be caught toiling at the tub.[45] Household soaps were positioned as a decisive help to housewives in their struggle against dirt, but such marketing reveals much about perceptions of women and their roles.

VOLUNTARY WORK AND OBSESSION
ABOUT HYGIENE

Middling and elite women discovered from the 1850s that the new public emphasis on hygiene offered them opportunities. They sought roles helping the disadvantaged towards better living conditions, reforming the habits of the dirty poor, and campaigning against adulterated household goods. In 1857, an earnest group set up the Ladies' Sanitary Association to promote sanitary knowledge and distribute cleaning products to the needy. They established branches in major cities and produced tracts for the working classes on such subjects as 'The Power of Soap and Water' and 'The Worth of Fresh Air'. Wealthy women donated money for prizes in hygiene studies at university level. Others became acknowledged reformers and teachers of hygiene, sanitation, and public health. The Women's Imperial Health Association, founded in 1908, took the crusade against dirt and disease to women living in the countryside. During the summer months, they travelled from village to village in a horse-drawn caravan, giving lantern slide shows and lectures on health and the proper feeding of children. In towns, this group followed in the footsteps of the Ladies' Sanitary Association and campaigned for free public lavatories for women.

The Women's Imperial Health Association was so successful that members proposed to extend its work throughout the Empire. In British colonies, hygiene was regarded as a discipline through which the bodies and minds of indigenous workers, mission converts, and pupils could be improved; their personal hygiene and household practices became the focus of bureaucratic scrutiny. In southern Africa especially, many white colonists from the 1890s maintained that indigenous peoples had lived in a state of filth before European influence. Fears about poor sanitation and disease became an aspect of colonial racism.[46] In South Asia, colonists were impressed by the regular bathing habit of Indians but still used standards of Western hygiene to suggest that Indian civilisation was inferior.[47]

Women's voluntary work to promote hygiene generally led to professional employment in health inspection and domestic science, as these new fields became established. But the link between women and hygiene education also increased discrimination against women in other professions. Those who had trained to become doctors and surgeons faced objections that their proper sphere was 'the hygiene of female and infantile life' and that their highest aspiration should be to teach mothers how to manage their health and that of their offspring.[48] Male doctors sought to guard their expertise from what they regarded as amateur female interest in germs and unhealthy smells.

Women's involvement in hygiene education encouraged them to engage in politics. For example, when key food adulteration bills went through the United States Congress in 1900, the legislation was hailed as 'of greatest importance to the women as the dispensers of household economy and of family hygiene'.[49] The particular status that the field of hygiene offered women was quickly appreciated by African Americans and reflected in their newspapers. In the early decades of the twentieth century, the *Chicago Defender* carried a weekly column on hygiene, sanitation, and preventative medicine, mostly for female readers. Louis W. George, advertising manager for the *Messenger*, also touted the 'sound hygiene and sanitary advantages' resulting from the use of cosmetics.[50]

Hygiene concerns became so prevalent that many products aimed at women were advertised as 'hygienic' just to increase sales. A food range including biscuits and liqueurs was labelled hygienic because it was prepared with allegedly health-preserving sea water; self-help medical guides included 'friendly advice on hygiene'; dieting was termed 'hygiene for the stout'.[51] The term was also used euphemistically. The Hygienic Stores Ltd, established in 1850 at 95 Charing Cross Road and still going strong in the 1930s, was an outlet associated with birth control and abortions. From 1900 or so, it sold Dr Patterson's Famous Female Pills for 'irregularities of every description'; lady customers were to communicate with the manageress.[52]

By the end of the nineteenth century, some free spirits were already arguing that hygiene had become a fetish. They complained that bigots were trying to impose restrictive notions of hygiene on others, basing their ideas on nothing more than an amateur course of reading, and that diehards thought nothing pleasant could ever be hygienic. 'You will ruin your health!' had become a tiresome refrain.[53]

Cleanliness was often held to be more important to health than nutrition and exercise. Wallpaper was to be replaced with sanitary, washable distemper, which was available in seventy shades by the early twentieth century. Carpets were considered a refuge for micro-organisms and feared 'as the plague'. Street dirt swept up by women's long skirts allegedly contained millions of tuberculosis germs. Slipshod housemaids with crude notions of hygiene were reckoned to be such dangers that prudent housewives kept a slate in the kitchen listing rules that maids must follow in the sanitary care of food. Car accessories in the 1920s included washing cabinets, 'a perfect boon' after changing a wheel or fiddling with the carburettor. Ironically, despite claims in fashionable magazines that hygiene had become a paranoia, quirky columns on health, disease, and home treatments were exactly what helped to increase sales.[54]

FEMALE DRESS

The emphasis placed on hygiene influenced women's dress. It provided ammunition to the upper classes who wanted lighter, looser garments which would allow them to exercise more freely, or just to socialise comfortably with others in contexts other than the drawing room. Dress reformers in the United States led the way. They tried to abolish corsets, garters, and high-heeled shoes. They insisted that heavy garments be suspended from the shoulders. In the 1860s, Lexington's Hygienic Educational Seminary for Young Ladies gained publicity on both sides of the Atlantic because pupils' waists were measured at the beginning and end of term to prevent competition for tiny waists. The average increase in girth over this time was two and three-quarter inches, which was thought a great improvement to the girls' health.[55]

In England, the Professor of Hygiene at the newly founded Girton College, Cambridge, lectured female students on such topics as thin boots, high heels, and small bonnets.[56] The National Health Society, established in 1871 to promote public health, held an exhibition of antiseptic dress, and organised lectures. Some women appreciated the comfort of 'the hygienic boot', which, unlike the narrow-soled, pointy-toed kind, rarely deformed feet. (In the 1880s, Clarks were the first company to bring out a range of hygienic boots and shoes designed to fit the shape of the foot.) Yet, in this over-draped era, the hygienic, functional costume of loose-fitting trousers and short overdress which activists favoured never caught on – not until the 1890s, when a similar outfit appeared for riding bicycles. Female clothing became a focus of culture conflict. Women who walked fast, swinging their arms, were accused of bad manners, or looking like they had been trained in a turnip field; traditionalists complained that the hygienic boot 'would make a strong man shudder'.[57]

Oddly, the trend towards hygienic dress for women sometimes became a means of control. In the male view, the most striking outcome of a woman's hygienic training would be her 'repose': both her figure and her behaviour would display an absence of extremes; she would maintain perfect self-control.[58] As late as 1914, the Council of the Institute of Hygiene thought it perfectly proper to appoint a committee of leading male scientists and medical men to consider whether women should or should not wear corsets. It ruled that the demands of modern civilisation seemed to require some form of corset but, for health reasons, the garment should be constructed on hygienic lines. It issued a memorandum giving precise instructions to guide manufacturers and corset wearers.[59] Yet a corset-free bust-supporter, or bra, had been patented in the 1870s.

The hygienic concern with ventilation soon extended to mackin-toshes and undergarments. The Victorians set great store by warm flannel underwear all year round, to protect against diarrhoea, dysentery, and even cholera. It is true that, in the 1850s, the fashion for the crinoline introduced the steel-hooped caged petticoat, which was lightweight. But afterwards, mishaps with the swaying skirt encouraged women to wear drawers, too. When the summer of 1858 proved unseasonably cold, Jane Welsh Carlyle complained, 'I cannot dispense with a fire all day long; and am wearing *two* flannel petticoats besides flannel drawers and shift!' December 1860 proved worse: 'I wear *all* my flannel petticoats *at once!* and am having two new ones made out of a pair of Scotch Blankets!'[60] She particularly recommended the Scotch blankets, as being much warmer than even flannel. But all these petticoats had to be kicked forward or dragged behind with every step.

By the 1880s, reformers of underwear were advocating lightness, warmth, and ventilation. The Rational Dress Society recommended that women's underclothing should weigh a maximum of 7 pounds, which still seems ridiculously heavy today. The bustle of the 1880s was a crucial factor in reducing the bulk of underclothing; the fashion demanded a severely tailored figure in front and clinging skirts. By now women could buy all types of ready-made underwear; plain sewing was a dying accomplishment. Only the fastidious with money to spare had underwear made to measure. Trends in underclothes were influenced from 1880 by the medical eccentric Professor Gustav Jaeger, who insisted that only rough animal fibres, such as undyed wool, should be worn next to the skin, both summer and winter. Wool, he said, encouraged and absorbed perspiration better than clammy cotton and linen, drawing 'poisons' from the skin.[61] His teachings prompted a new clothing business, 'Dr Jaeger's Sanitary Woollen System', established in 1884. Soon there was a craze for wool-jersey long johns and combinations (chemise and drawers in one garment), considered hygienic because they hung from the shoulders.

The fine-spun woollen or chamois under-suits recommended by sanitary experts were totally beyond the reach of the poor. If they had underclothes at all, they rarely washed them. One doctor thought it a great mistake that millions of English people had rushed to wear flannel next to the skin. It might encourage sweating and absorb 'animal effluvia', but 'the filth and stench often submitted to the nostrils of a medical man' was overwhelming.[62] Other doctors and leisured women doing charity work were just as ready to complain that poor women spent money on tawdry finery that would be better spent on comfortable flannel.

One Edwardian remembered the torture of woollen combinations as a child, which always tickled once washed, and the prevailing doctrine of warm underclothing. Over her combinations, she wore bloomers with an unbuttonable seat lined with flannelette, stays with suspenders to hold up thick stockings, a woolly bodice, blouse, and gym tunic. She recalled, 'Oh, we were simply smothered in clothes, and I used to say to my mum, oh do I have to wear these horrible combinations? You'll be sorry if you don't, she said, you'll get rheumatism.'[63]

Layers of underwear could prove useful, as one American survivor from the sinking of the *Titanic* discovered. When the ship struck the iceberg, Margaret Brown was dressed for warmth in extra-heavy Swiss woollen bloomers, two jersey petticoats, woollen golf stockings, cashmere dress, chinchilla opera cloak, and sable muff, in which she put her Colt automatic. In the lifeboat she shared her layers with shivering older women and children. Then, stripped to her corset and unmentionables, she took hold of one oar and directed her pistol at the men gripping the others. 'Work those oars', she yelled, 'or I'll blow your guts out!'[64] Ever afterwards, she was known as the 'Unsinkable Molly Brown'.

For most women in everyday situations, underwear meant a battle between looking slim and being warm. Medical men solemnly debated the suitability of different fabrics for women's undergarments: linen and cotton could be washed at high temperatures; silk was warm and porous; some swore by unshrinkable wool. Women themselves preferred to wear less and less. By the 1920s, some Parisians wore evening dresses over nothing other than a pair of lace panties – a fashion that would have been unthinkable earlier. The conflict between comfort and seductiveness continues, with Bridget Jones-type big knickers apparently gaining popularity during Covid lockdowns.

THE DEODORISED BODY

Today, bodily hygiene is inescapably linked to the purchase of deodorants, a market that has seen remarkable growth. In 1916, only an estimated fifth of North Americans bought any toiletries or cosmetics at all, despite the United States being in the vanguard of marketing ideas and practice.[65] Well-dressed women wore rubber-lined, under-arm dress shields that could be detached and washed, as in Europe. But by the 1920s, there were cream deodorants, and North American newspapers were counselling businesswomen to use them after their daily bath.

Advertisements for personal hygiene products were mostly aimed at young women. Soon perspiration was viewed as 'an unforgivable transgression', but deodorants of the early 1930s, such as Odorono, were tricky to apply because they did not work if the skin had been washed with soap.[66] No wonder Marjorie Joyner, a haircare entrepreneur and educator who wrote a beauty column for the *Chicago Defender* in the 1930s, assured readers that a five-cent box of baking soda was as good a deodorant as any other. From this time, 'daintiness' became the word commonly associated with female hygiene. It marked the unimpeachable standard that women had to reach.

As more women worked in offices alongside men from the late 1930s, or in settings where there were different ethnic groups, personal hygiene became an even greater concern. Manufacturers of toiletries fuelled fears that without deodorants people would lose friends, sour intimate relationships, and miss out on promotion because they unwittingly emitted offensive body odours. Research chemists stoked these anxieties to sell new products. They warned that bathing merely removed external odours and that a person's individual scent seeped through the pores over time; only a water-soluble pill of concentrated chlorophyll could neutralise these internally created odours. One African American office manager, careful to point out that she wrote as a friend and fellow worker, candidly advised women to pay attention to personal hygiene if they wanted to blaze a trail for those who came after them and heighten others' life chances.[67]

By the mid-sixties, the market for deodorants in the United States was growing by 15 per cent a year on average, while over half of British women were using deodorant each day.[68] All deodorants worked in much the same way, but manufacturers brought out separate ranges for men and women. Brands were designed to be popular for years because they were marketed as indispensable. Body odours and bad breath, issues hardly confined to women, were now covered without embarrassment as part of public discourse about health and hygiene.

It was the same with menstruation, hitherto treated far more coyly. In the late nineteenth century, menstruating women were still perceived as ill and vulnerable, an attitude even medical experts encouraged in their advice books for women. Yet from at least 1881, British magazines had regularly accepted advertisements for feminine hygiene products. In that year, Southall Brothers & Barclay of Birmingham advertised a disposable sanitary towel for the convenience of female travellers. German and North American firms followed suit. Most women still made sanitary pads at home, washing them each month. Few could afford Southalls' towels at 3s a dozen, only to throw them away after use. But within a few years the towels came down in price: in 1888 a dozen of the smallest cost 1s. Southalls claimed that this price was the same as the laundry cost of the cloth kind, although it was still beyond the means of working-class women.

In the twentieth century, feminine hygiene became enmeshed in the forces of consumer culture. Male-led advertising campaigns presented menstruation as a fundamental biological difference that would limit women's participation in public life. Whereas Southalls' sanitary towels had been advertised as an antiseptic product for health as well as convenience, Kotex towels, introduced to American women from 1921, were chiefly marketed as a scientific solution to a problematic aspect of female biology. Advertising campaigns for Kotex towels reinforced sexual and social inequalities while ostensibly offering a product that would help women to compete on equal terms with men. The initial advertisement read, 'Insure poise in the daintiest frocks', while early promotions announced that Kotex towels were popular with women 'in the better walks of life'.[69] Sanitary products have since become a focus of political campaigning for menstruating people's rights, with many arguing that they should be exempt from consumption tax and freely available to the poor. Ironically, while the manufacturers of Kotex early dismissed previous makeshifts as unsafe and unsanitary, homemade, reusable pads are making a comeback because they are kinder to the environment.

The advertising of feminine care products encouraged public acknowledgement of menstruation but exaggerated the shame and embarrassment involved in order to boost sales. Advertising also implied that periods are somehow offensive, which chimed with centuries-old beliefs that women harboured venereal diseases. Even in the 1960s, women were advised to take internal deodorant pills to stop body odours at the source during their periods.[70] Manufacturers next introduced scented female sanitary products, which themselves proved a source of irritation and infection. Then, in 2015, Gwyneth Paltrow, promoting her Goop brand, recommended vaginal steaming for a super clean uterus. 'V-steaming' soon became a popular beauty trend, though it carried risks: after one zealous attempt, a woman was hospitalised with second-degree burns.

Spas continue to offer V-steaming and body smoking for cleanliness and health, selling them as traditional, non-Western practices which promote wellbeing. In fact, fumigation of the uterus was used in medieval Europe to alleviate minor disorders, until male surgeons superseded medically skilled women. And the practice continued in some form into the seventeenth century.[71] Fumigating sulphur baths were prescribed for skin complaints and venereal diseases in the eighteenth century. Another related development was the portable vapour-box bath. These were sold for home use after Turkish baths became fashionable in England from the mid-nineteenth century. The user sat in a wooden box on a cane chair over hot coals. The box had a hole for the neck, so the head was lifted above the fumes. These low-cost sweat baths were said to prevent and cure a range of illnesses, forcing impurities through the skin's pores. Those who purchased them could self-medicate in private. An advertisement in one African American newspaper claimed that the vapour bath guaranteed health, strength, and beauty, but specifically recommended it for 'women's troubles', among other disorders.[72]

Women were also encouraged to practise vaginal douching for personal hygiene, though some used it to prevent pregnancy. It is an old practice, advocated in women's manuals from the eighteenth century to cure discharges then collectively known as 'the whites'. Women with such conditions were reluctant to consult doctors. They feared intimate examination, and discharges were linked to venereal disease which carried a social stigma. In any case, doctors did not have a good understanding of yeast infections until the 1960s. Women often resorted to home remedies for such common ailments, shaping their own routines for health and hygiene.

Douching for cleanliness alone took off from the late 1890s, and self-contained douching kits 'with no hooks, clamps or hoses' were advertised into the 1950s as a lifetime investment to preserve 'feminine daintiness'.[73] Only from the 1970s were women warned that regular douching was not required for hygiene and could itself cause infection.[74] Sensible advice about vagina health, partly stemming from better medical understanding, still has to compete with seductive advertisements for unnecessary toiletries. The so-called feminine care market is massive and in 2021 was set to nearly double by 2030.[75] Even manufacturers who insist they give full information about their products and empower women of today still have their eye on a defined market segment. Users can always turn to social media for self-help but will need to sift through conflicting discussions.

Female hygiene rituals relate to a larger story of changing cultural values, but most depend on the basic convenience of running water. By the mid-1820s, it was possible to find domestic baths in London attached to a small boiler. Water could be heated by a handful of coals, provided there was a window or chimney for a flue to carry off the smoke. Some feared such contraptions were unsafe but they soon spread to the provinces, where a basic boiler and tin tub could cost six guineas. In Britain, separate bathrooms were not common in middle-class households until the 1880s, and even in 1950 only 46 per cent of all households had one; in France and eastern Europe, the situation was worse.[76]

The dubious hygiene of the British working poor shocked Caribbean immigrants in the 1950s, accustomed to the standards of privileged white people in the colonies. Middle-class immigrants particularly resented the fact that, owing to racism, they were regarded as inferior to Britain's white working class, even though their views on hygiene were more fastidious. Hygiene was a key area where differing perspectives led some Black people in Britain to revise the matrix in which whiteness was aligned with authority and beauty.[77] In their view, people who rarely took baths and who were content to wrap their fish and chips in old newspaper were not socially superior. In Britain's racist, class-structured society, Caribbean immigrants began to place value on a specific Black identity.

In the United States, piped water was already plentiful in cities by the twentieth century. Yet inefficient drainage and fears about lethal sewer gas briefly caused some to forgo a supply of hot water in bedrooms during the first decade. Hygiene in North America improved rapidly after the First World War and by the 1940s the 'American look' was already one of scrupulous cleanliness. Slowly, most of Europe followed this example and had shifted from the weekly bath to the daily shower by the end of the twentieth century. But habits mutate: a survey in 2022 showed that 25 per cent of French people no longer wash every day, partly for ecological concerns and partly because they consider it unhealthy.[78]

Hygiene is an area where care for personal health and beauty extends beyond self to family and community, which resonates strongly with women. Yet it has proved a battleground on many fronts. The marketing of soaps and other cleansers has reinforced gender prejudices and social hierarchies. The advice of medical experts has patronised women. Hygienic female dress attracted a bizarre level of male attention. In 1922, the principal of the Institute of Hygiene drew on his scientific knowledge of textiles when lecturing on this very issue. He recommended kilts as the most hygienic type of skirt: 'There are three layers of material when the wearer is standing still, making it unnecessary to throw off so much heat from the body, and one layer when the wearer walks, thereby enabling heat to be thrown off rapidly.'[79]

Developments in hygiene certainly changed concepts of femininity. The opulent but pale and physically delicate woman who ornamented a Victorian drawing room gave way to the healthy, more sportive, and slimmer beauty of the twentieth century. An army doctor wrote in the 1930s, 'The over-dressed, over corseted and under-washed women of the last century were neither pure nor pleasing. The lightly clad, loose waisted and well-washed young women of to-day are clean and wholesome.'[80] Yet the path towards greater hygiene has been uneven: today the lack of public toilets remains an issue; personal care products can contain chemical allergens; and advertisements for toiletries continue to exploit and reinforce differences in gender status and education. At the same time, developments in hygiene have proved life-enhancing, offering women new career opportunities, and helping many to own and celebrate their bodies.

TEETH

Today, the Hollywood smile sets an enviable standard. Pearly teeth may be costly, but a flawless set is attainable. This was not always the case. Tooth decay affected rich and poor, and little could be done about it. Even Elizabeth I had to pad out her cheeks with wads of cloth to disguise tooth loss. Sugar was the main culprit. In the seventeenth century, only the rich could afford this imported luxury, but sugar consumption increased hugely in successive centuries and extended to the lower ranks. Poor diet was another factor. Scurvy was endemic in Britain, leaving the afflicted with spongy, bleeding gums, stinking breath, and loose teeth. No one understood that the illness was triggered by a lack of vitamin C, so the elite suffered as well as the destitute. Sarah Churchill, Duchess of Marlborough, made the arduous journey from Windsor to Scarborough in 1732, hoping that its spa water would cure her scurvy along with her gout. Quack medicines for scurvy were touted in newspapers well into the 1830s, long after people had discovered it could be prevented by fresh fruit and vegetables. The gnawing pain of rotten teeth was an inescapable fact of life.

People's sense of time was closely bound up with their dentition. A baby's teething was a great milestone, not least because it brought fevers and stomach upsets. Death registers from the eighteenth and nineteenth centuries frequently give 'teeth' as a cause of infant mortality. Survival was evidence of a mother's care and judgement in providing the right teething aid. In the early eighteenth century, a wolf's canine set in gold was thought to be best. It was hung around the neck so that the child could chew on it and rub their gums with it to relieve discomfort. One mother attributed the death of her eldest child and the painful teething of her second to the fact that she had not provided them with a wolf's canine. Her later children teethed easily, she said, 'for I had one for al[l] the rest'.[1] The emergence of adult teeth was another milestone. In Britain, when reformers proposed a law to limit child labour, they thought it could be enforced by an examination of a child's teeth as a test of age. In adulthood, tooth loss was a constant reminder of mortality, while old age meant a diet of pap.

Tooth decay had social as well as personal consequences. The stench of rotting teeth and tainted dentures commonly made company unbearable. People complained about the smell in enclosed spaces, such as shared carriages. Tooth problems especially affected women: not only did their teeth seem to decay quicker but they also experienced more pressure to keep their looks. Dentists did occasionally warn men that broken, tobacco-stained teeth and stinking breath would not recommend them to the ladies, but mostly they urged women to safeguard their teeth. This pressure increased from the late eighteenth century, as society became more conscious of hygiene. Manufacturers of dental products began to insist that good teeth, healthy gums, and sweet breath were essential to beauty and cleanliness.

In Victorian times, a gleaming smile became linked to the feminine ideal. One dentist wrote, 'It is more especially to woman that fine teeth are necessary, since it is her destiny first to gratify the eyes before she touches the soul and captivates and enslaves the heart.'[2] The perception that women's teeth were an ornament to beauty meant that women were rarely associated with unpleasant toothy idioms such as grinding, gnashing, gritting, and clenching. The whole subject of teeth is riddled with casual misogyny. This chapter explores women's response to tooth decay, its effect on social behaviour and etiquette, and the changing expectations of women's oral health as dentistry advanced.

EARLY DENTISTRY AND TOOTH LOSS

In Britain, dental progress was negligible until the end of the seventeenth century. The situation was little better in the rest of western Europe, and yet people had made false teeth for centuries. The ancient Egyptians struggled with gritty bread, and mummies have been found with implanted ivory teeth in their jawbones. The Etruscans deftly secured artificial teeth to sound ones with highly visible gold bands; they were probably a status symbol. In western Europe, interest in dentistry grew from the mid-seventeenth century, following a dramatic increase in tooth decay as more sugar and refined flour entered the diet. Physicians warned that sugar blackened teeth and even claimed it was bad for digestion. An early eighteenth-century comedy, mocking the mingling of classes in the spa town of Tunbridge Wells, advised any man marrying a London dame to inspect her teeth beforehand as if she were a horse, because, what with drinking hot liquors and eating sugar plums in church, not one in ten had a tooth left.[3] Women were easily criticised for drinking sweetened tea and eating candies. Yet sugar was addictive. Consumption in Britain alone increased five-fold in just sixty years from 1710.[4]

There were many traditional remedies for toothache, commonly supposed to be caused by a worm that fed on the teeth. The theory was ridiculed in the 1750s but not finally disproved until the middle of the nineteenth century. Women prepared and shared long-established remedies. One involved burning rosemary stems and holding the cinders in a linen parcel between the teeth to kill the worms. Another poultice for the teeth contained yarrow, trefoil, and primrose leaves. Women also shared recipes for improving the look of teeth. They could be whitened with vinegar or lemon juice and scrubbed with ground pumice or cuttlefish bone. Gums could be dyed red to enhance the whiteness of teeth – a trick used in some tooth-whitening products today. But acids and abrasives damaged tooth enamel, while cleaning with sponges, textured cloths, or poorly designed brushes was barely effective.

Some put their trust in folk practices which seemed to link the living and the dead. A tooth taken from a skull uncovered in a graveyard was a valued object. Kept about the person or applied to an aching tooth, it might ward off pain. The Victorian novelist Anna Eliza Bray recorded that in Devon this superstition continued into the 1830s. Women there were in desperate need of some remedy for toothache. Bray noted that most had no sound front teeth, a calamity she ascribed to their daily drink: acidic cider.[5]

Dental problems exposed sufferers to extreme quackery. Early eighteenth-century 'dentifrices' – powders and pastes for cleaning teeth – were touted as miraculous cure-alls. Advertisements falsely claimed that such products would heal scorbutic gums even when almost eaten away, whiten teeth however yellow or black, stop decay and rot, relieve pain, fix loose teeth in their sockets, preserve teeth into old age, and cleanse and cure a stinking breath.[6] But commercial dentifrices and mouth washes mostly contained strong acids, or abrasive ingredients that damaged tooth enamel. Many were sweetened with honey or sugar. And when scaling to remove tartar became fashionable from the 1750s, patients were often at the mercy of amateurs; experts warned that scaling damaged teeth if botched. When sea bathing became popular, some sufferers placed their hopes in the antiseptic qualities of salt water, only to be disappointed when bathing in and drinking sea water did nothing for their aching teeth.

Those with money had access to professional dental care from the 1660s. Samuel Pepys's wife, Elizabeth, suffered with her teeth and gums. She went to one of the first dental specialists in London, called an 'operator for the teeth', and had them scraped. Pepys thought the effect 'pretty handsome' but underlying problems remained; a few years later her face 'mightily swelled' with the toothache.[7] She was in agony for days until the abscess burst. People suffered tortures with their teeth even when they had access to expert help. Lady Mary Wortley Montagu, living in Italy in the 1750s, became so afflicted with scurvy-related gum disease that she was not expected to live. As she explained to a female friend, a surgeon was summoned who 'immediately apply'd red hot Irons to my Gumms' to cauterise them.[8] Then he spread caustics over the wounds to halt the infection, a painful treatment she endured for several days. Women's letters, right up until the mid-twentieth century, are riddled with accounts of excruciating tooth pain. The author and social reformer Hannah More, strong-minded though she was, avowed in 1813 that toothache had brought her to the edge of delirium.[9]

Extraction was the routine treatment for tooth decay. In cities, sufferers could go to professional dentists or lowly barbers to have teeth drawn. In the countryside, they might have to rely on itinerant tooth-pullers or local blacksmiths. The chief extraction tool was the dental pelican, so called because the claw that fitted around the diseased tooth looked like a pelican's beak. Even when used proficiently, the leveraging could result in laceration of the gums, serious blood loss, or, if the patient was unlucky, a fractured jawbone. The procedure itself was often humiliating. Before the invention of the reclining dental chair in 1832, the operator usually placed the patient on a low seat with the head tilted well back; to prevent any struggle, some liked to hold the patient's head firmly between their thighs.

Dentists might extract multiple teeth in one sitting. In 1797, the pioneering French dentist Nicolas DuBois de Chémant boasted of extracting twenty-eight from the mouth of a duchess (tact prevented his naming her). Probably he did not exaggerate. Having perfected the process of making porcelain dentures, he needed elite customers to make them fashionable, so it was in his interest to extract many teeth. But it was not unusual for teeth to fail together. Hannah More lamented that she had had fourteen extracted in a little over a year. In 1865, Sarah Andrews, a teacher in Hudson, Wisconsin, wrote to her brother, 'I do not know as you will believe me for I can hardly believe it myself. I actually had all my decayed teeth out yesterday, only eight. Wasn't I brave? I have not felt as well for some time as I have today.'[10] Unfortunately, it was not always clear which teeth were giving pain and dentists could draw the wrong ones. In 1853, Jane Welsh Carlyle had the dentist pull out two molars but returned to have a third drawn when her toothache failed to subside.[11]

Many put off visiting a dentist from fear or to avoid expense. In the late eighteenth century, one dentist described how a middle-aged woman with inflammatory toothache had repeatedly lanced the swelling caused in the roof of her mouth with her own scissors. By the time she consulted him, she had already lost part of her soft palate. Another dentist described how a young woman came to him after a botched extraction some two years earlier. The infection in her gum had caused a suppurating wound in her cheek, which she disguised with a piece of black ribbon. She was left with a depression in her face that permanently disfigured her. The details of such traumas give insights into women's intimate lives, although dentists obviously cited extreme cases to promote their careers.[12]

Great care was needed when choosing a dentist. There was no dental school in England until 1858, and no register of dentists restricting those who could practice until 1879. Many were charlatans whose tricks included offloading badly fitting false teeth that did not suit the wearer. The author Maria Edgeworth spared no effort when her half-sister, Honora, needed dental care in 1818. She took Honora to all the principal London dentists before deciding which one to trust. Each offered different opinions about how long Honora's failing teeth would last, suggested different treatments, and quoted different prices. Eventually, the two women fixed on 'a filer and stuffer' who abhorred 'artificial teeth and rivetting' and who came highly recommended.[13]

Tooth loss caused practical problems with articulation and digestion. Eventually, speech might be reduced to an unintelligible scramble of mumbles and whistles. One woman marvelled how an acquaintance 'spoke with her gums and chin, not with her toung [sic] and teeth'.[14]

Lack of teeth was socially isolating and hampered the ability of women to entertain polite company by conversing or singing. It also restricted their ability to eat in public. After the surgeon John Hunter published his study of human teeth in 1771, people accepted that mastication was the vital first stage of digestion. Yet contemporary dentures were of little use as far as chewing was concerned. Wearers often took them out before meals. The toothless resorted to specially invented hand tools to help them crush food, including apple-scoops and masticators resembling pliers.

If the elderly eventually resigned themselves to a liquid diet of broth, jellies, and milk, younger people with missing teeth seemed all set to damage their system by gulping down poorly chewed meals. In 1843, a dentist in Philadelphia recorded that rotten teeth and gums had ruined one young woman's digestion: 'Her symptoms of dyspepsia were general emaciation, pale countenance, pain in the region of the stomach, nausea, and rejection of food at all times by that organ.'[15] He explained that the patient had paid for expensive medical advice and drunk the mineral waters at Saratoga Springs, but to no avail. The cause of her health problems were her teeth, which she refused to address.

Women also feared tooth loss because all agreed it aged the face by as much as ten years, changing its contours and reducing the shape of the lips. Lady Mary Coke, a sharp-eyed observer of London society in the eighteenth century, kept track of the physical changes to all the women in her circle. After one social event in 1772, she recorded a marked difference in Margaret Bentinck, dowager Duchess of Portland, writing, 'The loss of her teeth makes a great alteration: She looks very old.'[16] The duchess, aged fifty-seven, was the richest woman in Britain, but money could not fix her teeth.

Women could be forgiven for making teeth an obsession; a pearly smile helped to determine their life chances and was one of the first things noticed by friends and lovers. The visible upper teeth are also central to a sense of self. Jane Welsh Carlyle, struggling with tooth problems in middle age, received an unwelcome reminder of the importance of teeth when her husband sent her an update on old friends in the 1840s. He wrote, 'Poor Mrs Johnstone has lost all her teeth, except a melancholy remnant or two, and those she employs her lips, in a painful forcible manner, visibly to *cover up*'; her sister '*sings* her speech' through missing teeth.[17] Carlyle also dwelt with sadness on his mother's loss of her upper teeth, which, he noted, greatly altered her appearance.[18] She could not be fitted with false ones due to the limitations of Victorian dentistry; the one stump she had left would not be enough to anchor an upper set.

ETHICS, ETIQUETTE, AND PROPRIETY

Society early connected teeth with female morality, and specifically with sexual morality. In 1664, Samuel Pepys complained that his London neighbours, the Turners, were not to be trusted. Mrs Turner in particular was 'a false woman, and hath rotten teeth and false, set in with wire'.[19] As far as Pepys was concerned, her artificial teeth, fixed among the rotten ones, were on a par with her character. An obvious reason why loose teeth were associated with loose morals was because mercury and salivation treatments for venereal disease easily rotted the teeth. But face creams and makeup often contained mercury, too. One dentist, examining a young woman's painful gums, was sure that mercury was the culprit. Given the link between mercury and syphilis, he hesitated to suggest it to her. Eventually, he traced the problem to the pomatum she used on her hair. The hairdresser routinely added mercury to the cream in order to destroy bugs.[20]

At the end of the eighteenth century, a notorious divorce case reinforced the easy connection often made between false teeth and immorality. In December 1800, Mr George Duckworth, an eminent attorney in Manchester, accused his wife of having an affair with her dentist, Mr Bott. Her teeth had been 'uncommonly bad' and at last Bott took them all out.[21] He made her an artificial set and afterwards it seemed that he had to visit the house often to clean and adjust them.

Duckworth successfully proved that during these visits Bott supplied more than professional dental services; he won his divorce.

The terrible state of most people's teeth in western Europe influenced social life and manners. Society valued well-preserved teeth not only as an enhancement to beauty but also as a sign of health. Early tooth loss implied a weak constitution or some underlying condition. Visibly healthy teeth signalled good digestion and careful hygiene. Consequently, some women were ashamed to show their imperfect teeth in public. They screened them behind the ornamental fan many carried, which survived as a fashion accessory into the twentieth century.

Polite society was also quick to make a virtue out of a necessity. Until people began to value sensibility and signs of emotion in the mid-eighteenth century, laughing in polite company was bad manners. Toothy laughter was held to indicate a lack of self-restraint, frivolity, improper sensuality, or just low birth and a total ignorance of etiquette. Partly it was frowned upon because social commentators interpreted laughter as a display of condescension rather than affability. Yet those who did have good teeth found a way to display them. In 1776, the artist and letter-writer Mary Delany commented on a new affectation among fashionable ladies, 'twisting their mouth, and *spreading it* out' when speaking, to show their white teeth.[22] By the end of the century, the feminine ideal was to offer a gentle smile with a glimpse of teeth. This was how women were shown in the popular portraits of the French artist Élisabeth Vigée Le Brun.[23] In the next century, Victorian women who could not match the standard continued to hide their teeth in public. Mothers encouraged their daughters to eat in their rooms before dining in company so that their teeth might not be noticed. It prompted the false notion that young women lived on little more than air.

As dentistry improved, the torture of those who could afford complex treatment only increased to begin with. The term 'dentist' was borrowed from the French and first used in London and Edinburgh around the mid-eighteenth century. It referred to a new kind of practitioner who was skilled in a range of operations in addition to cleaning and drawing teeth. Dentists were prepared to treat diseased gums with leeches, deaden exposed nerves with red-hot wire, and stuff opiates into cavities. By the 1780s, with Parisian dentists in the vanguard, the emphasis was on tooth preservation. Expert practitioners made crowns, attaching each with a gold or silver screw, and filled decayed teeth with a range of substances, including gold, the natural rubber gutta-percha, and lead. They also used mercury amalgams from 1830, although these blends were unstable compared to the kind used today. The novelist Fanny Trollope complained to her son in 1850 that she had suffered much at the hands of her expert dentist. She had to postpone a fitting for false teeth because her face was too swollen and inflamed to be touched. And she was shocked by the cost of her treatment. Conversion into modern values is always hazardous, but in today's money she had spent at least £5,000.[24]

From the late eighteenth century, because the upper ranks could afford dentists and had better advice about tooth care, visible misman-agement of the teeth suggested sloth, slack discipline, and even stupidity. The stakes were raised in the late 1770s after the Swiss physiognomist Johann Lavater maintained that clean, regular teeth indicated a generous, honest disposition. Teeth were used to judge character all the more. Poor hygiene was an easy target. Detractors of Marie Antoinette added to her other supposed faults by whispering that she never cleaned her teeth well.[25] Commentators also began to be more critical of national dietary preferences that might have an impact on oral health. One dentist worried about all the acidic gooseberry pies the English ate.[26] Mary Wollstonecraft, visiting Scandinavia in 1795, complained that women there flagrantly ruined their teeth with coffee and spices.[27]

The link made between propriety and oral hygiene soon touched the aspiring middling sort. One household medical work of 1781 insisted, 'those who permit their teeth and gums to become foul, commit an offence against decency'.[28] Dentists gave women specific advice: having long advised that quill toothpicks were safer than metal ones, they warned them not to pick at their teeth with pins and other metal objects, not to break off threads with their teeth when sewing, and not to use their teeth as nutcrackers. Victorian beauty manuals and fashion magazines for women echoed Lavater, reaffirming that teeth gave clues to character.[29] Contemporary newspapers applied additional kinds of pressure on women to preserve their smiles. Society pages noted that, since the management of teeth had become an easy matter, discoloured teeth were more likely to be noticed; humour columns offered witticisms explaining that women's teeth decayed earlier than men's due to the friction of their tongues on them; advertisements for dental products carried narratives in which men commented on a woman's beauty and shared their regret that it was marred by poor teeth.[30] But because sugar consumption had extended to all classes, the state of people's teeth had never been worse.

FALSE TEETH

Artificial teeth were a rich person's ornament in the eighteenth and nineteenth centuries. The Bluestocking and historian Catherine Macaulay was ambivalent about them. Writing in the 1780s, she blamed women's tooth loss on 'warm liquors, warm beds, and warm night-caps'; she remembered a time when women had no choice but to hide the flaws of age and lifestyle: 'When women had attained the age of thirty-five, they were obliged to give up every pretension to beauty, and vanity under the appearance of decency.'[31] Now she saw them veering to the other extreme, adopting implausible ornaments to beauty, like dentures, which only seemed to heighten the defects of age. And it was true that false teeth were mostly worn for vanity since they were of little or no use in eating. She may have been influenced by contemporary satires about women, which mocked them for wearing wigs, padded stays and rumps, and false teeth and eyebrows. Men even claimed that they lived in fear of marrying an *artificial* woman', and contemplated a law that would punish women who deceived men in this way, annulling any marriages made.[32]

Yet eighteenth-century artificial teeth fooled no one. Walrus tusk was the preferred material, although ivory and hippopotamus bone were also used. None were the same colour as human teeth, so they never looked natural. And it was possible to see where the base of the denture met the gum unless this part was covered by the lips. Artificial teeth did fill out the face but tended to distort the jawline because constant effort was needed to hold them in place. They also prompted jokes and caused embarrassment. In 1779 a newspaper reported that one woman laughed so immoderately when at the theatre that her upper set sprang out of her mouth and into the pit. The teeth were valuable, 'curiously mounted with gold springs', but since they landed in the cheap seats they were never found.[33]

The rich had a limited choice of dentures: the base plate could be made of ivory or gold; the teeth could be ivory or composed of assorted human teeth. From the mid-eighteenth century it was possible to have a full upper and lower set attached by springs. Even so, the upper row had to be anchored to at least two remaining teeth, while the lower row was essential to give it something to rest on. A full set of dentures made with human teeth could cost over £100.[34] It was an enormous sum when only about 7 per cent of families in England and Wales had a yearly income of £100 and above.[35] All the same, there was a healthy market for human teeth, supplied by grave robbers and battlefield scavengers. Ivory teeth were cheaper but still beyond the means of most people.

Women with a few missing teeth could improve their appearance by getting partial dentures, but a strip of artificial teeth had to be fixed at each end to sound teeth with thread or gold wire. Over time, these ligatures loosened sound teeth, which wearers could ill afford to lose. Poor hygiene made all false teeth offensive. Ligatures were hard to undo, so partial dentures were rarely removed for cleaning. Food was trapped in crevices and springs, and dirty ivory or bone decomposed with the action of saliva. Dentists feared that denture-wearers always inhaled such rotten air that their health would suffer. Anyone near them reeled from the fumes. Records of unusual casework included one woman fitted in the 1830s with a denture composed of natural teeth on an ivory plate. Embarrassment caused her to keep it a secret and she never removed it. In a few years the plate was cemented to her mouth with tartar. The teeth were 'in a high degree offensive' but tartar had at least preserved the colour of the ivory base.[36]

Many wearers also suffered pain from ill-fitting false teeth. Few outside major towns had access to good dentists, and it was hard to take accurate measurements of the mouth. In 1823, Dorothy Wordsworth, based in the Lake District, contemplated getting a new set of teeth from Mr Wallace, a dentist in Edinburgh; her London ones gave her no comfort. But she was not sure that he could make the dentures without seeing her in person. In the end, she decided that, unless she was going to Edinburgh soon, she would ask a friend to take her false teeth to Wallace for repair and adjustment. The result was likely to disappoint.

Another option for those who lacked teeth was to find a dentist who would transplant teeth straight from another person's mouth. This had been tried off and on since the 1680s; operators for the teeth had even experimented with the fangs of dogs and sheep. Dental transplantation became popular in the late eighteenth century when patients aimed to receive 'live' teeth drawn from donors on the spot. These teeth had a better chance of 'taking', especially since dentists usually transplanted only front teeth which had single roots. Critics objected that it was cruel to extract healthy teeth from poor donors, but no one could blame the desperate for getting money in this way. There was a darker side to the practice: donors were often children because smaller, younger teeth were easier to fit; some newspaper reports linked this trade in teeth to the abduction of young girls.

All understood that donors could pass on diseases like syphilis; at least the human teeth used in dentures could be boiled first. Despite the risk, transplantation remained popular with women on both sides of the Atlantic into the nineteenth century, which shows how desperate they were to have good teeth. Success was always a matter of chance. One diarist in Tennessee, who received three teeth in 1862, fell into a fever afterwards and kept to her bed for a fortnight. Then one by one, the newly planted teeth began to loosen and 'rise'. She wrote despairingly, 'I am not able to do anything hardly. Have got another tooth rising. I am nearly worn out with my teeth and other ailments.'[37]

Porcelain or 'mineral' teeth proved a major breakthrough. Invented in France in 1787, early mineral teeth gleamed with an unnatural whiteness and never looked real, but they did not discolour like ivory or decay offensively in the mouth. Full sets were difficult to make, expensive, and soon discontinued, but single porcelain teeth became widespread from the mid-nineteenth century. In this period, American dentists overtook the French. Factories in North America improved the glaze and churned out vast quantities of porcelain teeth in a range of colours. Victorian beauty handbooks gave helpful advice about artificial teeth. One explained that porcelain was best used when replacing molars, while 'natural teeth' were best for replacing incisors, whether screwed to a stump or fixed to a palate.[38] Mineral teeth had some drawbacks. They could have an abrasive effect on a person's remaining teeth. They also made a tell-tale clicking sound. In the twentieth century, when more young Americans had good teeth, this sound helped to mark the tension between generations. A young housewife praising the bravery of American soldiers in the Second World War added sharply, 'I hope the old ladies, who have been clicking their store teeth over the softness of this generation, will relax a little.'[39]

TEETH AND SOCIAL CLASS

Tooth care was an indicator of social class as well as mere propriety, because professional services for the teeth, other than simple extraction, were the preserve of the rich until the late eighteenth century. As dentistry improved and clean teeth began to denote class as well as a disciplined approach to the body, the middling sort adopted ostentatious habits of dental care. Frances Nelson, wife of the admiral, boasted to him that she had visited a dentist in anticipation of his return from sea: 'When I expected you I went and had my teeth put in order and wish I had done it some years back they look much better than you ever saw them.'[40] There was a growing market for tools to help clean teeth, not least because some feared that a build-up of tartar might work to eject them. People bought metal scalers. These varied in price, with the more expensive having a bespoke case with a mirror fastened to the inside lid. But in the 1820s, the diarist Anne Lister still preferred to clean the tartar from her teeth with a penknife.[41]

Toothpicks were a familiar item but prompted ambivalence. Some kept them in ornate cases, and this seemed to indicate extravagance, idleness, and frivolity. In England, picking one's teeth in polite company could appear rude. Fanny Burney, teased into giving her opinion on the matter, told a French acquaintance in the 1770s that it was permissible 'provided you have a little *glass* to look in before you'.[42] Yet the French were happy to pass round toothpicks and mouth-rinses at the end of each meal into the 1860s.[43] The ritual was too bold for the diffident English, however good for the teeth.

In contrast, toothbrushes became something of a status symbol. They were proof of refinement, whereas bad breath suggested dirt and disease. William Addis is credited with the mass production of the toothbrush from 1780. Jailed for causing a London riot, he watched prisoners cleaning their teeth with a sooty rag and reasoned that there must be a better way. He did not invent the toothbrush, which had made its way to Europe from China. Devotees had used brushes of hog bristles or horsehair on their teeth from the seventeenth century, although dentists warned that they were too rough. But Addis's version soon caught on. His brushes were made from animal hair set into bone or ivory. A toothbrush and tooth powder helped to convey wealth and prestige because, until the mechanised production of plastic tooth-brushes with nylon tufts in the 1930s, few could afford them. On the rare occasions when the lower classes were seen wielding a toothbrush, it was taken to be a sign of social pretention. In the 1770s, a pedlar's wife was cruelly mocked for taking up her toothbrush several times a day.[44]

In the navy, where scurvy was an enduring problem, toothbrushes helped to mark an important boundary between officers and the lower deck. Poor diet at sea meant that officers contracted scurvy just as their crews did, and even in the early stages this meant bad breath and rotting teeth. In 1758, Lady Anson described a visit that Captain Rodney and other captains made to her husband, then First Lord of the Admiralty. She complained that their company 'was so offensive from the state of their health, as to make it but just possible to bear the cabin with them, not even almost after they were gone'.[45] By the time of the Napoleonic Wars, naval officers at sea were asking their wives to send them toothbrushes, even though lemon juice had been issued in the British Navy to help prevent scurvy since 1795. Similarly, naval wives who travelled with their husbands wrote home for their favourite tooth powder in an effort to maintain standards abroad.[46]

The toothbrush became more widely used in the nineteenth century. Some women continued to fear that bristles would damage tooth enamel; in 1876, Madame Marie Bayard, in her *Art of Beauty*, recommended using the finger instead. And perhaps women were right to be cautious. Expensive toothbrushes had ivory, shell, or sandalwood handles; some came in silver-plated cases to protect the bristles. They were made to last for years and harboured germs. Even so, by the end of the century, regular use of the toothbrush was a firm ritual among the upper ranks. White smiles and fresh breath were signs of gentility. The way was open for the lower classes to emulate the same standards of oral hygiene to get on in life.

MOTHERHOOD AND DENTAL CAREERS FOR WOMEN

Given the link between oral hygiene and social class, it soon became a mother's duty to ensure that children were trained to use a toothbrush. Once Frances Nelson had visited a dentist in 1794, she eagerly passed on his advice. She wrote to Nelson asking him to make sure her sailor son brushed his teeth upwards and downwards, not crossways.[47] Fanny Kemble, travelling in North America in the 1830s, was particularly incensed by a mother in the same railway carriage stuffing her child with pound cake. She challenged the woman, whose excuse was that she gave the cake to 'keep her baby good'. Kemble 'looked at the woman's sallow cheeks and rickety teeth' and could not resist pointing out how much she was injuring her child's health.[48] It was a trivial incident, but Kemble described it at length in a letter home. It served to underline her own diligence as a mother, especially as she declared that she never permitted her own daughter to eat heavy cake.

This duty of care was soon enshrined in advice manuals. Harriet Martineau, noted for her writings on society, explained in her 1849 work, *Household Education*, that, if parents wished to spare their children pain and tooth loss, they had to make sure the children scrubbed their teeth. For the upper sort, this duty of supervision extended to offspring placed at boarding school. Dentists cautioned parents that a child's teeth could be ruined by inappropriate dental work; it should never be the case that the first that parents knew about a child's tooth problems was the dental bill on the list of school charges. One Victorian dentist pointed out that good oral hygiene was often a matter of custom; he observed that, while respectable white British tradesmen left their teeth 'disgustingly dirty', Black people were particularly careful of them.[49]

The pressure of tooth care on middle-class Victorian mothers was soon unrelenting and women took to virtue signalling in this respect. Magazines included patterns for how to decorate and embroider toothbrush racks. Home furnishings included toothpick racks trimmed with silk tassels and strung beads. Just before the First World War, one London doctor even asserted that childhood illnesses could be traced to the bad teeth of the mother.[50] When Britain eventually followed other European nations and introduced dental inspections into state schools in the first half of the twentieth century, a parent was expected to attend. Parents deeply resented this, since any fault found with their child's teeth was felt to be a criticism. Toothbrushing as an indicator of good motherhood has proved to be long-lived. When Reese Witherspoon was interviewed in 2019, she explained how she juggled the demands of family and a film career: 'As a mom, I'm kind of goofy. I like to dance around and tell jokes. But I'm pretty strict about bedtimes and making sure everybody brushes their teeth twice a day.'[51]

Although tooth care placed added burdens on women as mothers, dentistry did widen their job opportunities. In the eighteenth century, women worked as toothache curers, artificial tooth makers, and dentifrice sellers, often continuing their husband's trade when widowed. A widow in Leeds combined hairdressing, tooth-drawing, and ear piercing. Her business thrived and she advertised for assistants.[52] In the 1770s, one female dentist toured the Midlands, promising to fill, scrape, and extract teeth 'with matchless Skill and Tenderness'.[53] She occupied a gap in the market because most expert dentists practised in capital cities and spa towns. Later she did establish herself in Soho, London, where she set out to attract genteel customers, offering to attend ladies and gentlemen in their own homes.

Advancements in dentistry meant that women increasingly found employment in making dental apparatus. There were also jobs in factories making porcelain teeth. By the first decade of the twentieth century, porcelain teeth could be colour-matched to existing teeth. Women were trained to do this careful work and also to weed out flawed products. But dental-related work could be dangerous. From the 1870s, celluloid was used for dental plates and later for toothbrushes. Large teams of women were used in the early stages of manufacture, recycling cotton waste. Factory explosions and fires were a common hazard because celluloid is highly flammable.

The first female dentist qualified in England only in 1895, some thirty-five years after dental qualifications were introduced. Contemporaries noted that, while the profession might at first seem to suit women, since it called for manual dexterity and an orderly mind, it was doubtful whether women had the physical strength to draw teeth or the cool self-possession to act fast in an emergency. Perhaps, after all, women were better suited to act as assistants to some competent man?[54] Once anaesthetics came into general use, male dentists actively sought women assistants; their presence reassured female patients who would otherwise be unconscious and alone with them.

GAS AND RUBBER

In the nineteenth century, levels of tooth decay continued to increase with each generation; it was usual for the teeth of the daughter to be worse than those of the mother. The explanation was that ill-trained dentists tinkered with patients' teeth – a case of 'over doing' rather than neglect.[55] Because multiple extractions were so common, discoveries that lessened the pain of dental treatment made a huge difference to people's lives. Dentists had tried hypnosis for pain relief since the 1830s, but it could take thirty minutes to put patients into a trance-like state and for many dentists this was not practical: time was money. Some continued with hypnosis into the 1890s but meanwhile a speedier method of numbing pain had been found: inhaling ether. The gas was first used for extraction in 1846 by an American dentist, William Moreton, and rapidly trialled the following year in Britain. The method seemed ideally suited to women. Dentists announced that 'ladies of delicate frame and quiet habits' were more easily prostrated by the gas than men who drank strong liquors.[56] Not all practitioners were well trained in giving anaesthetics, and some women died from overdoses. But, by the end of the century, patients could at least face tooth extraction knowing that it was not bound to involve pain.

Around the same time, dentures were transformed by the discovery of vulcanite, a rubber–sulphur compound. An improved process for making vulcanite was patented in 1851 and the material was quickly used for denture bases worldwide. It could be moulded to the mouth and was much cheaper than ivory or gold. Well-fitting, artificial teeth now came closer to the reach of the masses. Dentists proclaimed the folly of keeping decayed teeth when they could be extracted painlessly

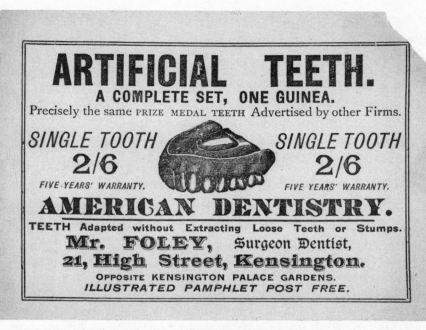

10. *A card advertising dentures, c. 1896. Foley's false teeth came with a five-year warranty.*

'at lightning speed', leaving people to 'enjoy the pleasure' of dentures.[57] Some dentists produced upper and lower sets costing from as little as one guinea, up to fifteen guineas, and even supplied dentures on a weekly payment system, although sets costing less than £5 were very inferior. Vulcanite plates adhered to the gums by suction, so there was no need for springs. The effect was totally new. In 1871 a young woman from east London, boasting of her teeth, was asked if they were natural or artificial. 'Neither', she replied; 'they are gutta percha'.[58] But despite improvements in dentures, gum-coloured plumpers were still sold for thin faces to the end of the century. Just as in the reign of Elizabeth I, plumpers helped to round out the contours of older faces and disguise fine lines around the mouth.

As dentures became less detectable, paradoxically the embarrassment of wearing them increased. Some women hesitated to remove a plate with just two or three teeth attached, and there were tragic cases of women who died from swallowing their teeth when eating or asleep. In the case of one woman who swallowed her teeth, a dentist fed her pieces of woollen cloth, having observed owl pellets and noticing that hard indigestible bones were wrapped in the skin of the mice it had eaten. Eventually, she safely expelled her artificial teeth. Others were not so fortunate. False teeth with sharp points and hooks might become impacted in the oesophagus. Vulcanite plates posed additional problems because early X-rays could not detect them.

High-end sets of false teeth, especially those mounted in gold, remained a valuable commodity. There were cases of women in domestic service who seized opportunities to steal expensive dentures and sell them to dealers and curiosity shops. Others were caught when they tried to pawn stolen dentures. A fraudster working as a domestic cook was sentenced to twelve months' hard labour for crimes that included ordering false teeth in her mistress's name for all her fellow servants.[59] This Robin Hood crime shows how much ordinary people needed false teeth.

THE MARKET FOR TOOTH CARE

Throughout the nineteenth century, the pressure on women to have good teeth intensified. Branded dentifrices began to be advertised with the image of a woman displaying a perfect smile. Advertisers targeted women because they understood that wives purchased most household toiletries; such tactics may have made women even more sensitive about their teeth. All the same, the message was increasingly one of hope. Whereas seventeenth-century household manuals had included recipes for aching teeth and stinking breath, nineteenth-century beauty guides offered advice about the prevention of tooth decay. In North America, pundits credited women with helping to improve dentistry. They alleged that the coquetry of Frenchwomen had spurred early French supremacy in the field, while the good sense of American women would hone the market for dentures: 'The time is not far distant when a lady will evince as much judgement and shrewdness in bargaining for a set of plate teeth, as she now manifests in the selection of any ordinary article of dry goods.'[60]

But if women were supposedly more alert to dental advice, they had long been victims of incorrect and contradictory information about tooth care. Sometimes they were told that alum mixed with cream of tartar and tartaric acid could safely be used to clean and whiten teeth; at other times, they were informed that alum was wholly destructive. Sometimes they were warned that acids harmed teeth as much as sugar; then, in the 1880s, they were urged to eat acidic strawberries to remove tartar. Sometimes dentists recommended hard toothbrushes and at other times soft ones. At various times they told patients that it was best to brush horizontally, or up and down, or with a rotary motion. Some denounced using charcoal as a tooth cleanser; others recommended it as safe and effective.

Some misapprehensions were scotched once and for all. By the end of the nineteenth century, all agreed that snuff, which American women had favoured as a tooth cleanser in the 1840s, was just an addiction. And the consensus was that harsh pumice stone damaged teeth. Other advice remained fanciful. Women were told that toothache could be caused by sitting on damp grass or remaining out among trees with the head uncovered after nightfall.[61] And seductive marketing still encouraged sugar consumption. In the 1930s, one advertisement told women to 'Eat more sweets.' It claimed that candies kept women looking young, made the mouth seem prettier, and entranced a future husband; the lover saw his gift becoming part of his beloved: 'It was a symbol of the future when he might be privileged to supply her with permanent nourishment.'[62]

Teeth were never just a vanity or a health issue. They had economic value. A fine set of teeth could help a woman hook a wealthy husband. Good teeth were essential in occupations where individuals needed to speak clearly – on the stage, for example, although in the 1790s critics noted that 'a ballad-singer without teeth' and a voice 'as hoarse as the raven' could still delight the common people.[63] Women in business found that teeth helped to create a good impression. Betty Bentley Beaumont, who emigrated to North America and became a successful merchant, returned to 'black and smoky' Liverpool in 1866. She broke two teeth on the voyage, eating 'sea-crackers as hard as boards', and one of her first tasks was to visit the dentist with her father:

> My plate being finished, it was put in my mouth; it felt very awkward and uncomfortable; it seemed to me that every one could observe that I had false teeth.
>
> Father was delighted, saying that my appearance was so greatly improved he was quite willing for me to go about and attend to business and pleasure.[64]

A businesswoman had to maintain her appearance.

In the early twentieth century, dentists promoted their wares through the women's suffrage movement, claiming, 'We are in business to make women equal as far as their teeth are concerned.'[65] Employers still discriminated on appearance when hiring staff, which especially affected women. In response, cut-price establishments like the London Tooth Institute provided cheap dentures to servants and working women (but not to the destitute), and there were rare cases of workhouses paying for a poor woman's dentures so that she could earn a living.[66]

Toothcare was vitally important for women who worked in dangerous industries. Hatters and fur-pullers suffered mercury poisoning, which loosened and blackened teeth. Across Europe, matchgirls exposed to white phosphorus were known to be at greater risk of contracting phossy jaw if their teeth were in poor condition, because toxic particles entered the system through cracks and holes in the teeth. Bryant & May, Britain's largest manufacturer of matches, tried to conceal the prevalence of the disease in its factories. If a woman appeared with a swollen face, she had to have her teeth out on pain of dismissal; an in-house dentist might supply dentures to those forced to have extractions. But fear of both the dentist and the sack encouraged matchgirls to hide symptoms.[67]

Many sufferers in advanced stages of phossy jaw lived as social outcasts in London's East End due to disfigurement and the foul odour of suppurating abscesses in the mouth. When the scandal was exposed, in the 1890s, dentists called for more preventative measures at match works. These included regular dental inspections, the provision of mouth washes, and appropriate measures to prevent workers with defective teeth from continuing in the trade. After the First World War, at the Bryant & May factory in Bootle, all the women were given a toothbrush and a box of powder for cleaning their teeth.

SLOW PROGRESS

At the turn of the twentieth century, public health concerns about teeth increased. A 1904 advertisement for the dentifrice Rubifoam reminded readers that in the past people had been duped by all kinds of pastes and tooth powders which had proved to be harmful. But 'in the present age ... of the wireless telegraph, of the telephone, the cablegram', Rubifoam offered the ideal toothwash. 'The men and women who would lead in the world's progress must have good teeth', the advertisement continued; pioneers on the road to a better life would have the sense to use Rubifoam for health and beauty.[68] By 1915, in North America especially, there was greater faith in the ability of dentists to save teeth. Beauty manuals aimed at the middle classes no longer advised having teeth extracted as soon as they became troublesome, as they had earlier.

Even so, for the bulk of the European population, progress in dental health was slow. It was common for young women even in their early twenties to have few teeth.[69] The school inspections that several Western nations introduced at the turn of the twentieth century revealed that around 80 per cent of schoolchildren had dental decay due to neglect and poor diet.[70] Parents took little action until teeth had to be extracted. Behind such statistics lay awful suffering. As late as 1914, a London labourer's daughter died of septic teeth, and similar conditions contributed to the chronic ill health of many working-class women; some doctors thought that severe neuralgia in pregnancy could be due to poor teeth.[71]

In Britain, working-class children simply did not clean their teeth even in respectable families. George Orwell, in his searing account of life in Yorkshire and Lancashire before the Second World War, noted that 'various people gave me their opinion that it is best to "get shut of" your teeth as early in life as possible. "Teeth is just a misery," one woman said to me.'[72] The ill-fitting dentures on offer might lead to further disappointment. One woman hanged herself in the 1930s because she thought false teeth had spoiled her looks.[73]

Meanwhile, in the United States, use of the toothbrush had become part of the sanitary behaviour expected of a full citizen by the early twentieth century. African Americans early recognised that the toothbrush had a part to play in their determination to achieve social equality, and shared the latest scientific advice on oral health. White slaveowners had routinely withheld toothbrushes and tooth powder from the enslaved, an easy means of maintaining perceived racial differences. But as these dental products became more affordable, African Americans briskly adopted them to help challenge white perceptions of their ethnic group.[74]

African American newspapers played a part in spreading the word that oral hygiene was an indicator of status and character, and that poor teeth signalled an absence of the discipline needed to follow hygienic habits and eat the right foods, not just a lack of means. This message was implicit in the advertisements they carried for dental products. A promotion for Odol mouthwash, for example, claimed that it 'ought to be found in every house where good teeth and healthy mouths are valued as they should be'.[75] The *Chicago Defender* gave African American readers firm advice about selecting the right toothbrush and effective brushing, and also promoted a calcium-rich diet for healthy teeth. In 1931, the newspaper teamed up with the Lincoln Dental Society to promote good mouth health, inviting questions about dental care and printing answers in a regular column. Enquiries from female readers allowed it to scotch a long-held misconception that it was unsafe to have extractions when pregnant, and to insist on the importance of tooth care for health and a long life.[76]

In Britain, sustained attention was paid to the nation's dental habits only in wartime. During the First World War, the appalling condition of the nation's teeth became a public issue. Bad teeth meant poor health at a time when the nation had to be strong. One dentist insisted, 'On our teeth depends the whole future stamina of the nation', although he was ready to admit that for women and girls natural beauty was also a consideration.[77] The Ivory Cross National Dental Aid Fund was founded to fix the teeth of soldiers and sailors. When the War Office started to provide dental care for the military, the Fund widened its remit to cover the poor, including mothers and children. During the Second World War, it specifically targeted the wives and children of men serving in the forces.

On both sides of the Atlantic, a wife's oral hygiene became implicated in her duty to maintain a stable family in wartime. In *The Waste Land*, T. S. Eliot includes a pub conversation between two women at the end of the First World War. They talk about Lil, whose husband is about to be demobbed. He had given her money for false teeth but, so far, she had done nothing about it. Her friend had urged her to get her teeth done: 'He's been in the army four years, he wants a good time, / And if you don't give it him, there's others will, I said.'[78] Lil was only thirty-one, but a hard life had already made her look 'antique'. In 1942, a female doctor in North America gave the same advice to a nervous, unhappy woman, 'fifty-six years old and minus all of her teeth'. Her husband had begun 'running around'; home life had fallen into 'tears and quarrels and recrimination'. The doctor gave the woman medicine for her nerves and told her to 'Stay at home and make her husband comfortable and stop nagging at him. First of all, she must get some teeth and fix herself up.'[79]

In Britain, there was a rush to get dental treatment after the introduction of the National Health Service in 1948. In its first year alone, the NHS supplied two million sets of false teeth. Many people preferred dentures to having teeth drilled and filled. Nineteenth-century fillings, which often led to horrible pain, had given fillings a bad reputation, and dental drills were primitive compared to the high-speed models of today. One woman described her ordeal in the 1930s: 'The pain of the drilling was terrible, I squirmed and wriggled; a moustache of cold sweat formed on my lip and I dug my nails into Betty's hand that I was holding tight. Dr. Goldsmith said for God's sake keep still, I can't do my work.'[80] Although multiple extractions became less common after 1948, many women still had all their teeth pulled, even healthy ones, as a twenty-first birthday present or before marriage. The aim was not to 'burden' future husbands with dental bills. Among poor communities, the practice was still current in the mid-1990s, by which time the process was free under the NHS.

When so many women had dentures, at least there was less shame in wearing them. But by the end of the Second World War, perfect natural teeth already characterised the 'American look' which seemed so hopeful and forward-looking. Hollywood had been influential in fashioning the American smile. Any misalignment of the teeth threw a shadow on film so had to be fixed with a porcelain cap. In contrast, the British at this time were stereotyped as having biscuit-coloured, irregular teeth. Women were always more likely to be disparaged. For example, in anti-smoking campaigns, women who smoked were more heavily criticised for stained teeth than men.

Clean, healthy teeth owe much to culture and economics. Zadie Smith in her novel *White Teeth*, about post-war, multicultural Britain, deftly mocks the notion that snowy teeth are an ethnic characteristic: Clara, a central character who is of mixed heritage, wears false teeth following a road accident. People of colour exposed to a faulty or inadequate diet are no less likely than white people to suffer dental decay and tooth loss. And toothcare was part of their fight for equality; not until the mid-1970s did people of colour have access to false teeth that looked natural. The breakthrough came when a student at Tufts University School of Dental Medicine, Sylvellie R. Cloud, developed a way of using commercial stains to tint the false gums. Before that, the sensitive issue of appearance had been neglected.

Despite huge advances in dental care in the last fifty years, including fluoridation, remineralising toothpastes, invisible braces, and precise, reliable implants, new forms of quackery have emerged. Some dental practices attract readers to their websites with clickbait about the dental problems of historic celebrities like Joan Crawford, or 'before and after' pictures of contemporary Hollywood stars. Then they encourage viewers to think that they, too, need invasive dental treatment to improve their looks. The moral imperative to take care of teeth is no longer uppermost: such websites normalise dental issues, explaining that, in the world of show business today, hard partying and drug use can take its toll on teeth. No matter: the latest procedures can be transformative.

Cosmetic dentistry holds out the promise of confidence, success, and reinvention with style. Customers book a 'smile design consulta-tion' as a first step towards a more youthful look, to be maintained by tooth whitening and other procedures. Although the stories and images on some websites cannot always be verified, the demand for cosmetic dentistry is growing. Demand is highest from young women under the age of forty-five. After all, good teeth also enable fashion statements in dentistry such as inserting jewels into teeth or wearing decorative mouthware like grillz to match a particular outfit. As with false teeth of old, grillz usually need to be removed before eating, although Madonna has boasted that she has learned to eat with hers in place.

Despite the slight risk of lisps, misalignment, and infection, cosmetic treatment is no longer regarded as simple pandering to vanity; personal appearance is understood to be bound up with psychology and general health. The flight of dentists from the NHS in Britain is therefore all the more regrettable. Parts of England, particularly rural and coastal areas, are 'dental deserts' where it is impossible to get NHS treatment. Just as in the nineteenth century, when sufferers were tempted to fill their own teeth with products sold by chemists, some now resort to DIY dentistry and Super Glue. After seventy years of progress, when the state of the nation's teeth improved and dentists even feared that the sophisticated art of making acrylic and porcelain teeth would be lost due to lack of practice, we may be going backwards. No woman wants to return to a time when female mentors advised that just four things made life worth living: a good husband, good shoes, good corsets, and good false teeth.[81]

HAIR

Hair is one of the most powerful bodily means of expressing identity. It can be curled, straightened, dyed, cut, extended, styled in myriad ways, sculpted, or left to stir with the wind. It can signal age, gender identity, sexual orientation, class, ethnicity, wealth, personality, and even political affiliation. Various hair colours have been popular at different times. In seventeenth-century England, lustrous dark hair was favoured. Today, blonde hair dye outsells all others and women with fair hair expect to be asked if it is natural. Absurdly, hair colour and texture are associated with different temperaments. Red hair is the most problematic, linked in medieval times with lust or treachery and still taken to signal a feisty character. Curls commonly suggest vivacity, while smooth, straight hair implies an even character and strength of purpose. Hair carries such an emotional and sexual charge that strict patriarchal religions try to make women cover it up, although many women choose to do so as part of a modest dress code. Hair enables the discussion of large issues but the starting point is usually at individual level.

The politics of hair is a study in itself. Women were mostly excluded from political life before the twentieth century but sought to influence opinion. Hairstyles helped them to do this. One approach was to wear hair ribbons in political colours. The elite had more options. In 1756, when war broke out with France, British women displayed their military zeal by fixing model warships to their hair.[1] In 1769, a London hairdresser gave customers forty-five ringlets to support the politician John Wilkes, who famously published a radical piece in number 45 of *The North Briton*. In France, Marie Antoinette used hairstyles to help construct her queenly identity and assert her will. When revolution came, insurgents denounced her extravagant fashions, powdered wigs, and false curls as deceitful and unpatriotic. In prison, her hair seemingly went white overnight and, after the king was executed, she kept it dishevelled as a mark of grief. It was roughly cropped before she was taken to the guillotine. British newspapers reported these dramatic changes to the queen's hair as symbolic of revolutionary barbarity. Some worried that the French revolutionary spirit would spread to Britain. In this febrile atmosphere, whether from misogyny or political bias, women could be abused in London's streets for the way they wore their hair.[2]

The politics of hair extends to sexual, class, and racial issues. The phrase 'Don't touch my hair!' expresses a common female reaction if some elaborate updo is about to be tousled; something like it has echoed down the centuries. But for Black women this is an unmistakeably activist response. Black hairstyling culture is closely associated with the fight against racial oppression. Some Black women spend a lot of money on hair products and many hours in the salon to achieve the look they want. They also have to deal with inept white curiosity about their hair texture – unwanted touching of braids and Afros is an offensive and all too commonplace microaggression.[3]

Hair health is a well-known marker. Shining tresses indicate general good health over a period of time. Hair becomes dull and falls out when we are stressed or unwell, as sufferers of long Covid have experienced. Luxuriant hair is pleasing, perhaps because humans are genetically wired to seek out healthy mates, so women have usually cosseted their locks. Seventeenth-century household manuals contain numerous recipes to colour, preserve, increase, or restore the hair. One extreme remedy for hair loss used burnt pigeon dung mixed with thickly tufted perennial plants. Fortunately, it was scented with rosemary.[4] Victorians reckoned that magnificent, waist-length hair was a young woman's dowry. Hair was to be nurtured from childhood because it could be life-changing on the marriage market.

Hair excites curiosity too. Kept dry, it lasts indefinitely and even seemed to grow after death (though we now know it does not). Hair has long been used in witchcraft. It was a common ingredient in so-called witch bottles, made to release victims from a witch's spell; in folk magic, spells are still sealed into plaits and knots of hair. Yet hair was also the subject of early scientific enquiry. In 1665, the natural philosopher Robert Hooke published drawings of different types of hair examined under his microscope. The instrument had limited powers of magnification, so he was able to confirm only that hair was round and not hollow. His readers were more impressed by his detailed illustration of a magnified louse clinging to a human hair. After all, as Hooke acknowledged, lice intruded themselves into everyone's company at some time or other. Victorian scientists likewise detailed discoveries that pandered to curiosity about hair. They calculated that women bore forty or fifty miles of it on their heads; blondes had about 140,000 filaments to brush each day, redheads just 88,000 or so.[5]

Hair's powerful aura, and the scope for hairstyles to create illusion through artifice, may help to explain why some men feel the need to exert control over women's hairstyles. Samuel Pepys clapped a wig on his own shorn head as soon as wigs were fashionable but kicked up a fuss when his wife experimented with hairpieces. He only allowed her to wear extra curls made of her own hair. Medical men made weighty pronouncements about hair: fever patients should have their heads shaved; women should cut their locks in preparation for childbirth. The eighteenth-century physician George Cheyne declared that blonde women were more given to nervous complaints and went grey early, as if pale locks signalled a wan constitution. His assertions about blondes continued to hold sway into the 1860s.[6]

Regulations about hair can be a means of control. Women in Victorian prisons and workhouses could expect to have their hair shorn as an additional humiliation. They bitterly resented this as an assault on their femininity and sexual identity. The 1865 Prisons Act recognised that it was a cruel and shaming punishment, ruling that women's hair should not be cropped against their will unless verminous. The provision was a clear case of gender stereotyping since it did not apply equally to men; in any case, it was often ignored, and female inmates continued to be cropped without consent. Some employments today constrain the way women can style their hair, especially if a uniform is worn. Women of African descent face outrageous discrimination in workplaces whenever the style of their natural hair is deemed unprofessional. Yet hair is also strongly associated with creativity and defiance. Laetitia Ky, an artist from Africa's Ivory Coast, tackles issues of racism and sexism by dramatically sculpting her own hair. One of her remarkable hairstyles showed a uterus with a middle finger on each side instead of ovaries – a protest against anti-abortion laws in the United States.

This chapter explores the rich meanings of women's hair. How did people use hair to express status in the past? To what extent is hair an essential part of ethnic and gender identity today? It also covers practical matters, including historic methods of curling and dyeing, and various styling products, from greasy pomades to modern formulas with vitamins and oils that promise healthy hair and flexible control.

HAIR AND COMMUNICATION

All hair, real or false, makes a statement. The eloquence of hair is reflected in popular idioms, from splitting hairs to making hair stand on end, from letting one's hair down to tearing it out. Women have always styled their hair to express individuality, even when many possessed no mirror to help them. Yet hair is also a means of establishing common cultural identity. Lady Mary Wortley Montagu, visiting Vienna in 1716, noted the 'monstrous' hair fashion of local women: they piled their hair more than a yard high and decorated it with three or four rows of huge bodkins made of diamonds, pearls, and red, green, and yellow stones.[7] In nineteenth-century Varese, even the poorest women wore expensive pins in their hair, usually eighteen to twenty, in the shape of a half-coronet.[8] Women of African descent have preserved traditional hairstyles despite oppression. These styles are a link with ancestors where no written records exist, a mark of identity, and a source of great pride.[9] Cultural appropriation of African techniques, such as white people perming their straight hair frizzy to mimic Black hair texture, is a sensitive issue today.

Women are judged on the style and condition of their hair. Such appraisals are often infused with snobbery. The uncharitable Lady Craven, visiting Genoa in 1785, commented, 'The females among the lower class disgusted me much by their head-dress – their hair is strained up to a point on the top of their head, and fastened to a pin – judge what a figure an old greyheaded or bald woman must make.'[10] A modern linguistic equivalent of her snobbery might be 'the council house facelift', which describes a working-class style in which the hair is scraped back into a ponytail so high that it stretches the skin. Even so, hair is usually central to women's self-esteem at all social levels. A Victorian reformer, investigating London's deprived East End, was surprised to find impoverished women busy curling their hair. A bonnet-maker explained why she made time to frizz hers after a long day's work: 'It's the only thing I ever do for myself from week's end to week's end; it's the only pleasure I have in my life.' A laundrywoman claimed, 'if it wer'n't for doin' up her hair at night, she'd drown herself or worse'.[11]

Good-looking hair is commonly part of an individual's power, or at least a source of confidence. Hairstyling reflects class and education; it alters with region and fashion. Women can therefore use hair to make and remake their identity. The sheer importance attached to hair in the Western world led to the denigration of African hair, viewed as inferior because it did not lend itself to fashionable European styles. Black women have faced criticism and exclusion as few other social groups have, so hair can be a complex concern. Due to mixed ancestries, Black hair varies, but some types can be dry, fragile, and easily broken. This hair needs exceptional care. The loose curls of people of mixed heritage also require some special maintenance. Every woman wants a hairstyle that will help her to feel more confident, especially when growing up, but, in the West, hairstyling for Black women navigates a difficult path between Western and African ideals of beauty and ethnic identity. On the positive side, this can prompt trendsetting originality. Black women's hairstyling is often at the forefront of innovation and self-assertion, setting a model for others and resisting easy definition.

Hair is both reverenced and fetishised. Lovers exchange hair, a practice that was widespread before technology improved communication, especially in wartime when lovers faced months and years of separation. Lockets and brooches were made with compartments for hair, kept close about the person. When hair oil reigned, such gifts had to be carefully dabbed: 'A lover is a little startled, when he finds the paper, in which a lock of hair has been enclosed, stained and spotted as if it had wrapped a cheesecake.'[12] Because hair endures, it was also fashioned into mourning jewellery symbolising the immortal soul of the departed. Commemorative pieces originally marked the passing of someone of high worth, but by the eighteenth century mourning jewellery had become popular and was rapidly commercialised. It had sentimental value but effectively drew attention to mourners themselves, underlining their grief.

Hair once had a kind of currency. The elite might send locks of hair to friends as a mark of favour. Public figures might receive a lock of hair from an admirer as a sincere tribute. In 1829, Jane Welsh Carlyle sent a tress to the polymath Goethe, enclosed in a letter from her husband so that there could be no misunderstanding. Women also gave hair to cement female friendships, exchanging locket strings, for example, made of their plaited hair. Victorian wives and daughters embroidered hair-pin cushions that, like other crafted items, signalled a loving home.

Women's evening haircare regimes invited the exchange of confidences. When the young Jane Welsh Carlyle visited her friend Eliza

Stodart, each evening the two girls said 'Goodnight' to their elders, then went to a bedroom where a fire was burning to 'do up' their hair and chat before going to bed.[13] Hair grooming still creates a supportive feminine space, most notably for women of South Asian and African heritages. The regular hair oiling and scalp massage for women of South Asian heritage, and the complex weaving and plaiting of Afro hair, provide opportunities to pass on rituals and techniques relating to hair-care, together with stories and gossip that help to bond communities together.

HAIR AND SEXUAL POWER

In England, women began to experiment markedly with hairstyles after 1660, when the restoration of Charles II brought more French fashions to court. They still had to observe propriety: a style suitable for a ball was not proper for church. They were also expected to arrange their hair according to their age, rank, and station in life. This form of signal-ling remains common in some cultures: in the Balkans today, there are hair-braiding styles for the different stages in a woman's life; in Senegal and other African countries where people retain traditional hairstyles, those styles differentiate childhood from adulthood and married from unmarried women. In the Western world, from classical times to the twentieth century, hair hanging loose down the back signalled a girl's virginity, modesty, and innocence. As she grew older, it took on conno-tations of sexual availability. Putting up one's hair for the first time signified maturity and marriageability.

Pinned-up hairstyles still needed careful judgement. In the 1750s, the artist William Hogarth used women's hair to help explain his theo-ries of visual beauty. He thought that flowing curls pleased the eye most but warned that a lock falling across the temples was 'too alluring to be strictly decent'.[14] There was a fine line between beauty and vulgarity. Young women were expected to wear fewer hair ornaments than older women. Updos carried layers of meaning, depending on whether the style was loose or tight. Neatness alone in a married woman was deemed elegance, particularly in Victorian times when the middle classes prided themselves on discreet, practical hairstyles.

By extension, the toilette set that took pride of place on a woman's dressing table in the nineteenth century had symbolic value. Often a bridal gift, it signified sexual maturity as well as respectability. After marriage, only a husband would see his wife's hair flowing down her back. The toilette set was rarely used; less expensive, washable brushes and combs were preferred for everyday use. Jane Welsh Carlyle professed to be wholly intimidated by the tortoiseshell brush and comb her husband gave her as a New Year's gift in 1844. The brush alone was the size of a pancake. But even aged fifty she was mortified when two male acquaintances made a surprise visit one evening after she had let her hair down. The modern phrase has a historical explanation!

Women with luxuriant tresses soon learned to use the power of their hair. The Victorian debutante Alice Miles was launched into society at seventeen to marry for money; her family was well connected but financially stretched. She eased her feelings by mocking eligible bachelors in her diary. Blonde and beautiful, she scoffed at the effect that unbinding her hair had on one aristocratic admirer: 'The way he stood motionless and stared at my hair was something fine to see. He was so struck dumb with admiration that he could not even bring out a compliment. An occasional "Oh my God" was the only vent it found in words. He looked so absurdly ugly too . . . it required all my good breeding to prevent me from bursting out laughing.'[15] She also thought men were idiotic to consider her angelic. She knew her good looks owed more to her mother sending her to bed by 10.30 p.m., and to her liking for healthy mutton chops, than to any angelic mindset.

Flowing hair was considered so sensual in an adult woman that it was almost never seen in polite society. Women who wished to show off splendid hair sometimes seized the chance to display it at fancy-dress balls, which were magnificent social events in the Victorian era. At a ball held in Shimla, Mrs William Bliss (Fanny Johnson) appeared as the White Lady of

Avenel, a ghost in Sir Walter Scott's novel *The Monastery*. Her hair touched the ground. One observer gushed afterwards, 'I never saw such hair.'[16]

Hair can be used to blur sexual boundaries. In the eighteenth century, fops ostentatiously aped women's tall hairstyles. When short curls became fashionable after the French Revolution, some women teamed masculine riding habits with a man's hat, worn over hair cut snug. It was a relief to jettison heavy riding wigs made to withstand sweat and weather. In the 1920s, when an androgenous silhouette was stylish, women again cropped their hair. By the 1960s, London and Paris noted that hair was no longer a prime marker of sexual difference as most young people wore their hair long: 'Every other boy-girl hippy-dipping down the rue in a tailored pant-suit, blue denims, Beatle boots and leather racing gloves.'[17] Hair remains a powerful sex symbol but the sexual significance of hair demands finesse; women with 'butch' hairstyles may be asserting their sexuality or repudiating social pressures to appear attractive to men. In any case, women do not style their hair exclusively to attract sexual partners. The hair salon itself, with its rituals and decor, offers a pleasurable escape and even community support.

HAIR AND SOCIAL RANK

Hair still indicates status today. Is it expensively cut and coloured? Obviously tinted at home out of a bottle? Eighteenth-century hairdressers flattered clients by declaring that they styled hair to match their clients' beauty, not their social rank. Yet hairdressers flocked to view aristocrats emerging from court events so that they could copy the latest styles. Elaborate coiffures took time and money. They were a sure sign of a woman's economic status because they could not be achieved without expert help. They also involved costly purchases, including hair powder, powder boxes, puffs, powder bags, powder machines, pomatum, orange-flower water, ribbons, pins, combs, and bear's grease.

Cleopatra is said to have been an early fan of bear's grease. Bears have strong, thick coats, so people assumed that rendered bear fat gave strength and vigour to the hair. It was advertised as a cure for baldness. From the mid-seventeenth century, Britain imported tons of bear fat each year from France; Russian bears were thought to yield the best. The fat was refined after import, mixed with beef marrow, and perfumed. The genuine article was often in short supply, so bear's grease was routinely adulterated with pig's fat or lard. Some retailers invited customers to see the fat cut from recently slaughtered bears to be sure of the genuine article. In the 1790s, Reeves Perfumery Warehouse and Ornamental Hair Manufactory in Holborn advertised that it killed one fat bear each month.[18]

Throughout the eighteenth century, hairstyles grew more extravagant among the European aristocracy as they became a mark of high fashion and refinement. By the 1770s, updos were very tall as women claimed more physical space in their bid to assert status. Some wore wigs. Otherwise, hairdressers piled heart-shaped pads of horsehair on a woman's head, stuck them together with scented pomade, then covered this tower with her own hair. They dusted the work with powder to add bulk. The total edifice could weigh as much as fourteen ounces and was so stiff it could bear the weight of jewels, flowers, wax fruit, and even wooden models.

This hair fashion soon crossed the Atlantic. One Bostonian woman complained in 1773 that it made the head 'itch, & ach, & burn like anything'.[19] In 1774, Georgiana, Duchess of Devonshire, took extravagance further by wearing a full-sized ostrich plume drooping in an arch over the front of her hair. Her next display was a hair tower fully three feet high, decorated with preposterous ornaments. The tower might take two hairdressers and several hours to complete but that did not stop imitators. It was also expensive. In the 1770s, if a hairdresser came to a London house, his 'dressing' might cost 2s. He would also use as much as two pounds of costly powder.[20]

A richly dressed headpiece, adorned with costly jewels, pompoms and aigrettes, was a target for thieves. In 1785, a London gang went after a group of aristocrats getting into their carriages in Tottenham

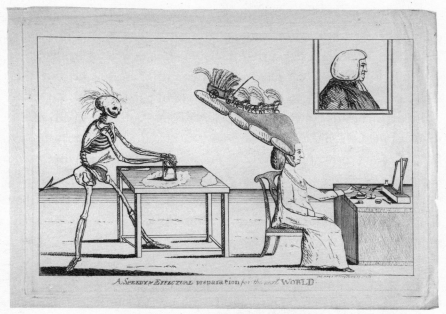

11. A satire on 1770s fashions and female vanity, especially in old age.

Street after a concert. One lady, whose headdress displayed several diamonds, had it torn from her head.[21] Yet female travellers found that elaborate hairdos could equally be good hiding places for their valuables. Female thieves and smugglers also routinely hid booty in their hair.

Towering hairstyles incited misogyny and social division. Men began to object to the greasy stacks as early as 1768, claiming that they stank. One critic described a supposed visit to his elderly aunt just when she was submitting her head to the celebrated hairdresser Peter Gilchrist. Her hair had not been 'opened' for above nine weeks, which, as Gilchrist confirmed, was as long as a head could well go in summer. The writer claimed that he was not so much repelled by the odour when his aunt's hair was undone as by the tiny organisms that swarmed out. He asked Gilchrist if the bugs were not liable to invade other parts of the body, but the hairdresser assured him they could not; the powder and pomatum formed a glutinous matter that clogged them and prevented their migration.[22] While such accounts may be coloured by misogyny, even Gilchrist admitted in his manual on hair that perspiration and a lack of ventilation caused current hairstyles to smell disagreeably.[23]

Some British men objected to women's hair fashions because they disliked male hairdressers, and foreign ones in particular. In the earlier eighteenth century, both male and female hair cutters had advertised their services. Hairdressing was even considered a suitable profession for reformed prostitutes. Yet by mid-century commentators were reporting that aristocratic women, and imitators from the middling sort, now preferred male hairdressers. This disadvantaged working women. The prolific author and actress Eliza Haywood sensed the mood of the times when she wrote:

> There was a time . . . when a virtuous woman would not, except in case of great necessity, have suffer'd her head to be uncover'd in the presence of any man; much less have endur'd that her hair should be handled, stroak'd, and twisted round the fingers of a foppish foreign barber . . . but fashions alter, – and what would forty years ago have been look'd upon as highly indecent, is now polite, because the mode.[24]

Haywood noted that husbands went along with the fashion because they did not want to be thought jealous, but they remained suspicious. Some had just cause: wives ran off with their hairdressers, as contemporary adultery trials show. After a hairdresser's visit, servants were always on the lookout for tell-tale patches of hair powder on the carpet. In any case, hairdressers easily became confidants, and husbands worried about the spread of scandal and gossip in the intimate setting of a lady's dressing room.

The business of keeping hair pest-free caused women great stress. Poor women and lower-class prostitutes often had dirty, verminous heads. In the 1780s, the radical tailor Francis Place noted that the hair of such women 'was straight and "hung in rat tails" over their eyes, and was filled with lice'.[25] The better classes were assumed to be cleaner, but fashion and contemporary hair products worked against this idea. Pomatum was largely grease, sometimes from vegetable oil but usually from animal fat. 'Persian Rose Pomatum', for instance, claimed to be made from 'clarified Bear's Grease, Buffalo's Marrow, and Odour of Roses'.[26] Such products attracted hungry pests. One woman recollected seeing a mouse peep out of the curls of a lady sitting in front of her at church, 'no doubt well fed with so much powder and pomatum'.[27] Mice were liable to enter the hair at night. This prompted the invention of bedside mouse traps and nightcaps made of silver wire that no mouse or rat could gnaw through.[28] Women used head-scratchers and put flea traps in their hair – tiny boxes filled with blood and glue. Hairdressers advised women who always wore their hair dressed to brush it out weekly, but few did because it was apt to tear when combed.

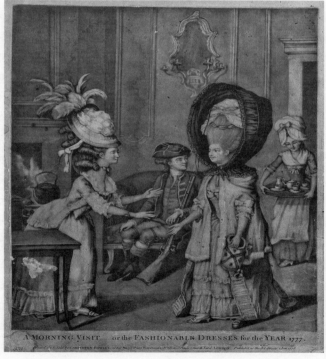

12. *A lady enters a breakfast parlour in an enormous calash protecting her hairdo, 1770s.*

The tall hairstyle was wholly given up in Barbados by 1788, where the heat made it unbearable, and it slowly died out in cooler climates. Whenever harvests failed and food was short, the rich were censured for using starch on their hair while the poor starved. In Revolutionary France, hair powder was shunned because it was associated with the hated aristocracy. In Britain, Prime Minister William Pitt taxed hair powder from 1795 to help pay for war against France, so most stopped using it. Instead, women adopted fresh-looking styles and dressed their hair with flowers. At the same time, suspicions of French hairdressers hardened; some feared they were spies. More women now advertised for maids who could dress hair, and London's hairdressing academies eagerly taught servants the latest techniques.

HAIRCARE AND RESPECTABILITY

Social opinion of women's hair was subtly influenced by the fact that most upper-class men received a classical education, a practice which waned only in the twentieth century. It was an easy step for them to make an unflattering connection between a woman with loose, unkempt hair and the Furies of Greek myth, usually depicted as crones with snaky hair, out to punish men for wrongdoing. For instance, *Cocker's English Dictionary* (1715) defines the Furies as 'Three imaginary hellish Spirits, with Snakes on them instead of Hair', and describes female defenders of Anglesey in Roman times as 'Women running about with their Hair about their Ears . . . like Furies of Hell'.[29] Newspaper reports consistently mentioned dishevelled female hair in connection with street brawls, domestic arguments, and street protests, when women were likely to be grabbed by the hair. This negative view of untamed hair may also owe something to male insecurities: in the Medusa myth, the only way Perseus could regain power from Medusa, cursed with snakes for hair, was by cutting off her head. In reports of adultery trials, disordered hair indicated illicit sex. Dishevelled locks were also a sign of madness: the heroine in the opera *Nina, or The Love-Distressed Maid*, first staged in 1786, signalled that she had become insane by appearing on stage with her hair unbound. The uncoiling of her hair electrified the audience.[30]

In contrast, neatly dressed hair was a sign of respectability and good taste, as Jane Austen knew when she praised the hair of Charlotte Craven, a family friend: 'She looks very well & her hair is done up with an elegance to do credit to any Education.'[31] Dressing the hair remained expensive: by the 1820s an acclaimed hairdresser could charge 10s for each person.[32] In the nineteenth century, hairstyling became ever more monitored among the well-to-do; fashion magazines recommended styles for morning, afternoon, and evening, depending on event. The upper classes, when commenting on the distress of the poor, were tempted to blame slatternly wives rather than poverty wages. They advised poor women to keep their hair neatly dressed, claiming that ragtag looks could drive husbands to the pub as much as a slovenly home.[33]

As the pressure to appear respectable increased, so did the number of hairdressers in major British cities. By the 1850s, it was already common for wealthy women to pop to a hairdresser before a dinner party. In London, most stylists were still men; when women of the middling sort went to have their hair cut, they might take a companion as chaperone. Then, in 1868, London hairdressers went on strike. One canny West End hairdresser, Robert Douglas, employed women as strike-breakers. It pointed the way to a business opportunity. The following year he set up a ladies' parlour; it proved so popular with female clients that increasing numbers of women went into hairdressing. George Eliot had a female acquaintance who set up on her own after being treated shabbily by her employer. She was expected to make a fortune.[34]

Cultural codes of modesty dictated that respectable women covered their hair in public, unless attending a formal evening event like an opera or ball. In the eighteenth century, women of all classes and stations wore a cap, though its quality varied with a person's wealth. From the 1780s, women might even wear their hat on top of the cap. Modesty aside, head coverings were protective and helped to keep hair free from grime. They also saved time. Jane Austen wrote, 'I have made myself two or three caps to wear of evenings since I came home, and they save me a world of torment as to hair-dressing, which at present gives me no trouble beyond washing and brushing, for my long hair is always plaited up out of sight, and my short hair curls well enough to want no papering'.[35] Marriage had passed Austen by and she aimed only to make her hair neat. The cap indicated propriety. When a nurse married a soldier and ditched her cap at once, appearing in her own hair as a married lady, other women were quick to pass censure.[36]

The link between loose hair and potentially loose morals was familiar to all. A young woman's first grown-up hat was a milestone, and it was 'improper' for adult women to venture out of the house bareheaded. But headdresses could be troublesome in themselves. Women's hats were a cause of complaint in church if they blocked people's view of the parson. In the nineteenth century, some theatre managers tried to ban women's hats, which obscured the stage. (Unlike men, they did not check them in at a cloakroom.) The bans proved unworkable. Once dressed, her bodice fastened up, a woman simply could not reach her hat. One reporter confirmed, 'she can no more put on her hat with her corsage buttoned, or take it off, than she can stand on her head'.[37]

Married women in orthodox Jewish communities are still expected to cover their heads with a wig or hat. The dress code for conservative Muslims requires women to cover their heads, and the modest dress movement appeals to a range of Muslim women who opt to wear head-wear. But for most women in the West, the habit of covering at least the top of the head weakened from the 1920s. The hat or head covering began to feel like a symbol of the conventions created by men to govern the bodies of women; growing numbers of women who wished to make a statement about their modernity and independence simply left it off. There were practical considerations, too. Hats did not always suit the latest hairstyles, or women's busy routines. Sunglasses also became more affordable from the 1940s, so a hat was not needed to shade the eyes. That said, women commonly wore hats into the 1950s.

GREY HAIR AND DYES

Today, hair is usually on show. The ageing of hair causes anxiety, and the modern haircare industry reveals how these concerns can be exploited. Yet hair has always affected women's sense of self. In 1828, the poet Caroline Bowles complained wittily, 'It is very hard one cannot be permitted to grow old and ugly without one's very identity being called in question . . . I never meet with any person who has not seen me for years, without being questioned (after a few oblique glances) as to what I have done with my hair.'[38] She joked that, since few believed her hair had ever been glorious, she would get the few surviving witnesses to sign a certificate as proof. She was only forty-one.

For women, grey hair is generally an unwelcome sign of age. Sarah, Duchess of Marlborough, noted for her rich blonde hair, preserved its colour by washing it in honey water. She loathed the fashion for hair powder. Hairdressers routinely had to reassure women that it would not actually colour the hair grey. But women who tried to preserve youthful hair risked pity and ridicule. Maria Edgeworth commented in 1830 that Lady Charlotte Bury might have been beautiful once but 'she dresses too young and is not well made-up – her own gray [sic] hair coming here and there into view between the false – too evidently false masses of brown'.[39] When, in the 1830s, older women in France were said to be wearing their own grey hair to evening parties, without hat or cap, Emma Willard, who campaigned for female education in North America, was so impressed by this liberated stance that she commented, 'the hair, the complexion, and the figure each suit the other; and why should ladies conceal grey hairs more than gentlemen?' But few dared admit to fading hair. Bury also learned that 'there are persons in Paris who earn their living by plucking the white hairs from ladies heads'.[40]

Grey hair was socially downgrading for women. Jane Welsh Carlyle revealed as much when she railed at the expectation that women would 'wear caps at "a certain age" for all that one's hair don't turn grey!'[41] But time takes its toll, although genetics, health, lifestyle, nutrition, and exposure to chemicals all play a part. Madame Bayard, in her beauty manual of 1876, advised readers to hide thinning hair and bald patches under a pretty cap, even though the young no longer wore caps. Women's magazines were already promoting suitable hairstyles for different life stages. Even in the twenty-first century there are debates about how hair should be styled in later life, including whether women can wear long hair over forty.[42]

Many grey-haired women resort to hair dye. After all, women have dyed their hair for centuries, often just to obtain a fashionable colour. During the Renaissance, Venetians bleached their locks with strong alkalis, then sat in the sun for hours to turn them blonde. In seventeenth-century England, fair women brightened their tresses with a decoction made from turmeric and alum. Because red hair was vilified, some of the earliest dyes claimed to turn it brown. In the 1760s, advertisements for Clarke's Liquid said that, if used on redheads from childhood, the world need never know their natural hair colour.[43] When hair powder was commonly worn, white powder concealed grey hairs pretty well, and coloured powders were available from the mid-eighteenth century. Women could also buy black pomatum to stain grey hair. But such dyes rarely produced good results; brown colours for red or grey hair left purple tints and stained linen. A lead comb gradually darkened hair but the effect was often streaky.

Outwardly, Victorians held that no respectable woman would dye her hair, but clearly many did. Sometimes they used the pretext of needing to revive the hair after a period of illness. Recipes for convalescent hair washes included cochineal to give an auburn tint. And temporary hair dyes might be advertised as acceptable. In the 1880s, a North American beauty catalogue offered Persian Khennaline Hair Stainer for instant results, 'free from the usual odium' attached to lasting hair dyes.[44]

The difficulty for women who needed to colour their hair was that, even in Victorian times, commercial preparations contained ingredients such as lead, sulphur, mercury, or nitrate of silver which damaged health. Strong chemicals caused skin irritation and hair loss. Critics claimed that ironically such products themselves turned hair prematurely grey. Beauty manuals offered safe dyes using nuts and roots, but these organic preparations had little effect, so the same manuals also offered recipes that called for dangerous white lead and quicklime. There was no safe way to bleach hair; beauty advisors warned that repeated use of hydrogen peroxide made hair brittle.

In any case, Victorian dyes fooled no one. In the 1860s, a brash yellow was produced using arsenic; the colour was associated with prostitutes. There was no good brown dye – most gave the hair a greenish tint. Black dyes left a purplish hue. And the colouring process was so onerous, taking two to three hours, that ladies were known to faint. Bizarre deaths were traced to poisonous hair dyes. The renowned French actress Mademoiselle Mars (real name Anne Françoise Boutet) is said to have died in 1847 from too liberal a use of hair dye. But the fact that women took such risks underlines the strong incentive to change hair colour.

The French chemist Eugène Schueller developed safer synthetic hair dyes from 1907 and founded L'Oréal two years later. To help sell the dyes, he launched a women's hairdressing magazine. During the 1920s, it contained many articles about the need to conceal grey hair, said to disadvantage women at social events and in the workplace.[45] Women began to spend more money on hair restorers and dyes, not least because in the early twentieth century there was increasing competition in the labour market. Now women with greying hair not only feared for their marriage but also worried that they would be replaced at work or find it harder to get the jobs they wanted. Advertisements for hair products played on these fears.[46]

The prejudice against dyed hair lessened markedly once the Hollywood star Jean Harlow became platinum blonde in the 1930s. Few admirers knew that the bleach treatments damaged her hair so badly that she had to film in wigs until it recovered. Fortunately, hair colouring today seems to have few health risks, although one common ingredient, paraphenylenediamine, causes digestive troubles and other allergic reactions in susceptible individuals. It has been used since the late nineteenth century since no alternative has been found to colour grey hair so well. Today, the creation of hair dyes is increasingly a science, while remedies for ageing hair are more sophisticated than ever, ranging from food supplements to hair transplants. Women can change their hair colour on a whim and some dramatically contest ageism, flooding Twitter feeds with selfies showing hair dyed fuchsia or arctic blue.

FALSE HAIR

If grey hair causes stress, hair loss has always been terrifying for women. In the days before permanent waving, hot tongs were mostly used to curl hair. Beauty experts warned that tongs injured hair follicles, and caused hairs to split, grow brittle, and fall out. Although curling fluids were touted as having all sorts of benefits, including strengthening the brain, many proved destructive. Even if women tried not to scorch hair, hot tongs took away its natural gloss. Women of African descent and others who straightened their hair with a hot comb and hair relaxers risked severe damage and breakage. Yet in centuries gone by, when few people washed their hair, and scalps accumulated dirt and scurf, hair loss resulted as much from neglect as from dangerous treatments.

The truism that a woman's hair is her 'crowning glory', endlessly repeated in the nineteenth century, reinforced unrealistic expectations of the abundance of women's hair. Even a radical suffragette newspaper stated, 'Without a fine head of hair no woman can be really beautiful.'[47] Yet due to poor diet or ill health, many women would never have good hair. Victorian beauty manuals agreed that it was harder to obtain luxuriant hair than to get a fine figure or clear complexion.

There were various home remedies for thinning hair. Eighteenth-century pundits recommended rubbing the scalp daily with vinegar or a raw onion.[48] Dr Campbell's Red Blood Forming Capsuloids offered a more complex solution. Launched in 1897 as a general tonic, this quack medicine was soon rebranded as a cure for baldness. It claimed to work through the bloodstream, killing off germs surrounding the hair follicle and allowing it to get the nourishment needed. After seven months, hair would be four feet long. Manufacturers of the product had to scotch rumours that it would also increase facial hair; depilatories for whiskers and bushy eyebrows have as long a history as hair restorers.

From 1850, the pressure to have 'big hair' led to a surge in the use of hairpieces. Sales rose by 400 per cent between 1855 and 1868.[49] There were switches, tufts, curls, and braids to suit every purse and hide every flaw. Since fashion called for unrealistic quantities of hair, women plaited false tresses into their own, or just pinned on 'borrowed locks' to save time and trouble. False hair became so common than many no longer denied wearing it. Yet it was one thing to add a few braids and quite another to disguise bald patches, so some still maintained that their hair was all their own. Women's hair tends to thin around the mid-scalp and frontal areas. Styles which constantly strain the hair back, particularly around the hairline, can lead to baldness. In Victorian times, continual frizzing aggravated the problem. Many opted for 'invisible fronts', or toupees worked on hair lace, which proved useful under hats or bonnets. But, as in the case of women's corsets, the growing popularity of illustrated advertising gave the game away.

Some women wore toupees simply for convenience. In 1802, Lady Stanley sent some of her own hair to be matched for a false fillet 'as my front hair is always coming out of curl in the damp summer evenings, and as I find everybody sports a false *toupée*, I don't see why I should not have the comfort of one too'.[50] But she did want it to be deceiving as well as fashionable. In the early twentieth century, 'damp-proof cycling fringes' were popular for seaside wear, while those who wished to appear seductive in a skin-tight bathing hat sewed a fringe of curls around the edges.[51]

Trade in human hair has long been global. In the eighteenth century, high-quality false hair was so costly that shipments from Europe might be smuggled into Britain. Thieves targeted hair merchants because human hair could easily be turned into cash. Brittany was a major source; peasant girls grew their locks for money, though it might take several years to achieve a valuable length. As Breton women wore close caps, the loss could be hidden until the next crop. A good trade was also done in convents, where hair was shorn. But, by the 1880s, much hair came from China. Marseille was the centre of the French wig trade and as much as half of the eighty tons used annually came from China.[52]

Hairdressers promoted styles that needed false hair because they made more money from selling it than from styling alone. Wigmakers increasingly made almost undetectable hairpieces and naturally encouraged women to wear them. They were popular in nineteenth-century North America, where there was a brisk postal trade and rural women ordered styles from illustrated catalogues. Swatches of hair were routinely smuggled into New York to be sold to wigmakers. Once liners docked, customs officers looked out for female passengers who walked stiffly or could not sit: one smuggler had $2,000 worth of hair sewn into her underclothing; another wore an underskirt so loaded with hair it weighed forty pounds.[53]

Some wigmakers used hair that posed a health risk because it came from prisons or dead people, or from French and Italian rakers who cleaned gutters and retrieved combings to supplement their income. Combings were naturally shed hair, removed from brushes and discarded. Periodically, there were contagion scares. In the 1860s, reports circulated that hair imported from Russia was infested with gregarines, microscopic parasites deposited by lice. Cheap false chignons were often made of horsehair wrapped in human hair, and some worried they could harbour disease. (Workers in horsehair were known to die of anthrax.) Such fears proved unfounded, but women were advised to dip false hair into concentrated ammonia liquid to kill parasites. Some played safe, kept all their combings, and had hairpieces made of their own dead hair. The result lacked lustre but was always a perfect match. Toilette sets often included a hair receiver – a pot with a small hole in the lid for combings.

Black women, under pressure to adopt Western styles in the workplace, found that hairpieces offered ready solutions. African American newspapers carried advertisements for the false chignons and braids of an earlier era into the late 1940s. Today, Black women choose extra plaits and hair extensions to achieve a style of choice, not to conform to an ideal. Weaves, sewn into the hair, have been around since the 1950s, offering options for length, volume, and colour, although some of African heritage object that they are not culturally authentic. White women who choose weaves for fuller hair are advised to go to expert Black hairdressers for a longer-lasting result. Other types of hair extensions can be clipped, taped, or bonded to natural roots. These are safer than they used to be but can still damage follicles.

Full wigs conceal hair loss from accident or ill health. In the past, wigs had the added benefit of concealing ugly scalp conditions, or just greying hair. Those with a busy social life often found it easier to wear a wig; in the 1770s, women sporting tall hairstyles could spend three hours just undressing. Wigs could be a status symbol when coated with expensive hair powder, but the elite still wore wigs even after powder became unfashionable. Elizabeth Grant remembered that, around 1810, her mother shopped for wigs in London: 'every woman, not alone the grey and the bald, wore an expensive wig instead of her own hair', while at court the princesses had their heads shaved and wore wigs dressed for evening wear to save time.[54] Older widows almost always shaved their heads and wore a wig. Some women saw no need for pretence and might even wear different colour wigs on the same day. Not all men approved; Sir William Hamilton insisted in 1798 that Emma wear her own hair.[55] But full wigs were particularly useful in the countryside, where hairdressers were scarce. And wigs were worn at the seaside, either as a kind of bathing hat or because curls drooped in the damp air.

In the late 1960s, low-cost, synthetic hair brought full wigs into fashion once more; women could change their looks and personality at will or just give their morale an instant boost. Wigs remain popular with Black women; they are convenient, cover any hair damage, and allow quick alignment with perceived codes of dress. And, as always, wigs offer a chance to experiment.

CLEANING HAIR

Fanny Kemble, reflecting in 1831 on hairstyles of the Georgian age, concluded 'we are certainly cleaner than our grandmothers'.[56] No longer was hair caked for weeks in a thick paste of flour and grease. Yet washing the hair was still a matter of debate. In the 1770s, the hairdresser Peter Gilchrist had advised women who bathed that they should never wet their hair, unless for their health. He told mothers that the best way to clean a child's head was to rub it with a linen cloth dipped in pomatum or hog's lard.[57] Some still feared that washing opened the pores to foreign substances. Even in the nineteenth century, hair washing might be a seasonal event. Girls in the Highlands washed their heads in spring with a decoction made from the young buds of birch trees. The Presbyterian kirk would then be agreeably scented, not reeking from snuff and peat smoke.[58]

In Britain from the 1830s, as hygiene became a symbol of respectability, beauty manuals included more advice about how to clean hair. Madame Bayard, writing in 1876, thought 'perfect cleanliness' indispensable to preserving the health and colour of hair, and advised regular washing with tepid water and mild soap. But she understood the practical difficulties: 'Ladies, on account of the length of their hair, cannot altogether avail themselves of water to clean it.' Alternatives included brushing finely powdered bran through the hair, or moistening it with egg yolk and lemon juice, allowing the application to dry, and brushing it out again. Some writers recommended sponging long hair with rosemary tea or quinine water, or just cleaning the roots with soap and water, or hartshorn.[59]

The Victorian adage 'Wash the scalp, but not the hair; comb the hair, but not the scalp' indicates how finely balanced hair advice could be.[60] If some thought that washing the hair made it healthy, others said it made hair brittle and weakened the roots.[61] A monthly wash seemed adequate, although the edges of the scalp about the face and neck might have to be wiped more often if exposed to black train smoke. But inevitably there was a difference between advice and practice: women busy with housework might not wash their hair for six weeks or more; accumulated dust was blamed for hair loss before the age of forty. But since women needed three bowls of warm water to wash long hair, and all morning to dry it, the operation was a luxury.[62] The thrifty middle classes revived the custom of wearing hair powder, which helped to keep styles in place without grease and postponed the need for washing. The powder, allegedly superior to the meal used in the eighteenth century, was not supposed to form a paste or make the hair wig-like.

Some beauty experts made the best of a bad situation and emphasised the importance of ventilating hair rather than washing it.[63] Hair had to be well brushed and combed, strand by strand, to prevent it becoming stiff and filthy; it should be loosely plaited for bed. Vigorous daily brushing for hair health and lustre became a mantra. By the 1890s, hairdressers recommended thirty minutes a day at the very least.[64] Those who were too weary to give their hair a routine hundred brush strokes a day could have their scalps mechanically brushed at the hairdressers. Originally this sensational equipment was reserved for men: there were fears that the rotary brush would become entangled in women's long hair. But in 1865 another pulley was added to draw the brush downwards in an extended sweep, which solved the problem. The power source was a wheel turned by a child, or sometimes a dog, but large establishments used steam or water power.

It was also axiomatic that hair had to be nourished to promote youthful luxuriance. Women used pomatum, brushed through their tresses, or doused locks with hair restorers, which, in the eighteenth century, had included ingredients to deter vermin. By the 1890s, pomade had the reputation of being vulgar, perhaps because some brands added colouring agents. Lighter hair oils then held sway and Rowland's

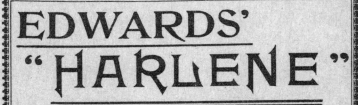

EDWARDS'
"HARLENE"

FOR THE

HAIR.

USED EVERYWHERE.
THE CERTAIN PROOF THAT
IT HAS NO EQUAL.

RESTORES THE HAIR.
PROMOTES THE GROWTH.
ARRESTS THE FALL.
STRENGTHENS THE ROOTS.

THE
Very Finest Dressing.
Specially Prepared and Perfumed
FRAGRANT AND REFRESHING.
Is a Luxury and a Necessity to every
Modern Toilet.

WITHOUT A RIVAL.

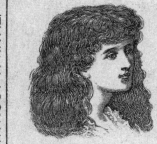
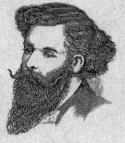

HEALTH TO THE HAIR.

AVOID IMITATIONS.

EDWARDS' 'HARLENE' Preserves, Strengthens and Invigorates CHILDREN'S HAIR.

It acts as a Tonic, and where it is used no other Preparation is necessary.

For Preserving and Rendering the Hair Beautifully Soft; for Removing, Dandruff &c.

1s., 2s. 6d., and (triple 2s. 6d. size) 4s. 6d. per Bottle, from Chemists,
Hairdressers, and Stores all over the World; or sent direct on receipt of
Postal Orders.

EDWARDS' 'HARLENE' CO., 95 & 96, HIGH HOLBORN,
LONDON W. C.

154=20

13. The reverse of a magazine insert, probably from the 1890s.
Plate 26 shows the other side.

Macassar Oil, allegedly from the Indonesian port city Makassar, cornered the market. The hairdresser Alexander Rowland had first sold it in London in 1809. The oil obtained royal approval and its fame spread to other European cities, North America, and Canada. Advertisements promised that it promoted luxuriant growth and prevented hair from turning grey (the darker version did have a slight colour). Consumers used it liberally, to the extent that house-proud women like Jane Welsh Carlyle worried about oily stains on cushions and furniture.[65] By the 1850s they had invented the antimacassar, a protective cloth for furniture. These drapes were visible proof of the centrality of luxuriant tresses to the Victorian ideal of beauty. Yet as Macassar Oil sullied clothes and bedding, it continued to compound the horrors of laundry day. Some mused that future generations would never understand the word antimacassar since the hair oil itself would have long disappeared, but it was popular well into the twentieth century until clean fluffy hair became desirable.[66]

THE HAIRCARE MARKET

The custom of making hair washes and conditioners at home persisted into Edwardian times, but from the 1880s they were increasingly being made on an industrial scale. Women were a target market because, with rising female employment, more had disposable incomes. The commercial development can be traced in meanings of the word 'shampoo'. It came to Britain from the Indian subcontinent and at first meant the massage element of a Turkish bath. By the twentieth century, a 'shampoo habit' signified a scalp massage, touted to improve mental powers, sooth the nerves, and promote hair growth. Women might shampoo their hair at home using ammonia water.

By the 1890s, hairdressers offered an 'antiseptic shampoo' for dandruff or just a regular clean, but these 'dry shampoos' used petrol as a solvent. The vapours seem to have been implicated in an explosion that caused a double fatality at a Soho hairdressers in 1909; subsequently, the famous hair tonic Petrole Hahn had to guarantee that it was non-flammable and non-explosive.[67] Next, there were powder shampoos to be mixed with water, then wet shampoos available in sachets. The first modern (no soap) shampoo, Drene, was only introduced in the 1930s.

Today, the value of the haircare market is heading towards £100 billion a year. Black women have played a prominent role in the growth of this industry. They found ways to build careers in hair-related commerce and, once successful, to help others in their ethnic group. In Britain, this trend came only with large-scale immigration from the Caribbean in the 1950s. But African Americans early used a range of products to condition and straighten their hair. Living as a minority in a white, racist society, they chose fashionable hairstyles to increase their life chances, not least because plantation slavery had brutally suppressed the intricate and symbolic hair designs of Africa. Commercial straighteners in the late nineteenth century were often spurious, if not harmful to hair, but Ozonized Ox Marrow and a related brand, Ozono, were advertised as safe and effective. Ozono was said to be the invention of a Mrs S. M. Moore, which may have helped to build trust. It claimed that without using injurious hot irons it could straighten 'Knotty, Knappy, Kinky, Stubborn, Harsh, Refractory hair', as if styling was a matter of discipline.[68]

Madam C. J. Walker, said to be the first American millionairess, did promote the hot comb alongside her hair softener and other beauty products, and as a Black woman she helped to sanction hair-straightening in the early twentieth century. Yet there was some resistance to it in the West Indies, where Walker expanded her haircare empire; most young Caribbean girls continued to wear their hair unprocessed into the 1960s.[69] The practice is controversial today because it implies continuing, unacceptable pressure to follow European standards of beauty, but Walker's aim was to boost the confidence of African Americans and raise their prospects. Her products for natural hair enabled women to choose whether to adopt European styles or not. After all, hair-straightening is not always a symbol of Black women's aspirations; many just enjoy the versatility of different hairstyles.

Madam Walker formerly worked for Annie Malone, who also thrived in the haircare industry. In 1918, Malone established a college in St Louis that was part school, part manufacturing plant, part retail business, and part community centre for African Americans. Malone was a multi-millionaire by the 1920s. Some used their hairdressing qualification as a stepping stone to a career in another field, as did Jane Gray, who in 1947 became the first Black laboratory technician at her local hospital in California.[70] South Korean Americans now dominate the retail side of supplying Black haircare products in the United States, as do people of South Asian heritage in Britain. But African American entrepreneurs continue to find specialist areas, such as natural haircare, where their expertise gives them an edge; and increasing numbers of Black British women think it important to support Black-owned hair brands.

When Black women began setting up haircare businesses in Britain, salons appeared first in London then in the Midlands, in step with the Caribbean diaspora. The businesswoman and hairdresser Carmen England paved the way. Born Carmen Maingot in Trinidad, she opened what is believed to have been Britain's first hair-straightening salon, in North Kensington in 1955. It was decorated with a mural by Althea McNish, a designer of African Caribbean descent who went on to achieve international recognition. The following year, the celebrity pianist Winifred Atwell used some of her wealth to open a hairdressing salon in Brixton. At this time, women who had emigrated from the West Indies were finding it almost impossible to get their hair commercially styled. Atwell, a trained pharmacist, had been developing new ways of caring for Black hair, but her public schedule meant that her hair needed to look immaculate most days. She realised that the only way to achieve this was to open her own premises. She launched her modern salon – which boasted rock gardens and television as well as the usual equipment – with tremendous fanfare; a second followed in Mayfair. These women effectively challenged racist policies in an era when many white salon owners barred Black immigrants.

By the 1970s, haircare was a lucrative career for Black women in Britain, and salon ownership a means to get on in the world. Such was the influence of Madam Walker that many Caribbean women went first to her beauty school in the United States to train as beauticians and hairdressers before setting up salons in Britain, even though there were similar opportunities in Britain. Forward-thinking Alfred Morris was training Black and white students in his school of hairdressing from the late 1940s.[71] About a fifth of his student intake came from abroad. Roy Lando, a Jamaican hairdresser, set up his school in north London in 1958.

Afro hairstyling received an enormous boost from the entrepreneurship of Len Dyke and Dudley Dryden, who established their London shop selling cosmetics and records in 1965. At first, they imported skin and hair goods from the United States but then they began to make their own. Dyke and Dryden's beauty products became a multi-million-pound business, stocked in high-street chain stores from the 1980s.

The hair industry in the West has been slow to realise that Black women are an important market. In 1980, the industry's leading international magazines began to carry information about the unique nature of Black hair. Manufacturers developed more products and services to meet the hair needs of a range of consumers of African heritage, also finding a new market in those who wished to celebrate their cultural roots. The number of Black-owned hair businesses has also boomed in recent decades, producing products and accessories for new trends in Afro hair, and responding to the demands of current lifestyle choices, such as the need to keep hair in condition and hydrated when working out. The market is so lucrative that some hairdressing chains in Britain, mostly attracting white clients, give staff extra training so that they can also cater for Black women. The signs are that mainstream salons are set to become more diverse; industry standards for hairdressing now insist that all trainees must learn to cut and style Afro-textured hair. Yet salons for Black hair, sometimes of multiple ownership, continue to be important.

THE TYRANNY OF HAIR

In 1969, the radical feminist Germaine Greer deliberately set fire to her hair in a London restaurant. She had a narrow escape; waiters rushed to put it out. She may have been bored, or out to shock, but the act neatly references the strong and conflicting emotions that hair excites. While it can signal identity and status, its care has long placed restrictions on women's freedom. In the 1770s, once a lady's hair was dressed, she could seldom take it down herself without extreme pain. Hair powder was often adulterated with plaster of Paris, chalk, lime, or marble powder, and could set hard. For elite white women, the hairdresser's punctual knock at the door was part of the daily ritual. Fanny Burney, who in 1786 accepted a position at the court of George III, grumbled about her hairdresser, 'Full two hours was he at work, yet was I not finished.'[72] She especially loathed drawing-room days at court, 'which begin with full hair-dressing at six o'clock in the morning, and hardly ever allow any breakfast time, and certainly only standing, except while frizzing'.[73] Wealthy women often read or wrote letters while their hair was dressed; the poet Anna Seward composed verses; others received friends.

Curls had to look effortless but, in the days before electrical appliances, frizzing with flame-heated tongs meant curling paste, papers, and pins, as well as great care. In the late 1790s, when short curls were in fashion, hairdressers left clients bristling all over with stiff curl papers before styling. Jane Austen claimed to be in two minds about the results: 'Mr Hall was very punctual yesterday & curled me out at a great rate. I thought it looked hideous, and longed for a snug cap instead, but my companions silenced me by their admiration.'[74] Curling papers and pins became a daily necessity. When Maria Edgeworth stayed with friends in 1813, she appreciated their thoughtfulness. On the dressing table she found 'hair-brush – powder pomatum – ivory comb – tortoise shell combs of different sorts – pincushions and even papers ready cut in abundance for curling the hair'.[75]

Victorians found their hair routine a trial too. They spent hours putting hair up in the morning, taking it down at night, brushing it for the recommended time ('a very irksome business until it becomes mechanical'), and curling it for the next day.[76] Pundits agreed: 'Woman will never be emancipated from her thraldom to brushing, combing, curling, crimping, and plaiting until her hair-burdened head is laid on its final resting-place.'[77] The effect sometimes repaid the effort; some even incorporated their nightly hair-brushing into sexual foreplay. Others found haircare affected their mental wellbeing. Doctors guessed as much in the 1880s, when they ascribed the increase in neuralgic headaches among women to tightly drawn back hairstyles.[78]

To minimise the use of damaging tongs, some Victorian women wore curling pins to bed each night. Then they worried about the dangers of sleeping in iron pins: the iron might rust with perspiration, damage or discolour the hair, or draw off healthy electricity from the head. Rubber crimping pins, invented in the 1870s, were clumsy but safer to sleep on.[79] By the 1890s, there were soft kid curlers. Comfort apart, there was always the problem of looking seductive in rollers and curling papers. Fluffy mob caps with lace and ribbons seemed the answer, and attractive nightcaps were recommended into the twentieth century.[80]

Hairstyles have long disrupted sleep. Before any grand ball, stylists were heavily booked, meaning that clients would have to accept any appointment offered. Fanny Kemble recalled the eighteenth century when court beauties had their heads dressed overnight for the next day's event and sat up in their chairs for fear of destroying the edifice by lying down.[81] If they slept at all, they might wear a protective calash of black silk which opened like a carriage hood.[82] Tight bands or fillet nets were other options. Advertisements in the 1760s claimed that nets would preserve dressed hair for a whole month.[83] Victorians wore finer, 'invisible' nets made of human hair to protect their 'front coiffure'. They judged hairnets to be safer than close nightcaps because they permitted more ventilation. Women continued to wear nets overnight into the twentieth century to safeguard perms and waves, and routinely wore protective headscarves when outside. Black women today might still opt for a headscarf or sleep bonnet to keep their hair for the night, and increasingly wear bonnets or headwraps in public. But the headwrap has multiple meanings within the African tradition. A sign of modesty, it also indicated social status and occupation. In the British colonies, it was a symbol of resistance and courage for free and enslaved women, besides being practical.[84]

When the expectation was that white women would have long hair, some did experience it as a form of oppression. George Eliot complained in the 1880s, 'I have all my life wished it were possible for me to have my hair cut short that I might wash it every day. But short hair is held by the many to be the worst heresy in a woman who has not had it ordered by the doctor.'[85] In New England, Fanny Kemble took matters into her own hands. Exasperated by her mass of hair, wet with perspiration in the summer heat, she cut it to finger length, writing, 'I only wish I could be shaved and go about bald.'[86]

To cut hair short was a statement. The act might signify deep mourning. It could also signpost independence, identity, and modernity. By the 1890s, short hair marked the 'New Woman'. Under the headline, 'the Newest of New Women', one newspaper told the story of a young lady 'of severe aspect, with short hair' who boarded a crowded tram. A gentleman offered his seat but 'the lady declined, saying, "Indeed, no! This so-called politeness on the part of mankind is only the gilding of our chains; they are polite because they think women inferior to them." '[87] Allegedly, this protest astounded some and amused others.

During the First World War, female hairstyles had to adapt to new pressures. German women allegedly gave their hair to be made into diving straps for U-boats. In Britain, women doing the jobs of men who had joined the forces, showed their professionalism and support for the war effort by styling their hair more austerely than for generations past. Long hair was a bother when it came to doing the chores that now fell to them, such as car maintenance; magazines recommended wearing a bathing cap for messy garage tasks.[88]

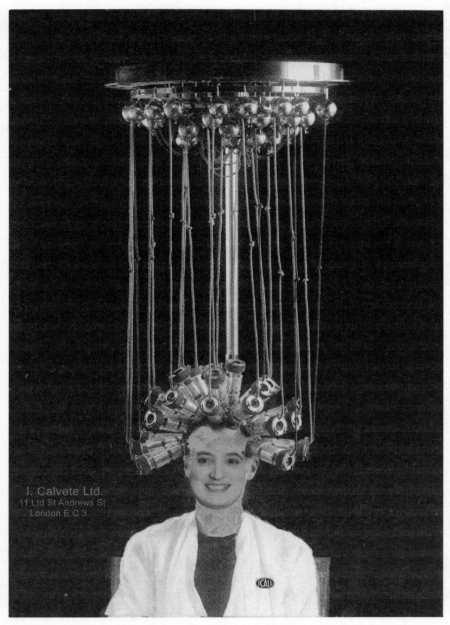

14. *A 1923 permanent-waving machine, patented by Swiss hairdresser Eugene Suter. It has twenty-two tubular heaters.*

Afterwards, the 1920s 'crop' indicated rebellion against the moral codes of the day. It was young-looking, convenient, and signified independence. But some merely followed fashion and regretted bobbing their hair. Anna Daly Morrison confided, 'My ears stood out in bold relief. I wanted to cry.' Her husband's reaction did not help. He 'took one look at me, and exclaimed, "My God, but you've made a mess of yourself." I feel like a criminal. Nothing more was said.'[89]

Short hair was easier to perm. In the 1920s, entrepreneurs improved equipment for permanent waving. Curls were achieved by heating the hair to a high temperature on electric rollers, suspended on a chandelier-type contraption to lift them from the scalp. A 'cold wave', using chemicals rather than heat, was invented in the late 1930s and gained popularity after the Second World War. As in chemical straightening, it involves breaking and reforming the hair shaft. Ironically, the concept of 'problem hair' was introduced just when advertisements for perms insisted that no woman needed to endure problem hair any longer. The concept proved so useful for selling product that it has never disappeared.[90]

Still, there has been a sea change in white women's hairdressing in Britain since the 1950s. The weekly wash and set, when women sat in rows under bonnet hair dryers, hair tightly clamped in rollers, died out once the revolutionary hairdresser Vidal Sassoon introduced the precision cut and blow dry. Moisturising shampoos and conditioners enabled frequent washing and looser styling, especially as more houses got a hot water supply. Women found that they could maintain their hairdo at home with little fuss, while the 1970s brought heated rollers and palm-sized hair dryers, displacing the heavy electrical appliances of earlier decades.

Hair is still a means of expressing conformity or dissent. The spiked mohawks of the punk movement from the 1970s were markers of a radical subculture; dramatic Goth hairstyles signpost a refusal to conform. In the Black experience, hair is crucially a matter of accommodation or resistance. In the mid-1960s, the Afro became fashionable; it was less damaging than expensive straightening treatments

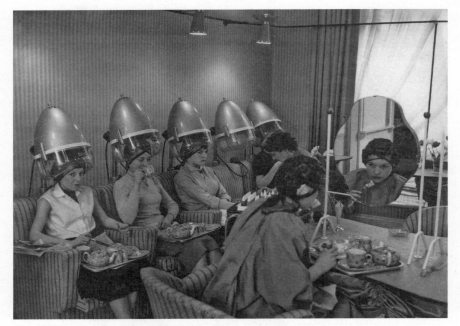

15. A hair salon in 1950. A row of women sit under hooded
hair dryers, drinking tea.

and a source of great pride. The Afro was not always a pro-Black political symbol but became one during the Black Power movement. When
Afros became heavily politicised (the taboo-breaking musical *Hair* was
advertised by an Afro in 1967), some turned to other natural hairstyles.
Combined with new fashions in dress, these trends were, and are,
hugely influential. They have in turn responded to world events such as
the independence of former colonies. Yet the element of resistance is
constant. The many creative productions by artists of African heritage
who reference their hair types have heightened public awareness of this.
Recent examples include Jay Percy's *The Three Mothers*, one of thirty-six
globes in the outdoor touring exhibition *The World Reimagined*, which
sets out to transform public understanding of the transatlantic slave
trade. Percy explores the theme 'Mother Africa' and uses traditional
hairstyles to summon up the richness of African culture before
colonialism.

Black women still face discrimination for their Afro-textured hair, in part because white people are ignorant of its properties. During the Covid pandemic, in England Afro haircare products were shockingly classed as non-essential, unlike general haircare products. For a time, Black women had great difficulty in obtaining the shampoos and conditioners they needed. And as many as 93 per cent of Black people in Britain today have suffered hair-related microaggressions.[91] In professions and workspaces, Black women have more trouble than white colleagues finding hairstyles that will help to signal their capability and ambition. Their freedom to wear their hair as they like remains a race issue that has complex links to perceptions of beauty and sexuality. Nevertheless, society is changing: in 2020, British campaigners launched a Black hair code to try to end discrimination in schools and workplaces, while in 2022 the International Swimming Federation finally approved a swimming cap for Afro hair.

The history of women's hair suggests that a choice of hairstyle can never be entirely without constraint. It will be affected by hair type and facial features. It will depend on what is technically possible. It will reflect what women have been conditioned to think of as fashionable or beautiful, and what they think appropriate to their situation in life. These influences are in continual flux, which helps to make hair so interesting. Afro hair is increasingly admired. In 2013, Antonia Opiah, entrepreneur and founder of Un-ruly, a website celebrating Black hair and women, staged a display to promote understanding of different types of Afro: three Black women held up signs inviting passers-by to touch their hair. The project backfired. Critics compared it to the scandalous exhibition of Sarah Baartman. Yet Black women are creating the freedom to style their hair as they please, bar the inherent constraints that limit all women. Afro-textured hair, long seen as low status, is being recognised as a versatile and dynamic hair type that promotes creativity since it can be sculpted in many ways. Hair has a remarkable power to encourage the appreciation of diversity and all kinds of beauty.

§8§

SPA TOWNS AND SEA BATHING

As a young girl in the 1790s, Elizabeth Ham was prescribed regular sea bathing for her weak eyes:

> I was bathed in the sea every other morning. Summer and Winter, heat and cold, I never missed the plunge, in the depth of Winter the guide used to come for me there was no other person bathing, and the reluctant nurse-maid used to accompany me. The bag and horse and guide were waiting, the rattling chains were soon hooked on to the machine. Oh, the misery of undressing! But, the plunge made all pleasant again, for the water was warmer than the air, but the indispensable walk after bathing generally chilled me again.[1]

For centuries, water treatments at spa towns and sea resorts were a key part of European women's pursuit of health and beauty. Spa and sea water featured prominently in doctors' prescriptions for a range of conditions but were thought especially useful for female disorders. Some towns, like Weymouth, were briefly both spa and seaside resort; but from the later eighteenth century the beach experience won out. Sea bathing was given a major boost by George III, who recuperated at Weymouth almost every year from 1789 to 1805, making it Britain's most fashionable health resort.

The rise of seaside towns at the expense of inland spas marked a significant social change, which strongly impacted women. Jane Austen had first-hand experience of the shift, which occurred in her lifetime. She lived for periods at the spa town of Bath and at the coastal town of Southampton, popular for sea bathing. When she died in 1817, she was working on *Sanditon*, a novel about an imaginary hamlet on the Sussex coast, undergoing transformation from fishing village to fashionable resort. It was a topical theme. Yet completed chapters show that Austen was mostly intrigued by what coastal towns offered women besides sea bathing. Her story has a disturbing undercurrent. It suggests that the economic pressures of developing a new resort had a parallel at the time in the mercenary demands of the marriage market.

Women's experience of spas and seaside towns was obviously shaped by practicalities such as where they could most easily travel. It was also affected by their age, affluence, health, and whether or not they were tied to an ailing companion. That said, spas and coastal resorts offered broadly different environments: the spa was an enclosed, mostly fresh-water offer, the coast an open, saltwater space. How did women maximise the possibilities of both in their pursuit of health and beauty?

TAKING THE WATERS

The beneficial effects of hot and cold water on the body had been known since antiquity but Europeans were slow to appreciate natural mineral waters. The waters at Spa, now in Belgium, only became famous in the fourteenth century. They were mostly drunk, proving diuretic and laxative. Physicians decided they were good for melancholy, sterility, gout, fevers, and a range of skin diseases. English travellers and scholars were among the first foreigners to appreciate Spa's waters and they helped to promote England's own springs, giving them the name 'spa' as well.

England's mineral springs grew popular in the 1600s. At this time, there were seven or eight known sources, including the thermal resorts of Bath, Buxton, and Bristol Hotwells. Bath was cramped and stinky; Buxton had a fine moor where ladies could take the air in their coaches; Hotwells was tiny but favoured by consumptives. The number of spa destinations proliferated after the Restoration of Charles II in 1660, extending into Ireland and Wales. They had their heyday in the eighteenth century, so an inquiry into the female spa experience naturally centres on this period.

At first, spa towns had little to offer beyond their waters; accommodation was likely to be poor. In 1716, Lady Marlborough visited Bath and complained, 'I never saw any Place Abroad that had more Stinks and Dirt in it.'[2] At night the streets were so noisy, she could hardly sleep. In the 1720s, she visited Scarborough. There she found that the invalids kept a common table, each paying their share, which at least meant they got to know each other. But communal living could be taken too far. She discovered that the ladies' assembly room had a separate chamber intended for shared use once the waters began to operate. It was furnished with about twenty holes over retractable drawers that could be emptied, 'and at the door . . . a great heap of leaves which the ladies take in with them'.[3] Horrified, she made a hasty retreat.

Later in the eighteenth century, spa towns near good roads became fashionable watering places, providing genial environments for the enjoyment of poor health. Bath and Tunbridge Wells (the latter smaller and relatively rural) each had a summer season, drawing crowds between June and late September. Bath raised its game and increased its popularity by having a spring and autumn season as well. These major centres were frequented by 'quality', but across Britain there were literally hundreds of small spas catering for the health of all classes, from minor country gentry to middle-class tradesmen and Pennine lead miners. And sometimes upmarket spas still allowed the poor to drink the waters for free.

In an age when the limitations of professional medicine encouraged people to manage their health actively, a regular spa visit seemed prudent if the cost of travel was not too great. Doctors investigated the properties of different spa waters, whether sulphurous, chalybeate, saline, or carbonated, and decided each type was good for different ailments. The pure waters at Great Malvern were recommended for skin and eye disorders. The hot springs at Bath, which were rich in sulphate and calcium, were said to strengthen the body against gout, arthritis, disorders of the nervous system, and heart disease, among other things. Spas were thought especially good for the nervous complaints to which women seemed liable; their waters were purgative, and doctors linked nervous disorders to digestive problems.

Spa invalids were always advised to consult the resident doctor on arrival to see if the waters were suited to their case. But the medical analysis of the day involved much guesswork. If patients improved, there was no way of checking what had given relief, whether the waters themselves, rest and a change of diet, or novel company and surroundings. Many were disappointed in their hopes of a cure: Lady Marlborough felt the gout return to her hand after a couple of weeks at Scarborough; Anne Pitt, a maid of honour at court, tried the waters at Bath, Bristol, and Tunbridge Wells in the 1750s but none reduced her swollen legs.

Londoners had springs in the capital. They went to Bagnigge Wells in Camberwell from the 1680s, when the source was called Black Mary's Hole because a Black woman, Mary Woolaston, lived nearby and sold the water. The site flourished from 1760 to the end of the eighteenth century, by which time it boasted a tea garden popular with citizens and apprentices. There was also Islington Spa, briefly patronised by royalty and people of fashion in the 1730s. Other springs within walking distance were at Hampstead and at the Dog and Duck in St George's Fields. But all soon attracted rough crowds, prostitutes, and swindlers. Ladies who valued their good name avoided them. In short, London venues could not be compared with towns famous for their spas alone.

Bottled English and Continental spa water had been available from the seventeenth century. Physicians often prescribed bottled waters and gentle exercise even if patients stayed at home. Imported mineral water was expensive: in 1706, water from Spa cost 14d a flask, or 12s a dozen.

The price did come down later in the century but purchasers had to guard against cheats and counterfeits. Given the established trade in mineral water, in theory the sick had no need to travel to a spa town. But resolute invalids could not simply rely on bottled water and take the cure in their own bathtub; the point of a spa visit was to leave the pollution and pressures of the city behind.

Other visitors to spa towns sought a wholly different body-centred experience. They went for pleasure, flirtation, to find a marriage partner, or even to arrange a discrete abortion. Spa waters were especially recommended for gynaecological problems, including failure to conceive. Cynics suggested that, if a woman did become fertile at a spa, the most likely explanation was an adulterous liaison not the mineral water. All the same, in 1781 when James Graham, a self-styled doctor and pioneer sex therapist, recommended two flasks of mineral water a day for sterile women, the price of bottled water in London doubled. A spa regime was also coyly prescribed for the 'Crime of *self-abuse*' among the young. The physician and satirist John Arbuthnot wittily complained of an early season at Tunbridge Wells, 'The company consists chiefly of *bon-vivants* with decayed stomachs, green-sickness virgins, unfruitful or miscarrying wives.'[4]

Spa doctors advised patients to drink the laxative waters before breakfast and then take moderate exercise to aid their operation. To fill the hours, spa towns soon offered some diversions. These gave wealthy women opportunities for self-presentation which were eagerly seized. Dress and display allowed them to assert their social rank and test the power of their charms. Women wore provocatively loose habits when drinking the waters; later they went walking or riding in tight costumes that accentuated their curves; if there was dancing in the evening, they dazzled the company with elaborate gowns and jewels. Multiple changes of dress each day attracted notice. In unfamiliar surroundings, a woman could display her personality, try out a new identity, and signal sexual preferences. Some adopted masculine riding habits even when not on horseback. Arguably the outfit was practical and economical when worn for several activities, but it also blurred genders. In 1782, when Fanny Burney went to the last ball of the season at Brighton, she noted, 'some of the ladies were in riding-habits, and they made admirable *men*'.[5] To add to the glamour of social engagements, both sexes had access to cosmetics, which were readily available to disguise the pallor of the sick.

RELIEF FOR THE MERCHANT CAPTAIN'S WIFE

Mary, the daughter of a Wapping apothecary, married Captain Thomas Bowrey in 1691, when he returned to England after a career in the Indian Ocean. They settled in Wellclose Square, Wapping, within easy distance of the wharves and shipyards along the river. The couple's household accounts show they regularly bought bottled spa water and a medicine called 'hysterick water'. As the daughter of an apothecary, Mary would have been familiar with common remedies; Bowrey also kept books on household medicine in his library. Hysteria in women was commonly thought to be caused by the womb moving from its natural position, but the condition was beginning to be linked more to the brain than to the uterus. This meant it could be diagnosed in men as well as women, particularly those given to study or oppressed by business. That said, hysteria was still chiefly associated with women who were nervous or emotional. It was a catch-all term for a range of vague complaints.

Whatever the couple's actual disorders, they journeyed to Bath in 1699 for the waters. Hysteria was certainly thought to respond to a spa regime: doctors recommended a change of scene, relief from polluted city air, gentle exercise, and cold baths. Bowrey and his wife were childless, which might have been another reason to go. They later made several summer visits to Tunbridge Wells. The Tunbridge waters were considered particularly good for hysteria, and after 1708 Tunbridge also offered a cold plunge bath. Any spa visit was a commitment; Bowrey complained in 1705 about their difficult journey to Tunbridge. Even mid-century, when the town was little more than four hours from London by post chaise, carriages were liable to overturn on the road.

Elizabeth Montagu, the author and literary hostess, had a hair-raising journey there in 1760. She described 'the danger I was in of such an overturn in my coach as would probably have been fatal'.[6] When Jane Austen chose to begin *Sanditon* with a dramatic carriage accident, the device was perfectly plausible.

Bowrey's account books confirm that spa visits were expensive; from the early days, spas were about the commodification of health issues and then beauty treatments. The couple travelled with fine clothes and jewellery to display their status. Spa visitors also expected to treat themselves to delicate foods in season, costly sweetmeats, and candy.[7] When in Tunbridge, the Bowreys bought much more refined sugar from Jamaica and Barbados than they ever did at home. Contemporary remedies did call for sweeteners – in electuaries or medicinal ingredients made into a paste with honey or sugar, and in lozenges and cordials. One well-known recipe for 'hysterical water' had to be sweetened to taste, possibly to disguise the flavour of other ingredients, which included dried millipedes.[8] English spas of the time created a supportive, feminine milieu in which women at leisure shared handicraft tips and indulgent recipes for sugared confectionary.[9] This aspect of a spa community might easily coexist with a shadier world of amorous intrigue and sexual licence – and might even serve to cloak it.

Physicians set out a routine for spa patients which helped to justify the expense of travelling for health. They specified when to drink the waters, how to prepare the body for their effect, what to eat, and when to exercise. Yet Bowrey's accounts reveal the tempting distractions also on offer. At Tunbridge there was a daily market, rural walks, and genteel shops, including milliners and 'toy shops' selling silverware, china, and other trinkets. Music was played every morning as visitors drank the waters. There were large coffee houses that served tea and chocolate too. The town had regular balls, rooms devoted to gambling, and innocent raffles for prizes such as books or gowns. But diversions and gambling losses had to be paid for. There was also an expectation that visitors would donate to local charities. In 1703, Bowrey spent £30 3s 6d at Tunbridge in just four weeks. For comparison, the master of an East Indiaman was paid £10 a month, although he would have traded on the side, too.[10] Quite simply, without money there was no enjoyment at Tunbridge.

In May 1704, Mary went to Bath by herself; Bowrey was too busy with his ship to leave London. She wrote asking him to send her a lacquered wooden bowl.[11] (In the pools at Bath, women tied floating bowls to their arms to carry handkerchiefs, lozenges, and perfumes that would combat the taste and smell of the water.) Bowrey wrote back advising her to stay the month or 'as much longer as you please, and if you want more money you shall freely have it'.[12] He added gallantly that he missed her, but would happily lose her company if Bath was doing her good. Perhaps after all he preferred his ship and a London quayside to a sulphurous thermal bath.

In the Bath pools, the sight of loosely dressed women, without stays, created a sexual frisson. Moralists had long complained about mixed bathing, and there was lewd talk of covert fumbling among bathers. But rituals helped to preserve decency. The sexes were partly segregated: men, in drawers and waistcoats, kept to the centre of the pools; women, guided by female chaperones, waded towards seating on the outer edges. They wore drab canvas or linen garments that billowed out in the water to conceal their shape and tended to sit with the water decently up to their necks. In 1741, when the tall dowager Duchess of Norfolk pulled rank and had the waters topped up to her chin, she nearly drowned a row of less important, shorter bathers. The prospect of flirtation might liven up the experience, but few looked their best in the water: no rouge or paint could withstand the sulphurous fumes, and hair drooped limply. Some women resorted to wigs, doubly useful because the mixtures they used to wash their hair tainted the water. On leaving the pool, a woman would go up some stairs, a door would close behind her, and in privacy female attendants would slip a dry flannel gown over her head before removing the wet one.

Spa towns catered for the well-to-do but created job opportunities for women who needed to work. Women were ever-present, as landladies, shopkeepers, cake-makers, washerwomen, musicians, performers, and prostitutes. They worked as guides in the baths and as pump attendants, dispensing water pumped to the surface specifically for drinking. Some became notable figures. At Tunbridge Wells, Bell Causey directed affairs from about 1725 until her death in 1734, ensuring that events ran smoothly and that visitors paid their bills. At Harrogate, Betty Lupton, 'Queen of the Wells', supervised the Royal Pump Room for fifty-six years until her death in 1843.

Mary Bowrey's lone visit to Bath shows how spa towns provided spaces where a woman might enjoy relative autonomy during her stay. Men often dominated households as much as workplaces, so a spa visit might offer wives a welcome respite. Spas can never have been thought too scandalous or women would not have risked their reputations by going there. Social protocols were strictly applied. In 1704, the year of Mary Bowrey's visit, Richard 'Beau' Nash became Master of Ceremonies at Bath, enforcing standards of social behaviour. When Bell Causey died, he appointed himself Master of Ceremonies at Tunbridge Wells too, installing Sarah Porter to advertise amenities and levy subscriptions from visitors. She acquired the title 'Queen of the Touters' because no one escaped her attention.

RETREATS FOR LEARNED WOMEN

Spa towns offered food for the mind as well as relief for the body. The larger spas had their own newspapers and published poetry miscellanies each season. Amateur writers submitted verses, which circulated in manuscript before being considered for publication. Female authors had to be careful: spa culture encouraged the writing of bland, complimentary pieces but the holiday atmosphere also nurtured erotic and scandalous verse. Still, the important point is the existence of a literary community. Spas inspired new dances and songs too, which were printed for circulation with the musical score. This lively material promoted spa towns in a way that increasingly appealed to women.

When Sarah Medley produced her *Descriptive Guide to Leamington Spa, Warwick, and the Adjacent Towns and Villages* in 1826, she catered for an established female market that not only wanted the usual practical information (such as local doctors or the prices of public baths) but also poems and details of where local flowering plants could be found.

For many women, the spa expedition was never a quest for health. Instead, it offered a welcome change from formal country-house visits, a wider social circle, and stimulating entertainment (by 1815, seven English spas had their own theatres). Part of the fun was the opportunity for different classes to mix more freely. The elite found the variety of characters in a spa town briefly amusing, while the lower orders got the chance to mingle with 'great folk'. All understood that a chance acquaintance made at a spa would not be recognised in more formal surroundings. At Tunbridge Wells in 1745, Elizabeth Montagu typically marvelled at the many nations and faiths she met. She added tartly, 'I never saw a worse collection of human creatures in all my life. My comfort is, that as there are not many of them I ever saw before, I flatter myself there are few of them I shall ever see again.'[13]

At a spa town, high-ranking visitors aimed to form an agreeable 'party' so that good company was ensured and excursions to nearby sights and country houses were easily arranged. Enjoyable conversation raised the spirits even if the mineral waters did not. Elizabeth Carter made a tour of the Rhineland and Low Countries with a party in 1763 that included Elizabeth Montagu and her elderly husband. They took in Spa, which at that time was cheaper than Bath or Tunbridge Wells. She found the formality at Spa tiresome, but fortunately had not bothered to pack a large hoop, which had to be worn when the formal dress code demanded wide skirts, so she was spared grand occasions when foreign aristocrats were present. As an aside, she disapproved of some English women who took advantage of the different customs at Spa, seizing the opportunity to plaster on rouge as the French did.[14]

The spa experience out of season could be dull. When Elizabeth Montagu visited Bath as a young woman, before marriage, she exclaimed: 'I went to the Ladies' Coffee House, where I heard of nothing but the rheumatism in the shoulder, the sciatica in the hip, and the gout in the toe. I began to fancy myself in the hospital or infirmary, I never saw such an assembly of disorders.'[15] Jemima Yorke, Marchioness Grey, who had wide cultural interests, also found Bath tedious towards the end of a season. Stranded there in October 1749 with her friend Lady Anson, she discovered that the library had 'no Books that give one the least Curiosity to read them', and wailed, 'What shall we do now?'[16] In bad weather, it was impossible to take a walk, while the poor health of many spa residents meant they cancelled engagements at short notice. It was easy to fall into a depression. But she also found Scarborough dreary in high summer, complaining that the resort did not have enough to fill the idlest day. Its social routine was determined by the laxative force of its waters: visitors kept London hours and dined late to leave a long morning for the waters to take effect.[17]

Learned women saw that many spa visitors just fancied themselves ill. 'Half of us come here to cure the bodily evils occasioned by laziness', Elizabeth Montagu wrote from Tunbridge Wells in 1749, 'the other half to remedy the mental disease of idleness and inoccupation, called l'ennui.'[18] All the same, the spa routine did chime with the latest ideas about preventative medicine, which recommended exercise. Spa towns had horses for hire and Montagu seized the chance to ride, insisting, 'I am convinced half of our faults arise from want of shaking the machine.'[19] For other elite visitors, the experience was just another form of lavish consumption: they purchased a variety of activities in search of wellbeing.

Intellectual women like Montagu used spas to create space for reflection. At Tunbridge, she explained to a friend, you could have 'the most retired, or the most public walks, as you are disposed'.[20] Later in life, she rented a house some distance from the wells so that each day she was guaranteed hours of retirement, never mixing with society except when drinking the waters. In London, alongside other educated women, she had built a reputation for hosting conversation parties during the winter season. Guests provided the entertainment by discussing literary and philosophical topics with verve and wit. These meetings, which became known as the Bluestocking Circle, were quite intense, and hostesses regarded a summer spa visit as recuperation and a means to prevent ill health. Carter wrote to Montagu, 'I rejoice to hear you are going to Bath, I always consider you there, as collecting a provision of health against the winter dissipations.'[21]

The Bluestocking Circle had its origins in casual breakfast meetings at Tunbridge Wells and other spa towns during the 1750s. It remained essentially a female salon, though it included eminent men who supported female learning. And the Bluestockings continued to use their time in summer spa retreats to discuss their literary projects. At Tunbridge Wells it was easier to avoid company than at Bath. It was at Tunbridge, in 1761, that Montagu persuaded Elizabeth Carter to publish a volume of her poems. Afterwards they shaped the project in correspondence. For women like Carter, of modest means, spas also offered a useful summer retreat when aristocratic acquaintances left London for their country estates.

If spa towns afforded lone women certain freedoms, the lack of a male escort could limit what they did. At Spa, Carter did not dare to leave the public walks, despite wishing to enjoy more scenery, because robbers were rumoured to lurk in the woods. In Bath, Jemima, Marchioness Grey, felt trapped 'like a Bird in its Cage' when she eyed the surrounding countryside: 'I have no adventurous Guide, no Fellow Explorers, & walking alone in this Place is impossible.'[22] But she reflected that, since she wanted to make a figure at the public breakfasts, it was probably best not to be seen tramping in shortened petticoats and heavy leather shoes. Lady Anson arrived to keep her company and later their husbands joined them. The women's routine now changed dramatically. They were no longer limited to receiving visits in their lodgings because their husbands escorted them to all the public places. Yet they did have a sneaking regret that they had lost these home visits, when they had been able to flirt and receive male flattery uncensured.

THE SPA MARRIAGE MARKET

In June 1700, Mary Clarke wrote from the family's Taunton estate to her husband, who was serving as a member of parliament in London. A neighbour, she explained, was taking her two eldest daughters to Bath. Doubtless she aimed to find them husbands since there were few eligible men in Taunton and her neighbour hardly needed to worry about her fertility, having children enough. Clarke joked to her husband that they should try to get their own daughters married first, if only to vex their neighbour. But perhaps she secretly longed for the distractions of Bath.[23]

As spa towns grew in importance, they became pivotal to the marriage market. By the end of the eighteenth century, the daughter of an affluent family who had been educated in dancing and playing the piano, and was ready to 'come out', knew what to expect. She was exhibited at a local ball. If no desirable suitor appeared, she was taken to Bath or to Cheltenham Spa, which had become popular thanks to royal visits. If she was of the highest rank, she would be given a London season. Those who failed to make an impression in fashionable society had no choice but to decamp to a narrower sphere, such as a summer bathing place.

Finding a marriage partner was for the most part a commercial transaction. At Tunbridge Wells, Elizabeth Montagu remarked, 'A beauty and a keeper of a toy shop, are always unhappy in an empty season.'[24] Beauty was a commodity with a price, just like the trinkets of inlaid woodwork sold in Tunbridge as souvenirs. A contemporary anecdote shows the desperation of some women to secure a husband:

The manner by which Miss Cumberland's match was brought about is rather curious. A very pretty Work Box was raffled for at Tunbridge, and Mr. Badcock was the fortunate winner. Miss Thrale happening to be in the Shop at the time, Mr. B. offered it to her; but as the Gentleman was an entire Stranger to her, she declined accepting it. She, however, related the Circumstance to Miss Cumberland, whom she met soon after, and who replied, 'Good Lord! How could you be

so silly? I am sure if he had offered to me I would have accepted it!'
This was told to Mr. B., who thought it probable if the Lady was so
willing to receive the Box, she might perhaps do him the Honour to
accept his Hand. He accordingly offered it directly, and She accepted
it most graciously.[25]

Single women of genteel status could not accept gifts from men without
being compromised. Ironically, an offer of marriage might be accepted
without hesitation; for some it was the whole object of visiting a spa.

Life in a spa town was something of a performance. The rules and
protocols observed at each venue were even printed in ladies' pocket-
books. Young people were continually rating members of the opposite
sex; meanwhile, their own behaviour was closely observed by older
women devoted to cards, scandal, and gossip. In Bath these critics were
known as 'the Cats'. Etiquette was so important in the marriage market
that, well into the nineteenth century, schoolmistresses in Bath had a
strangely elevated social position. They instructed young girls in the
skills needed to enter society with success, they maintained an elite social
network so that they could position pupils to advantage, and they acted
as the pupils' chaperones.

Girls at a spa in search of husbands were burdened with responsibility: their families would have paid hefty subscriptions to get them
into balls and select parties. No wonder Jane Austen disliked Bath,
despite its intellectual stimulus. Another author, Lady Louisa Stuart,
felt the same. In 1787, she prepared to take her ailing mother to Bath.
Disappointed in love and, at thirty, past the first flush of youth, she
knew she would be a misfit: 'I cannot say I am partial to the place . . .
or the life one must lead there.'[26]

In wartime, with many young men in the military, husbands were
especially difficult to find. Spa towns had an even higher female population. Yet Bath was popular with naval officers on leave and with their
families. Out of season it had cheap rooms to rent, entertainments, and
ready provision for invalids. It also offered a supportive refuge and

opportunities for naval women to connect with public life. Here they met military and political figures and soaked up the latest news for wider communication through their network of correspondents. Horatio Nelson's wife, Frances, wintered in Bath with her asthmatic father-in-law from 1794 when Nelson was at sea. Having grown up in the West Indies, she was keen to escape the family home near the Norfolk coast with its biting winds. Bath's streets were now segregated by class, aristocrats having withdrawn into exclusive circles. To ease her conscience, Frances assured her husband that she rented in the cheap, lower part of town. But at the same time, she planted the idea that she would have to move in summer: her Bath lodgings near the river would be stinking and too hot.[27]

LATER EUROPEAN AND NORTH AMERICAN INFLUENCES

The European spa experience, as it evolved in the nineteenth century, offered contrasting experiences for women. In Germany, especially, some spas grew rather staid. Governed by strict routine in accordance with medical advice, they attracted the middle classes, who, for three weeks or so in the summer, set about improving their health with the same earnest determination that they devoted to business. But Continental spa towns were also famous for their high-class gambling salons, offering a world apart from the water treatments and restricted diets administered to genuine health-seekers. The realm of roulette and rouge et noir exerted a dark fascination: fortunes were won and lost; there were suicides and scandals. By the 1860s, it was claimed that most visitors to German spas used health concerns as a cloak to gamble without restraint. Gambling licences were tightened up in the 1870s, but Continental spas retained their glamourous reputation for ostentation and excitement. Elderly aristocratic women were often blamed for fuelling the gambling addiction. This connection between women and gambling was long-lived: even in the 1960s, advertisements for Baden-Baden showed women gambling in evening dress.[28]

The North American elite praised state-run European spas for being strictly regulated. Back home, their privately owned spas offered such an excess of pleasure that any therapeutic effect was minimal. American spas like Saratoga Springs were tawdry and commercial by the 1860s. Critics blamed female extravagance and vanity for this state of affairs. They accused women of succumbing to 'domestic depravity' within the 'promiscuous herding' of North American spa towns, and reproached women, not men, for 'the demoralization of the watering places'.[29] Riled by activist women's organisations campaigning for the right to vote, critics challenged women instead to reform the spas and make them fit for the pure-minded. And the Women's Association of Greater Saratoga, formed in the 1890s, did restore the reputation of Saratoga Springs, lobbying hard to make it a national park.

In Britain and Europe, spas added more sports facilities to the experience. Some even included fashionable gymnastics. Female visitors therefore needed more outfits, for tennis and golf as well as for walking and riding. By the end of the nineteenth century, dressmakers could barely keep up with the demand for travel clothes in peak season. Women in gorgeous gowns added to the attraction of these resorts; even straw hats for spa wear changed shape each season. And beauty was literally on parade: at Spa, summer beauty contests were introduced in 1888, the first winner being an upper-class woman of mixed heritage from Guadeloupe. As personal display reached new heights, commentators in the 1890s noted with unease that young girls of thirteen or fourteen wore makeup in spa towns.[30]

Continental spas did help to revolutionise travel for single women and for wives seeking relief from difficult marriages. Earlier English tourists had expected to buy a carriage once they had crossed the Channel, then sell it for what it would fetch on return. But by the late nineteenth century, comfortable foreign travel was no longer the preserve of an elite few. Nor did women always need to engage travelling companions. Rail travel had made it easier for women of more modest means to visit Continental resorts, and to travel alone if they kept to familiar routes. Magazines carried advice on what to pack, and reassured women that 'in every Continental hotel one sees solitary ladies, or pairs of sisters or friends'.[31] A woman travelling alone no longer raised alarm or suspicion, and most hotels had English-speaking staff who could help with travel arrangements.

Meanwhile, in Britain, spa towns were becoming places of genteel retirement, attracting widows and spinsters, who sought the comfort of like-minded company and an abundance of local doctors. At Bath, mixed bathing in the pools ceased altogether. Spa towns did retain their individual character. For instance, military families returning from the East or West Indies favoured Cheltenham, where the waters were said to relieve tropical diseases. But rail travel and improved plumbing at destination hotels began to usher in the luxury 'spa break', which proved a more uniform experience. For example, the Spa Hotel at Tunbridge Wells, just one hour by rail from Charing Cross or Victoria in the 1890s, advertised 'Baths of every description, including Turkish, Electric and Swimming'.[32] It had experienced masseurs and masseuses; was heated to 60°C in both winter and summer; offered billiards, smoking, and reading rooms; and boasted a golf course and tennis courts. By the early twentieth century, the Clifton Grand Spa and Hydro in Bristol provided every form of hydrotherapy available in Europe, Turkey, or Russia. It also had duplicate facilities for women and men, so that all members of a family could take their bath at the same time with perfect propriety.

Although the promotional material for spa breaks still emphasised recuperation, this was about to change. In 1905, Helena Rubinstein was already researching the beauty treatments on offer in fashionable European spas and cities. Increasingly, spas would be viewed as health and beauty centres. They got a new lease of life by offering varied treatments to address skin conditions such as cellulite and other 'problem areas'. Spa towns like Bath had introduced Christmas entertainment to attract winter visitors, but soon realised that a menu of beauty treatments would attract clients all year round. During the First World War, German air raids frightened off visitors to coastal towns in the North of England, but Bath and Harrogate were thought secure and continued to flourish. The contemporary emphasis on a slim figure meant that a course of spa baths and waters could also be promoted to women who wished to lose weight. After the war, with Continental travel still depressed, those with money flocked to English spas offering the latest treatments. By the 1920s, medically trained staff at Harrogate even dispensed ultraviolet rays, labelled 'artificial mountain sun'.[33] The less affluent made do with branded salts, which claimed to turn tap water into a mineral water that was gently laxative and good for health; or effervescent salts for a home tub, which claimed to be as 'Exhilarating as a Bath of Champagne'.[34]

By the 1930s, German spas were again attracting English crowds; visitors were delighted to find them surprisingly cosmopolitan. Young people unexpectedly met many of their own age travelling with parents 'taking the cure', so spas continued to be places where marriage partners were found. During the Second World War, Continental spas suffered another setback; many closed or were put to military use. Yet to this day they give highly respected and disciplined treatments for specific disorders, and they have never really lost their reputation for ostentatious luxury. In contrast, the therapeutic provision of British spas transferred to the National Health Service after 1948. So-called spas offering beauty treatments, relaxation, and recuperation then began to open in major cities. In contrast, countryside destinations developed more rigorous programmes for a health re-set, typically including yoga, holistic treatments for wellbeing, exercise classes, and system-cleansing diets.

This new spa industry has seen amazing growth. Packages billed as 'escapes' and 'retreats' reflect the pressures of society today, with some spa centres blocking electronic signals to shield clients from emails and social media. Private health hydros and luxury spas continue to promise weight loss, stress reduction, and a pampering detox that will change how women look, think, and feel. Smaller, inner-city spas are mostly positioned as self-indulgent experiences, to be booked for a special occasion. A glance at Tripadvisor shows that popular venues can quickly become over-crowded, the bathing experience more like a pool party, leaving customers sweaty and stressed rather than rejuvenated. Negative comments about food, fellow bathers, cost, and cleanliness offer an uncanny echo of the complaints that spa visitors made in previous centuries, with one key difference: references to physical ailments are almost totally absent.

THE SEA AND HEALTH

Sea bathing for health at first offered an intense experience. As Elizabeth Hams discovered, a medicinal plunge into the sea left indelible memories. English physicians touted the health benefits of bathing in the sea with growing confidence from around 1750. Yet some had hit upon it earlier. Dr Robert Wittie was adamant that cold sea bathing at Scarborough had cured his gout in the late 1660s. Sir John Floyer, a firm advocate of bracing cold baths to toughen people up, took a leap forward around 1700, when he realised that the sea was not just a vast chilly bath but a saline, medicinal one. The seaweed body wraps that some spas specialise in today are a faint saline legacy.

Doubtless, the lower classes living near the sea were quite used to bathing in it. But Scarborough did not offer its spa visitors the option of immersion in sea water until the 1720s. The practice slowly caught on. A versifier of 1723 gave encouragement, urging women to toss their pills and potions aside, and jump into the sea to bring a healthy glow to their cheeks: 'Not Paris Rouge will make them shine / With colour half so charming'. The elderly Duchess of Marlborough, staying at Scarborough in 1732, noted that the Duchess of Manchester, still child-less, went into the sea every day.[35]

By the 1760s, sea water was hailed as a 'universal medicine', a natural cure for a range of disorders, whether sipped or bathed in.[36] Resorts sprang up around the British coast. These tended to be towns of some significance because they had to have passable roads. Even so, accommodation was often scarce; owners of houses near the sea could cash in on a growing market for summer lets. Coastal residents soon saw that money could be made. They looked for wealthy patrons or a doctor's backing to give their town competitive edge. Fanny Burney noted with amusement that Weymouth rushed to benefit from George III's patronage in 1789. Town authorities even hired a group of fiddlers to play 'God Save the King' when George dipped his head beneath the waves. The royal children had bathed at Eastbourne; the Prince of Wales favoured Brighton; now Weymouth wanted its turn. After all, its south coast was warmer than Scarborough; hardy bathers could visit all year round.

Some seaside towns thought to provide saltwater baths, so that health-seekers could still be immersed at low tide. As early as 1753, Harwich advertised seawater baths which could be emptied and refilled in case patients had contagious skin complaints. A 'crane chair' dipped those without the courage or strength to plunge straight in, and there were separate dressing rooms for men and women. Margate had a warmed saltwater bath by 1765, and Brighton had hot and cold seawater baths by 1769.

From the outset, doctors meant to control the new therapy. They explained which illnesses would respond to sea bathing (never those that affected the bowels). They defined the condition the body should be in before immersion (never too warm, or fresh from violent exercise). They prescribed how long to stay in the sea (rarely above a minute, or risk spasms). And they advised when to bathe (early in the morning, unless a patient had eaten or drunk too much the night before). Female attendants in flannel jackets and straw bonnets stood ready to help women make the plunge. They aimed to duck the patient's head under water as a wave broke, prolonging the shock for maximum benefit. Afterwards, patients could expect a tremor of exhilaration, 'a sudden and universal glow of the whole body'.[37]

Various forces helped to establish the new trend. Manufacturers of patent medicines for gout, scurvy, and venereal disease jumped on the bandwagon. They were quick to advertise their products as excellent preparation for this new treatment, or a prudent addition to spa water and sea bathing. The wives of prominent naval officers, frequent visitors to the coast, were in the vanguard of female bathers. Lady Anson, whose health was always delicate, dipped in the sea at Southampton in 1751, where her husband, then First Lord of the Admiralty, joined her; Lady Howe bathed at Exeter in 1759 while waiting for her husband's ship to return to Portsmouth. Their aquatic exertions were reported in newspapers and mentioned in female correspondence.[38] Sea bathing was recommended to women especially, because doctors thought it an excellent remedy for nervous disorders. But some satirists implied that self-diagnosed nervous complaints could be a pretext for a kind of holiday. Whole families seemed affected, and nothing could cure their affliction except 'spending the Summer Months in some dirty Fishing Town by the Sea-Shore'.[39]

Fanny Burney first experienced sea bathing at Teignmouth in 1773. She had been suffering from a heavy cold and was told to 'harden' her constitution. She wrote, 'I was terribly frightened, and really thought I should never have recovered from the plunge. I had not breath enough to speak for a minute or two, the shock was beyond expression great.' Afterwards, she did feel a glow, and enthused, 'It is the finest feeling in the world.'[40] She bathed again in the 1780s, when she visited Brighton with the diarist and author Hester Thrale and members of her family. Thrale could swim, which was rare for a woman of the time. She was a firm believer in cold-water baths for women, which she thought improved the complexion and made them better sexual partners, 'bracing up everything that frequent Pregnancy relaxes'.[41] Thrale had thirteen pregnancies, so spoke from experience. Burney recorded that the party rose at six: 'We went to the sea-side, where we had bespoke the bathing-women to be ready for us, and into the ocean we plunged. It was cold, but pleasant. I have bathed so often as to lose my dread of the operation, which now gives me nothing but animation and vigour.'[42]

From the first, fashionable bathing resorts encouraged a degree of licence. Elizabeth Carter grumbled, 'What can be so contradictory as a dip in the fine fresh cold sea in the morning, and going into a hot crowded ball room at night; no good can ever come of it.'[43] Yet bathing resorts offered women new sensations of freedom beyond temporary escape from the social round or confines of domesticity offered at a spa. Burney, at Weymouth with the royal party in 1789, described these sensations: 'I am delighted with the soft air and soft footing upon the sands, and stroll up and down them morning, noon, and night.'[44] At the seaside, on a breezy beach, no one could maintain the decorum of the pump room. When family parties took the air, it was often unclear whether girls were 'out' or not. Couples could form with less surveillance. That said, seaside assembly rooms still enforced rules of politeness, especially at Weymouth, where the connection with royalty ensured formality. Gentlemen were not allowed to appear in boots there, and they had to leave their swords at the door. Ladies could not wear riding habits. Neither sex could wear coloured gloves. No tea table could be carried into the card room; tea drinking was not to interfere with the serious business of playing cards.[45]

Daughters were taken to a seaside resort to find a husband, just as they were escorted to spas for that purpose. During the Napoleonic Wars, militia regiments were stationed at the coast in case of invasion. The presence of soldiers made sea bathing more attractive to mothers with marriageable daughters, but it also brought dangers. Elizabeth Ham recorded that, as she walked with two female friends on the promenade at Weymouth one evening, three officers appeared and seized each girl by the arm. She broke free and ran down a side street but got a fright and was scolded for being out late.[46] Less timid girls in seaside towns found plenty of opportunities for flirtation.

PEEPING TOMS AND TAMSINS

Public sea bathing was a magnet for prying eyes. A racy poem about Scarborough in 1732 describes male interest as women emerged from the waves: 'See kindly clinging, the wet Garment shows / And ev'ry

Fold some newer Charms disclose.'[47] At Scarborough there were early attempts to segregate the sexes. Women used two little houses on the shore, where they changed into blue linen shifts before female guides helped them into the water. Men hired local boats called cobbles and rowed a decent way out to sea before jumping naked into the water.

The invention of the bathing machine helped to preserve modesty. These were essentially wheeled changing huts. Most were horse-drawn into the sea, allowing bathers to step into the waves while the driver unhitched his horse and went in search of another fare. Liverpool had early models in the 1720s, but Benjamin Beale of Margate is credited with inventing the full-blown version mid-century. It came with a large canvas hood, which could be lowered over the steps for greater privacy. Most large resorts had adopted bathing machines of some design by the 1800s. There were rarely enough because men used them as well as women. Margate had a waiting room, with a piano and newspapers, where bathers entered their name in a book, then took their turn for a vacant machine. At Brighton, bathing machines were doubly useful: until the town's sewerage system was improved in the 1830s and 1840s, bathers otherwise encountered stinks and effluence from sewerage pipes on the beach. But at Kemp Town, further east, women were said to prefer being carried across the pebbles by brawny male attendants. They were dropped at bathing machines parked in the water.

Despite rituals to uphold decorum, seaside resorts offered easy opportunities to encounter the opposite sex in various stages of undress. There were numerous complaints about men bathing indecently among women. At Scarborough, a traveller in the 1750s noticed that some male bathers only rowed a short distance from the shore so that they could show off their physiques to women bathing nearby.[48] In the 1760s, a father who had taken his family to Scarborough protested that, as his wife and daughter emerged from their bathing machine, a dozen naked men exposed themselves to view. Worse still, other women on the beach seemed wholly used to such displays. He complained that, much as he wished his womenfolk to benefit from a course of sea bathing, given such outrageous behaviour he would as soon carry them to a brothel.[49] Accidents led to embarrassment too. At Ramsgate in 1801, a bathing machine overturned in the autumn winds. The two men in it lost all their clothes and ran for shelter to nearby bathing rooms. They were filled with women and 'a scene of much confusion ensued'.[50]

As sea bathing became more popular, coastal resorts tried to enforce segregation: the sexes bathed at different times or were asked to use different parts of the beach. At Brighton, in the early 1800s, women generally went into the water on the east side of town and men to the west. But well into the 1860s, men and women were found bathing near each other.[51] This was not so surprising because few people swam; most bathers were 'dipped' close to their machine. Problems increased when people did begin to swim for pleasure; men considered swimming drawers effeminate and entered the water 'in a state of nature'. Critics now grumbled that on British beaches there was 'not the slightest pretension to even common decency'.[52]

The situation was partly a class issue. Steamboats and faster rail travel meant that beaches were sometimes crowded with day-trippers. Working-class tourists were either ignorant of the conventions or had no money to hire a bathing machine. This was especially true in Margate. An easy sail from London, it had been fashionable in the mid-eighteenth century but went downmarket when faster, cheaper transport brought holiday crowds. The open-air, seaside experience was easier to infiltrate than an exclusive spa. That said, upper-class men who insisted on bathing in the time-honoured way remained a key problem. For one reason or another, regulations about mixed bathing were often ignored or unenforced.

Peeping Toms at the coast carried telescopes or lorgnettes, which they trained on women's bathing machines rather than on distant shipping. But women were just as likely to spy on naked men. At Margate in 1865, women were observed using their opera glasses to get a better view.[53] Even so, some ladies preferred to act as if male sea-bathers in the nude were invisible or simply not present.[54] It says much for Victorian double standards that female students were only admitted to life drawing classes at the Royal Academy late in the century and, even then, the models had to be partially clothed.

In contrast, the French had always allowed mixed bathing. They also preferred beach cabins to clumsy bathing machines with hoods. Because in France bathers had to walk down to the water, both sexes wore costumes extending from neck to knee. It was the same in the United States, where mixed bathing in some form of dress had long been the custom. Fanny Kemble described the scene in 1838, when, to escape the heat of New York, she took her children to Long Island:

> There are two little stationary bathing-huts for the use of the whole population; and you dress, undress, dry yourself, and do all you have to do, in the closest proximity to persons you never saw in your life before. . . . This admitting absolute strangers to the intimacy of one's most private toilet operations is quite intolerable, and nothing but the benefit which I believe the children, as well as myself, derive from the bathing would induce me to endure it.[55]

Decades later, Americans would complain about gross indecency on British beaches, where they found men sauntering practically unclothed just yards from 'mothers and nurses, with their companies of young girls'.[56] The ambiguity of British beach etiquette persisted until the end of the century, when nude and mixed bathing was forcefully suppressed in major resorts, and it became routine for men on mixed beaches to wear a costume. Meanwhile, Victorian women got an eyeful.

WELLNESS TOURISM

Health visitors to seaside resorts always expected to be diverted. At Margate, a notable attraction into the 1800s was the chance to buy smuggled goods at cheap prices from sailors. Seaside towns also copied

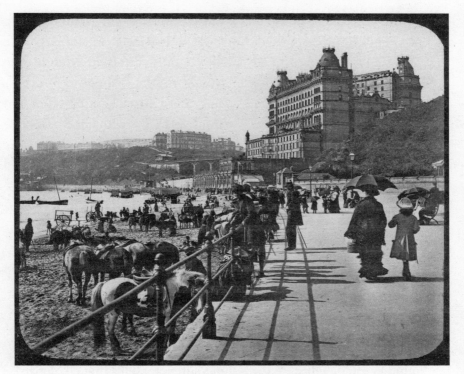

16. Foreshore Road, Scarborough, in the 1900s. The Grand Hotel, on the right, opened in 1867.

many of the legitimate entertainments that spas provided. There were assemblies, balls, theatres, libraries, markets, and raffles for trinkets. The chief entertainments soon moved from the town itself to the seafront. Seaside promenades replicated spa walks; yachts and carriages could be hired for pleasure trips to neighbouring villages.

Some thought that the craze for sea bathing would spoil life for coastal residents. Elizabeth Carter, based in Deal, was glad the town boasted no assembly rooms or public diversions: 'We can never become a fashionable bathing place, which is a very lucky circumstance for the natural inhabitants.'[57] She deduced that in fashionable resorts local businesses grew dishonest, unable to resist the temptation to overcharge visitors; residents then suffered when the cost of provisions increased.

Critics also objected to rakish behaviour at seaside towns: the mingling of ranks in public places, the late hours spent dancing and gambling. By the early 1800s, the novelist Lady Charlotte Bury dismissed Brighton as 'a sink for the lees of dissipation'.[58] Seaside visitors themselves noticed that they easily slipped into bad habits. Mary Figgens, at Margate in 1828, admitted that, freed from watchful neighbours, she had become lax about going to church on Sundays.[59] The lowering of moral tone in seaside places was something that Jane Austen was exploring in *Sanditon*. Families with daughters to marry off and businessmen eager to turn towns into money-spinning destinations shared the same mercenary outlook.

Remote, solitary beaches remained an attractive option if women could escape there. On the west coast of Ireland, Elizabeth Ham recorded splashing in the sea each morning with female friends for an hour or more. After a hearty breakfast, they were often so sleepy they had to fortify themselves with a glass of port wine.[60] But remote beaches were not always idyllic. In August 1870, on holiday in north Wales, Catherine Paget, daughter of the famous surgeon James Paget, recorded grimly, 'A very unpleasant bathe this morning: all on the stones & frightfully rough.'[61]

As major resorts became tourist sites, they held less attraction for those genuinely seeking recuperation. At Ramsgate's East Cliff in 1861, Jane Welsh Carlyle appreciated the sea air, which improved her appetite, but scorned the town below, 'The shops look nasty, the people nasty, the smells are nasty! (spoiled shrimps complicated with cesspool!)'[62] Even suburban East Cliff was too noisy for her, with its brass bands, groups of female fiddlers, and blacked-up entertainers, the beginnings of traditional seaside attractions. Her dissatisfaction may simply reflect passing feelings and the state of her tense marriage: she travelled alone, leaving her workaholic husband at his desk. Having insisted that her health demanded sea air, she could hardly admit to him that she was having a good time. It was the same when she went to Folkstone in 1865. There she complained of a superabundance of earwigs: 'They are found in your *hair-brush*! in *the Book* you are reading! in fact I defy you to say where they will NOT be found!'[63]

Yet burgeoning sea resorts, like spa towns, offered varied occupations to women who had to support themselves. The early feminist writer Mary Ann Radcliffe, infirm and widowed, tried to make a living by selling pastries during the summer season at Portobello in the early 1800s. It was the nearest beach to Edinburgh.[64] Sadly, she found that the cost of her business exceeded the money she could earn. Others, with more capital, set up coastal boarding schools for girls whose parents thought they needed sea air for their health. As in spa towns, some women became notable social figures. Martha Gunn, for example, brawny and rotund, was known as 'queen' of the Brighton dippers. Born in 1726, she dipped from about 1750 until ill health forced her to retire in 1814 or so. She was honoured in song and thought to be a reassuring presence during the Napoleonic Wars. She featured in humorous prints designed to quell invasion fears, shown repelling French forces with her bare hands.

Sea bathing, like spa visiting, brought genteel women into contact with resilient lower-class women doing hard manual work. At Teignmouth in 1773, Maria, a stepsister of Fanny Burney, wrote: 'You see nothing here but women in the summer – their husbands all go out to the Newfoundland fishery for 8 or 9 months in the [year] so the women do all the laborious business such as *rowing* and *towing* the boats and go out a fishing yet I never saw cleaner Cottages nor healthier finer Children.'[65] Teignmouth had few visitors, and local women were so poor they wheeled the town's bathing machine into the water themselves.

In 1791, Fanny Burney viewed women working the cockle beds near Exmouth:

Women scarce clothed at all, with feet and legs entirely naked, straw bonnets of uncouth shapes tied on their heads, a sort of man's jacket on their bodies, and their short coats pinned up in the form of concise trousers, very succinct! and a basket on each arm, strolling along with wide mannish strides to the borders of the river, gathering cockles. They looked, indeed, miserable and savage.[66]

Their appearance was so alien to her that she could only compare them to drawings of South Sea Islanders, published after Captain Cook's 1768–71 voyage of exploration to the Pacific. Burney was attuned to contemporary descriptions of unfamiliar peoples living close to nature. Her brother James had served on Cook's second and third voyages, and he wrote about voyages to the Pacific Ocean after he retired from the navy. If doctors used the robustness of coastal women as evidence of the sea's health benefits, genteel female visitors were keenly struck by these examples of female independence.

FASHION AND DISPLAY

In Victorian times, leisure seekers flocked to seaside resorts. A relaxing break with exercise did much good, but fun and entertainment mattered more to these crowds than the health benefits of sea water. On the beach, women sought new freedoms and displayed more of their bodies than ever before. Of course, there was a downside: bathing costumes became fashion garments that changed with the season; bodies had to be toned.

'Elegant' bathing dresses for women (some even with life-preserving cork jackets) were advertised as early as the 1780s, although most women still bathed in homemade woollen smocks.[67] Bathing gowns were made of heavy material that billowed out in the water. In the nineteenth century, these dresses became shorter and were worn over bloomers or trousers. By 1890, most costumes for women were bifurcated and high-necked, though often short-sleeved. The trousers came down to below the knees if women used a bathing machine; otherwise, they might be buttoned at the ankle. A skirt was still considered indispensable to disguise hips, and it was fastened by a belt over the one-piece costume.

Heavy twilled flannel was the recommended material, being warmer and less clingy than other fabrics. Navy blue was the fashionable colour, tastefully embroidered or trimmed in white. Fashion experts warned that coarse lace and fancy buttons were vulgar.[68]

Hair was an issue for women bathers. By the time that sea bathing grew popular in the 1790s, manufacturers of hair dye had to assure clients that salt water would not alter its effect. On the whole, it seemed best not to get hair wet. In the 1880s, Parisiennes were rumoured to wear wigs into the sea. In any case, they could be seen sporting wide-brimmed straw hats, taking care not to let the sea reach their hair. American women favoured close-fitting, oiled-silk caps under straw bonnets for additional protection. Allegedly, sea bathing could cause hair to fall out in clumps – a source of much anxiety. Doctors reassured women that it would grow back, but by the early twentieth century manufacturers had come up with restorative hair washes to 'remove the sticky feeling left by the sea', just as expensive soaps were marketed to repair the skin after sea bathing.[69]

For upper-class women, a key reason to visit French spas and beaches in summer was to get an early glimpse of dress fashions for September, which would be on display. In the late nineteenth century, society magazines began to carry pieces on beach fashion. This became much more important once mixed bathing was the norm. Navy-blue serge dresses were all the rage on promenades; they could withstand a splash of sea water yet still look smart. By the early 1900s, fashion dictated lightweight serge bathing suits and straw poke bonnets, which were making a comeback. Both items were quite unsuitable for swimming. As more women learned to swim, practical swimwear became a battle-ground because it exposed more of their limbs. Combination garments of stockinette came into vogue, daringly sleeveless but still knee-length. Yet all knitted bathing costumes sagged in the water and, until the invention of elastic yarn in the 1930s, threatened modesty.

Beach culture has proved both liberating and repressive for women. In Atlantic City in the 1920s, women could be arrested for revealing too much flesh, although a tan was fashionable by then. Ironically, the Miss America beauty contest began in Atlantic City in 1921. From the outset, the competition included a swimsuit round and some contestants dared to bare their knees. Racy images of women in close-fitting swimsuits appeared in newspapers from the 1920s; by the 1930s, women were sunbathing in two-piece costumes that showed their midriff. Yet the competitive element was always present: in the 1930s, when the British chemists Timothy Whites and Taylors Ltd brought out their holiday brochure, they prefaced the beachwear section with the ominous caption 'Look perfect in the water'.[70]

During the Second World War, many British beaches were fortified with barbed wire against invasion. Women who defiantly managed a semblance of the beach experience found it a comforting reminder of a way of life they hoped could be recovered. In North America especially, images of models in swimwear carried patriotic meaning and were used to boost morale. After the war, pin-up calendars became normalised, displayed in male workplaces and leisure settings such as public bars.

Beauty contests with women in swimsuits became a regular feature in Britain, helping to boost morale as part of the post-war recovery. Between 1956 and 1989, these were staged at the seaside in Morecambe, setting standards for the female beach body. The ideal was self-evidently white and European. In the United States, where beaches were racially segregated into the 1960s, women of colour were excluded from the Miss America competition until 1970, by which time feminists were protesting at beauty contests, throwing flour and tomatoes. At the same time, community-based Black pageants had a strong following. They offered a space where white ideals of beauty could be challenged, even if contestants were chiefly looking for fun and adventure.

Technological advances in materials, including the invention of Lycra in the mid-1970s, allowed the manufacture of swimsuits that kept their shape, helping to overturn expectations of female modesty on the beach. But mass media outlets increasingly imposed stringent beauty standards on the female beach body. The culmination of this trend was perhaps the infamous Protein World weight-loss advertisement that appeared in the London Underground network in April 2015. The poster read 'Are You Beach Body Ready?' It was repeatedly defaced. Women complained to the UK Advertising Standards Agency that the campaign was body-shaming for profit and objectified women. It was banned on the Tube, although later shown in North America; Protein World benefited hugely from the publicity. In 2018, the offensive slogan was reclaimed by the body positivity movement but the link between the beach experience and the objectification of women's bodies is hard to break. When, in 2021, the Olympic women's beach handball team complained about sexist uniform rules that required them to play in bikinis, the International Handball Federation conceded only that, from 2022, female beach players could wear 'body fit' tank tops and 'short tight pants'.

In Britain at least, the rage for sea bathing has dwindled, partly because increasing awareness of the level of pollutants in coastal waters has cancelled out any long-held association between water, health, and purification. Clearly, women's experience of spas and sea resorts has always been ambivalent. This was particularly the case when it was a chance to secure a marriage partner, not just improve health and well-being; a young woman's stay would be monetised and hedged by social expectation. That said, the desire for liberty and self-expression is shaped by the experience of repression. Spas offered visitors a wider circle; the beach could allow a complete subversion of social proprieties. Women at all social levels benefited from the opportunities afforded by these health trends and, in the process, they made a significant contribution to the economy and character of spa towns and coastal resorts.

EPILOGUE

Health and beauty remain urgent life goals today. After all, attractive women still have an advantage when it comes to finding desirable partners. And they still have an advantage when securing jobs, despite feminist activism which supports equal opportunities and challenges the sexualisation of workplaces. Admittedly, in some professions those with plain features may be rated more competent, but on the whole good looks are beneficial, not least because they increase self-confidence and help to produce a better impression.

The pursuit of health and beauty has taken countless paths over these four hundred years, but there are obvious continuities. Consumers remain susceptible to hyperbolic claims for beauty products. Women today are happy to use a range of hair preparations once intended for horses, Mane 'n' Tail. There is still unrelenting pressure to achieve whatever body shape is in vogue. Restrictive undergarments are by no means a thing of the past; the global shapewear industry is booming. Even corsets and waist trainers still have a following, despite predictable warnings about everyday use. And there remains widespread unease about appearance and reality when it comes to women's looks, even in this age of rampant photo-editing, semi-permanent makeup, and technology to develop personalised skincare.

Obviously, a woman's public image is unlikely to reveal her complete identity; the function of a created look is partly to disguise or enhance the real person. But as more women use virtual, try-on features to experiment with dress and makeup, their online image can become a counterpoint to how they look in real life. The experience of Covid lockdowns emphasised that, although personal care may be self-affirming, the visible result is chiefly designed to impress a person's status and role on an audience. Women who work online from home, at one remove from social situations and the judgement of peers and superiors, are prone to the charge of 'neglecting their appearance', a criticism once directed at suburban housewives. Yet some report feeling pressured to look their best online, when other means of influencing colleagues are drastically curtailed. There has been a rise in plastic surgery due to online networking software such as Zoom.[1]

Social media may fragment audiences, but it has had a great effect on the pursuit of health and beauty. Whereas in the nineteenth century women turned to beauty manuals, and in the twentieth century to magazines, young women today go online for advice and information about beauty issues. Role models have aways been influential: society belles, music-hall celebrities, femmes fatales, high-profile actors, and famous pop stars have all prompted fashions or helped to sell products. The effect of such cult figures can persist for decades: in the 1950s, girdles were still advertised as essential to achieve the seductive Mata Hari look, although the courtesan had been executed as a spy during the First World War. But now social media uniquely draws on the encyclopaedic information of the Internet and enables an immediate response. 'Influencers' offering beauty and exercise tips not only increase knowledge of products and techniques but also build trust, until viewers are ready to chance an online purchase. Top influencers create a demand that is continually updated.

Health and beauty are preoccupations which are increasingly affected by globalisation. A homogenised white beauty ideal, accentuating youth and slimness, is heavily promoted worldwide. This owes much to the United States, where historically the beauty industry has enjoyed large advertising budgets and where, due to social pressures, women spend large sums on beauty products. The image of the ideal modern woman naturally varies in different countries because of a layering of the local and global, but it is difficult to escape idealised body shapes. Women everywhere are bombarded with images of what, ideally, they should look like.

THE BEAUTY INDUSTRY

The commodification of beauty took off in the early twentieth century as hairdressing salons multiplied and more cosmetics and toiletries were produced on an industrial scale. Commercial societies brought freedom of choice but, increasingly, the female body became a site for competing economic and industrial interests. In 2019, before the Covid-19 pandemic, the global beauty industry generated an astonishing $500 billion in sales a year.[2] The creation of makeup, fragrances, and products for hair, skin, and personal care accounted for millions of jobs, directly and indirectly. Covid restrictions underscored the industry's economic value while exposing some of the commercial pressures women face. With the shift to home working and mask-wearing, sales of lipstick and other makeup plummeted. In 2020, retail sales in the beauty industry declined globally by 15 per cent in comparison to the previous year; colour cosmetics took the biggest hit, with sales falling by 33 per cent.[3]

The market for beauty products is expected to recover. That said, a survey in 2022 found that more women were choosing to go makeup free, which prompted story-sharing on social media. Some welcomed the trend, commenting that makeup was bad for the skin, harmed the environment, was overly tested on animals, and was liable to blatant greenwashing. They claimed that women were more comfortable in their skin and had no need of makeup to feel powerful or beautiful. Others contradicted this view, complaining that they were still expected to wear makeup for work and had no choice in the matter, while others insisted that they chose to wear makeup for themselves, even if home-working. Intriguingly, some wore makeup for remote working because they were treated better when they had it on. A few sceptics thought that the whole debate was a massive phishing exercise prompted by the beauty industry.

The quest for health and beauty, which affects multiple aspects of the body, is bolstered by an extensive web of influence that is hard to ignore or escape. These days, perfect teeth, a slender body, and stylish hair are better class signifiers than dress itself.[4] The desired look keeps changing, so the demand for improving products is always present. Yet the promised improvement is rarely attained, or not for long, because women age. The commercial motive is inescapable. For example, plus-sized models may feature in advertising but do so to reassure customers that a certain brand has their interests at heart; the 'authentic' body is used to increase sales.

BEAUTY AND MENTAL HEALTH

The Covid pandemic increased anxiety among the general population and inevitably affected women with body image problems. On the one hand, video conferencing and seeing their faces on screen made people more conscious of their appearance. On the other, mask-wearing and the chance to hide body contours in baggy clothing while home working encouraged camouflaging behaviour. Gym closures exacerbated mental health issues. Exercise for wellbeing is touted more than ever as a public health concept, but knowing that exercise is good for you and feeling good about doing exercise are different things. For many, fear of embar-rassment is a barrier to keeping fit.

The body positivity movement has done much to reclaim the word 'fat'. The word has even been excised from Roald Dahl's children's books. The fat-shaming so prevalent in the past is now less common. But women who are heavier than usual are still regarded as lacking in self-control, even if not plain lazy and stupid. Keeping fit, especially at a time when there is pressure on national health services, has become a moral issue. Those who neglect to exercise can feel guilty and may even experience hostility, although not all weight issues are due to a lack of exercise. Ironically, the road to self-improvement itself turns out to be emotionally damaging. Being fat can also be a sign of social inequality today. The dangers of overly processed, unhealthy food have been well documented, but food products are often made to be tasty and cheap. The actor and political activist Miriam Margolyes is typically acerbic on body image: 'The fashion industry compels us to be skinny, the food industry compels us to be fat. We are treated like a punchball between those two industries for money. That's what capitalism does.'[5]

In another paradox, today's emphasis on wellbeing and the advice to accept one's body shape sits uneasily alongside the ideal of slim beauty. Advertisements for iconic brands routinely tell women to embrace their flaws.[6] Yet, as with many aspects of health and beauty, such advice can be turned on its head. Some women are unable to come to terms with their appearance. They feel that they have doubly failed and experience the body positivity movement as toxic. Beauty is obviously related to an individual's physical health and mental wellbeing, but health itself is increasingly commodified in the beauty market. The concept of well-being is co-opted to sell products designed for bodily care.

These ambiguities and the manipulation of consumers help to explain why the pursuit of health and beauty can be experienced as both empowering and oppressive, both creative and deadening. Wellbeing and preventative medicine seem to be matters of personal responsibility. Health and beauty products give people choices about their appearance but also make them responsible for how they signal their identity. Cosmetic purchases do enable many women to obtain the so-called beauty premium but some baulk at the expectations imposed on them. The singer-songwriter Billie Eilish has explored body-shaming for her Generation Z fanbase. Her short film *Not My Responsibility* is a response to the double standards placed on young women regarding appearance – she got negative comments when she promoted body positivity and wore oversized clothes to conceal her shape, and still more criticism when she wore corsets that revealed her curves. Some women spend so much on their looks that their beauty habits can be termed a lifestyle. It may be a personal decision to opt for plastic surgery and beauty treatments, despite cultural pressure. But those who pursue youth and beauty above all else risk losing control of their lives.

A view of women's health and beauty over four centuries helps to explain why, with regard to personal grooming, women find it hard to attain the self-confidence needed to resist manipulation. In the past, they had to fight to wear makeup overtly. Consequently, they are susceptible to the argument (often used in marketing) that makeup is a right and allows them to create their own identity. Health and beauty are bound up with women's activism. Many who campaigned for women's suffrage were also active in the dress reform movement, demanding practical, comfortable clothes that permitted healthy exercise. Similarly, aspects of the pursuit of health and beauty are linked to women's fight to contribute to the political life of the nation. In the case of women of colour, health and beauty practices are also linked to their struggle to be free from racial oppression.

BEAUTY AND SOCIAL VALUES

Attitudes to female health and beauty illustrate changing social values and how we think about modernity. The 'New Woman' who emerged in the late nineteenth century and campaigned for rational dress was eager for social and political reform. The 'Modern Woman' who succeeded her in the 1920s and 1930s, with some overlap, was just as independently minded but more concerned with refashioning her body to mirror the aspirations of a new age. Thanks to networks of world trade and faster transmission of cultural influences, the Modern Woman emerged as a recognisable figure across continents, with local variations.

Her svelte athletic outline, her precise makeup, and very often her distinctive short hair signalled a determination to grasp the opportunities of modern life, whatever the dangers. As the image of the Modern Woman permeated the global marketing of cosmetics and toiletries, it contributed to the ethnic formation of beauty in different nations, although, in colonial settings, women of European descent had long monopolised the category of 'beautiful women'.[7]

Across the world, the twists and turns of cultural change are played out and reflected on the female body. In open cultures, the latest grooming practices and trends rapidly become the norm. It is now unremarkable to see women in trousers, although, as noted, in 1930 one commentator thought that women would never wear male dress since it was not beautiful. The pursuit of health and beauty can be both enslaving and modernising to different degrees. But it would be a mistake to wish for a static standard; the world would be confined to a narrow appreciation of beauty.

Physical expressions of health and beauty can be moulded to convey gender-fluid identities. The use of cosmetics is a way for gay men and those of fluid gender to connect with femininity. This is nothing new: the Chevalier d'Éon wore makeup and wigs in the 1770s. In recent years, increasing numbers of heterosexual men have started to wear makeup, aiming for the flawless skin tone associated with cosmetic use. The growth of unisex and men's products is a profitable trend in the beauty industry, and many brands are staking a claim to gender inclusivity, using trans models and developing genderless makeup lines. In 2021, Unilever announced that it was dropping the term 'normal' in its messaging about beauty products. (Typically, the term had been used to describe products for the hair and skin.) The beauty industry chiefly wishes to appear responsive to consumer issues to sell more product, but in defining brands as socially responsible and inclusive it also helps to shift cultural norms.

Early on, the pursuit of beauty became infused with national pride, which enabled the racialisation of beauty aesthetics. Among both Black and white people, advertisements for beauty products were chiefly aimed at the leisured upper or middle classes. In the African American press of the early twentieth century, advertisements for Madam C. J. Walker's skin creams were infused with a politicised celebration of Blackness. They appealed to bourgeois ideals of hygiene and deportment and were shaped by the notion that it was the duty of African American women to promote 'racial uplift'. Into the 1940s, newspapers in the United States, Europe, and the European colonies marketed creams to preserve skin from tanning in ways that tacitly implied that white skin was superior.

Historically, the beauty industry has promoted white supremacy and been limited in product range and brand messaging when it comes to diversity and inclusion. In the wake of Covid, the Black Lives Matter movement, the success of Black celebrities, and growing support for the LGBTQ+ community, this is changing. Many beauty brands are responding to consumer demand worldwide for products that reflect all ages, skin tones, genders, and body types. This trend towards diversity and inclusion also means that there is greater representation of minorities in brand videos, advertisements, e-commerce photography, and among social media influencers. And because liberal consumers often seek out brands that align with their core values, some companies insist that their inclusive products are supported behind the scenes by an equitable workplace. The beauty industry seems to be moving towards the promotion of shared values as a force for social cohesion, rather than fabricating national beauty types.

A study of contemporary health and beauty shows the increasing impact of consumers' environmental concerns. Some ingredients from endangered species, such as spermaceti and baleen, have long been superseded. The civet is now a critically endangered species, so certain perfume manufacturers use synthetic civet oil rather than the fluid extracted from its glands. The beauty industry, constrained by the availability of raw materials, is bound to monitor some environmental concerns. It is also aware that consumers often consider sustainable approaches to cosmetics when making a purchase. Customers become attached to brands that appear symbolic of their own values, allowing them to project a particular self-image through consumption. Arguably, mass-produced cosmetics manufactured with harsh chemicals and toxins no longer find such a ready market. Younger consumers call for sustainable, natural ingredients, minimal packaging, and fair working conditions, all paving the way for new industry standards.

Makeup is therefore increasingly linked to social conscience. The use of animals to test cosmetic ingredients, which energised the 'beauty without cruelty' movement of the 1970s, still prompts outrage. Animal testing was banned in the UK and in member states of the European Union. Then, in 2020, an EU agency ruled that companies could test cosmetic ingredients on animals if there were safety concerns for workers during the manufacturing process. In the UK, public opinion is still against the practice. Most say that they would not buy a cosmetic product if they knew it had been tested on animals; in 2023, the government had to promise that it would grant no more licences for animal testing of chemicals exclusively used in makeup.[8]

Sectors of the beauty industry readily target scrupulous, eco-conscious consumers, by touting natural, organic ingredients and 'pure' or 'plant-loving' products. In this context, the terms 'clean' and 'natural' are not well defined, and the green marketing of beauty products has led to the demonising of perfectly inert substances and to the overuse of botanicals which, in high concentrations, can irritate the skin; after all, 'natural' does not necessarily mean 'safe'. But revenue from the natural and organic cosmetics market is growing worldwide as women prioritise products that are advertised as sustainable or vegan.

Responsible consumers are seeking to reduce their environmental impact in other ways, by choosing hygiene and cosmetic products in solid form rather than liquid versions which are mostly sold in plastic containers. Fashion commentators have extended the term 'utility chic' to cover cosmetics that combine two or more uses in one, such as a hand cream that also serves as a lip balm, or soap that also works as shampoo.

The beauty industry thrives in a value system that links human worth to what we look like, but to some extent individuals are prepared to alter consumption patterns for the good of the environment.

GROWING OLD

Any exploration of health and beauty throws light on women's experiences of growing old. The body is a mark of time and, while some societies esteem older members, Western cultures idealise beauty and youth. The double standard applied to ageing men and women means that older women are more likely to be socially marginalised and more at risk of losing their jobs. The physical changes of later life not only pose a challenge to older women's social status but can also affect their earning power. In this light, the pursuit of health and beauty is anything but a subjective or trivial matter for older women, and many aim to mitigate the social consequences of looking old.

Some brands tout their inclusivity by extending ranges to older age groups. Yet the assumption is always that female consumers will wish to appear younger and aim to reduce the signs of ageing rather than accept them. One thing is clear: everybody gets older, so the treatments on offer yield diminishing returns. Mature women are less likely to be swayed by the latest trends; they know how they wish to present them-selves. But they can still fall prey to advertisements for miracle skin creams. In this field, the beauty industry often implies that the signs of age are somehow medically abnormal. Dark-spot correcting creams, for example, are marketed for age-onset blemishes. These high-end, 'anti-ageing' creams contain skin-bleaching properties and other ingredients to brighten, lighten, and tighten the skin, addressing an issue coyly described as 'uneven pigmentation'.

In societies that define youth as a standard of beauty, how does the ageing process affect individuals? Diaries and letters reveal how women have reacted to the natural process of growing old, and how, at different periods, they have sensed how the passing of time is written on the body. For example, in 1808, Sarah Collingwood, who had not seen her admiral husband for five years while he was serving at sea, wrote to confess that she had become 'immoderately fat'.[9] In 1850, Jane Welsh Carlyle learned that her mother-in-law could not be fitted with the upper false teeth needed to improve her speech and appearance: Victorian dentistry lacked the technology.[10] This revelation affected Carlyle's attitude to her own dental problems and sharpened her sense of ageing. Tooth decay impinges disproportionately on women because of social expectations. This helps to explain how toothpaste and gum products are advertised today, and the importance of teeth in advertising generally.

Older women who wear a lot of makeup, or who appear excessively disciplined in matters of diet and exercise, have long prompted derision as well as censure. Charlotte Charke, author, actor and noted cross-dresser, wrote in her autobiography of 1755 that her estranged elder sister was of an age when she should cease to paint her face and instead consider her soul.[11] Aware of such attitudes, some women have attempted to forestall criticism. Elizabeth Cady Stanton, an activist in the women's rights movement in the United States with much influence in Britain, professed to welcome old age. 'The hey-day of woman's life is the shady side of fifty', she wrote, averring that the time had come when she could devote herself to the inner, higher life, for 'who would be forever young, to dwell always in externals?'[12] But Stanton was notably vigorous in old age. Others, less fortunate, find that ageing means not just wrinkles and grey hair but years of poor health. An older Fanny Kemble was particularly distressed by her lack of energy, 'a greater sign of age than white hairs, wrinkles, or loss of teeth'.[13] She had spent a lifetime travelling and crossed the Atlantic seventeen times, but as an old woman baulked at even a short journey.

Most disguise the ageing process for as long as possible. After all, as a famous eighteenth-century hairdresser noted, beauty and virtue have great advantages over virtue alone.[14] Wrinkles bring their own set of judgements, particularly for women. Do they look older or younger than their years? Are their clothes age-appropriate? Are they age-defying or growing old disgracefully? Since the signs of age are influenced by lifestyle, many such judgements are implicitly moral ones. From this viewpoint, if you look old and fat you have only yourself to blame. Yet a youthful appearance often depends on income and whether an individual can afford expensive treatments. Social media now attracts numerous mid-life influencers (who generally look nothing like their years). That said, some older women defiantly post online images of themselves as they begin to look their age and worse.

Many social media posts reflect women's conflicted response to ageing. Typical comments include, 'It's all very well for the lucky ones, but what about those whose looks have been devastated by age, who have lost all confidence and self-esteem but are never allowed to admit it and have to pretend that old age is wonderful and liberating.' Or, 'We get told that it's wonderful to be invisible because now we can do whatever we want because no one cares. How is that supposed to make me feel good?' Women's reflections in contemporary magazines are equally illuminating. One author expresses relief at the prospect of letting go, of leaving off the hair dye and the makeup that has ceased to flatter an ageing face, of no longer having to pretend to be anything but what she is. Another, at ninety-one, feels shame if she does not walk at least five thousand Fitbit steps and swim forty lengths of the pool each day.[15] Some with grey hair opt for rainbow-hued 'fairy strands' or tinsel extensions, although the very name suggests a wish to believe in the power of magic rather than technology.

There is an element of doubling and contradiction at the heart of the debate about health and beauty. Some feminists argue that the beauty industry exploits women – that, in order to make women feel good about themselves, it first has to make them feel bad about themselves. Others maintain that women have choices in society and can use the opportunities afforded by the current beauty culture to personal advantage. The very existence of such contradictions adds to the anguish some women feel about their appearance: they sense that they are trapped, whether they follow the latest health and beauty trends or ignore them. Even a woman as successful as Michelle Obama confesses to having trouble accepting herself as she is, and in her writing explores how best to cope with anxiety and self-doubt – although this helps, of course, to make her an appealing role model.

The pursuit of health and beauty is ultimately a quest for power and happiness, which is why it is important for the full range of Black beauty to be recognised and respected. It has always been bound up with a range of social, cultural, and medical developments. In the future, it will be implicated in a fresh round of creativity. But paradox is at the very heart of the subject. With the emergence of a more secular, consumer society, people bought into the notion of collective social improvement maximising opportunities for the individual. Yet ideas of beauty are inescapably tied to the degeneration of the body. Whatever perfection an individual attains can only be transient. The beauty industry is a major beneficiary of this paradox, profiting first from the youthful wish to attain an ideal and later from the need to delay the ageing process. It also profits from the contradictory relationship between the liberal idea of individuality and the pressures of social conformity, between celebrating varieties of beauty and seeking an empowering standard. This ensures a continually renewing market for beauty products and health aids. In a worldly age, there is little hope of escaping such contradictions and perhaps no strong desire to do so. The sense of optimism seems to have faltered badly in our times, but the quest for beauty continues to promise the world.

NOTES

BARS	Bedfordshire Archives and Records Service
BL	British Library
BM	British Museum
Bodleian	Bodleian Library, Oxford University
Carter, *Letters*	Elizabeth Carter, *Letters from Mrs. Elizabeth Carter to Mrs. Montagu, Between the Years 1755 and 1800*, ed. Rev. Montagu Pennington, 3 vols (London: F. C. & J. Rivington, 1817)
CL	*Country Life*
CLO	Thomas Carlyle and Jane Welsh Carlyle, *The Carlyle Letters Online*, ed. Brent E. Kinser (Duke University Press, 2007–16), https://carlyleletters.dukeupress.edu
E. Montagu, *Letters*	Elizabeth Montagu, *The Letters of Mrs. E. Montagu: With Some of the Letters of Her Correspondents*, ed. M. Montagu, 4 vols (London: W. Bulmer for T. Cadell and W. Davies, 1809–13)
HB	*Harper's Bazaar*
ILN	*Illustrated London News*
JE diary	John Evelyn, *The Diary of John Evelyn*, ed. E. S. De Beer, 6 vols (Oxford: Clarendon Press, 1955)
LMA	London Metropolitan Archives
Montagu, *Letters*	Lady Mary Wortley Montagu, *The Complete Letters of Lady Mary Wortley Montagu*, ed. Robert Halsband, 3 vols (Oxford: Clarendon Press, 1965–7)
NMM	National Maritime Museum, Greenwich, London (now part of Royal Museums Greenwich)
OBP	Old Bailey Proceedings Online, www.oldbaileyonline.org
SP diary	Samuel Pepys, *The Diary of Samuel Pepys*, ed. Robert Latham and William Matthews, 11 vols (London: G. Bell & Hyman, 1970–83)

TNA   The National Archives, London

UKDS   P. Thompson and T. Lummis, *Family Life and Work Experience Before 1918, 1870–1973* [data collection], 7th edn (2009), UK Data Service, SN: 2000, https://ukdataservice.ac.uk/app/uploads/guidefamilylifeandworkexperiencebefore1918.pdf

PREFACE

1. Olivette Otele, *African Europeans: An Untold History* (London: Hurst & Company, 2020), 182–3.

INTRODUCTION

1. *The Listener* (15 August 1946), 208.
2. *Lakes Herald* (24 November 1882), 4.
3. Lady Mary Coke, *The Letters and Journals of Lady Mary Coke*, ed. J. A. Home, 4 vols (Edinburgh: David Douglas, 1889–96), IV, 81 (6 June 1772).
4. E.g. Ben Child, 'Beyoncé's Rep Denies She is Making a Film About Freak-Show Victim Saartjie Baartman', *Guardian*, 6 January 2016, https://www.theguardian.com/film/2016/jan/06/beyonce-rep-denies-film-freak-show-victim-saartjie-baartman (accessed 21 November 2023).
5. Norma Myers, *Reconstructing the Black Past: Blacks in Britain 1780–1830* (London: Frank Cass, 1996), 18; *The Gentleman's Magazine*, 34 (1764) 493.
6. Charmaine Nelson, 'Venus Africaine: Race, Beauty and African-ness' in Jan Marsh, ed., *Black Victorians: Black People in British Art 1800–1900* (Aldershot: Lund Humphries, 2005), 47.
7. Dorothea Herbert, *Retrospections of Dorothea Herbert, 1770–1789, 1789–1806*, 2 vols (London: Gerald Howe, 1929–30), I, 64.
8. Susanna Cocroft, *Beauty a Duty: The Art of Keeping Young* (Chicago and New York: Rand McNally & Co., 1915), 270.
9. *The Listener* (31 December 1930), 1107.
10. *Beauty and Fashion: An Illustrated Journal for Women*, 1 (29 November 1890), 6.

1 BODY SCULPTURE

1. See Charmaine A. Nelson, *Representing the Black Female Subject in Western Art* (New York and Abingdon: Routledge, 2010).
2. Montagu, *Letters*, I, 314, LM to Lady — (1 April 1717).
3. SP diary, VIII, 193 (1 May 1667).
4. LMA ACC/1302/075, Dorothy Wood to her husband (undated but before 1704).
5. Francis Place, *The Autobiography of Francis Place*, ed. Mary Thrale (Cambridge: Cambridge University Press, 1972), 52.
6. Ibid., 78.
7. *London Daily Post and General Advertiser* (1 January 1736), 1.

8. Edward Ward, *The London Spy*, ed. Paul Hyland (East Lansing, MI: Colleagues Press, 1993), 198, 296.

9. E. Montagu, *Letters*, IV, 21–22, EM to Mrs Scott (28 May 1756).

10. Sir Charles Knowles, *The Trial of Captain G— for Crim. Con with Admiral K—s's Lady* (London: for H. Owen, 1757), 18.

11. Ward, *London Spy*, 246.

12. *Public Advertiser* (4 July 1775), 2.

13. OBP, 4 December 1754, trial of Elizabeth Maddox and Sarah Jenkins (t17541204-33).

14. See OBP, 17 January 1728, trial of Sarah Dickenson (t17280117-43).

15. Mary Delany, *The Autobiography and Correspondence of Mary Granville, Mrs Delany*, ed. Lady Llanover, 2nd series, 3 vols (London: Richard Bentley, 1861–2), I, 497–8, MD to Mrs Port of Ilam (1 March 1773).

16. *The Gentleman's Magazine*, 13 (1743), 430.

17. *Public Advertiser* (26 January 1788), 1.

18. Frances Burney, *Diary and Letters of Madame d'Arblay (1778–1840)*, ed. Charlotte Barrett, 6 vols (London: Macmillan & Co., 1904–5), I, 93 (26 August 1778).

19. Rebecca Gibson, 'Effects of Long Term Corseting on the Female Skeleton', *Canadian Student Journal of Anthropology*, 23, no. 2 (2015): 45–60.

20. *The Gentleman's Magazine*, 13 (1743), 430.

21. *The History of the Works of the Learned* (March 1743), 187; [Joseph Spence], *Crito: Or, A Dialogue on Beauty. By Sir Harry Beaumont* (London: R. Dodsley, 1752), 19.

22. Elizabeth Berkley Craven, *Lady Craven's Journey to Constantinople* (Dublin: n.p., 1789), 348.

23. *Public Advertiser* (16 September 1783), 2.

24. Maria Josepha Stanley, *The Girlhood of Maria Josepha Holroyd, Lady Stanley of Alderley*, ed. J. H. Adeane (London: Longmans, 1896), 58, MJS to Serena (5 July 1791).

25. Valerie Steele, *The Corset: A Cultural History* (New Haven and London: Yale, 2001), 16; Lynn Sorge-English, *Stays and Body Image in London: The Staymaking Trade*, 1680–1810 (London: Routledge, 2011), 3.

26. *Ipswich Journal* (27 March 1802), 3; *Bell's Weekly Messenger* (23 July 1815), 8.

27. *Westminster Journal and London Political Miscellany* (24–31 October 1772), 1.

28. *Bristol Mirror* (20 May 1815), 3.

29. SP diary, VII, 162 (12 June 1666).

30. *London Journal* (13 November 1731), 1.

31. John Breval, *The Art of Dress. A Poem* (London: R. Burleigh, 1717), 16.

32. Montagu, *Letters*, III, 12–13, LM to Countess of Bute (16 March [1752]).

33. Delany, *Autobiography and Correspondence*, II, 450, MD to Mrs Dewes (21 January 1747).

34. Lady Mary Coke, *The Letters and Journals of Lady Mary Coke*, ed. J. A. Home, 4 vols (Edinburgh: David Douglas, 1889–96), IV, 1 (1 January 1772), 178 (21 June 1773).

35. Horace Walpole, *The Letters of Horace Walpole, Fourth Earl of Orford*, ed. Paget Toynbee, 16 vols (Oxford: Clarendon, 1903–5), XII, 388, HW to the Countess of Orrery (7 January 1783); BL Add MS 75643 f. 129, Caroline Howe to Lady Spencer (4 June 1793).

36. *Morning Post* (4 September 1802), 2.
37. Mary Robinson, epilogue to *Nobody: A Comedy in Two Acts* (1794), quoted in Chloe Wigston Smith, *Women, Work, and Clothes in the Eighteenth-Century Novel* (Cambridge: Cambridge University Press, 2013), 186.
38. Maria Josepha Stanley, *The Early Married Life of Maria Josepha, Lady Stanley*, ed. J. H. Adeane (London: Longmans, Green & Co., 1899), 292–3.
39. Mary Russell Mitford, *The Life of Mary Russell Mitford, Related in a Selection from Her Letters to Her Friends*, ed. A. G. L'Estrange, 3 vols (London: Richard Bentley, 1870), 183–4, MRM to Sir William Elford (23 June 1824).
40. Mary Berry, *Extracts from the Journals and Correspondence of Miss Berry from the Year 1783 to 1852*, ed. Lady Theresa Lewis, 3 vols (London: Longmans, Green, & Co., 1865), II, 346.
41. Jane Austen, *Pride and Prejudice*, ed. Vivien Jones (London: Penguin, 2014), 55.
42. Lady Charlotte Campbell, *Diary Illustrative of the Times of George the Fourth*, 4 vols (London: L. Colburn, 1839), II, 82; I, 281.
43. *Lady's Own Paper* (24 June 1848), 2; (2 September 1848), 2; (25 August 1849), 16.
44. *Western Mail* (28 April 1885), 3.
45. *Daily Telegraph & Courier* (24 May 1881), 7.
46. Steele, *The Corset*, 52.
47. *Totnes Weekly Times* (25 December 1869), 3.
48. Mel Davies, 'Corsets and Conception: Fashion and Demographic Trends in the Nineteenth Century', *Comparative Studies in Society and History*, 24, no. 4 (1982): 611–41.
49. *London Journal, and Weekly Record of Literature, Science, and Art* (1 August 1896), 5–6.
50. *Chambers' Edinburgh Journal* (16 September 1848), 184.
51. *Fun* (29 August 1893), 88.
52. Caroline Bressey, 'Looking for Work: The Black Presence in Britain 1860–1920', in Caroline Bressey and Hakim Adi, eds, *Belonging in Europe: The African Diaspora and Work* (London: Routledge, 2011), 60–78, at 67, 69.
53. *Chambers' Edinburgh Journal* (24 July 1852), 49.
54. Emma Hope Allwood, 'Meeting Mr Pearl, Fashion's Most Notorious Corset Maker', *Dazed*, 15 April 2016, https://www.dazeddigital.com/fashion/article/30768/1/meeting-mr-pearl-fashion-s-most-notorious-corset-maker (accessed 22 November 2023).
55. *CLO*, 10.1215/lt-18341121-JWC-MAC-01, JWC to Margaret Carlyle (21 November 1834).
56. Steeve O. Buckridge, *The Language of Dress Resistance and Accommodation in Jamaica 1760–1890* (Kingston, Jamaica: University of the West Indies Press, 2004), 138, 176–8.
57. Patricia A. Cunningham, *Reforming Women's Fashion, 1850–1920: Politics, Health, and Art* (Kent, OH: Kent State University Press, 2003), 22.
58. *Illustrated Sporting and Dramatic News* (4 September 1886), 728.
59. *Rational Dress Society's Gazette* (January 1889), 2.
60. Leigh Summers, *Bound to Please: A History of the Victorian Corset* (Oxford: Berg, 2001), 50.
61. *Sheffield Evening Telegraph* (1 March 1890), 2.

62. *The Leisure Hour: An Illustrated Magazine for Home Reading*, 43 (1894), 671.

63. *Bow Bells: A Magazine of General Literature and Art for Family Reading* (9 October 1891), 346.

64. *Bath Chronicle and Weekly Gazette* (12 May 1814), 3; *Morning Post* (22 August 1821), 1; *Chambers' Edinburgh Journal* (15 August 1846), 102–4; Lady Isabel Burton, *The Inner Life of Syria, Palestine, and the Holy Land: From My Private Journal*, 2 vols (London: Henry S. King & Co., 1875), I, 305.

65. *Country Life Illustrated* (21 October 1899), xiii.

66. *Answers* (15 November 1890), 397.

67. Francis A. Walker, *The Wages Question: A Treatise on Wages and the Wages Class* (London: Macmillan, 1888), 179 fn 28; Norah Waugh, *Corsets and Crinolines* (New York: Theatre Arts Books, 1954; repr. New York: Routledge, 2015), 166.

68. *London Journal, and Weekly Record of Literature, Science, and Art* (27 September 1856), 63.

69. Bernard Smith, 'Market Development, Industrial Development: The Case of the American Corset Trade, 1860–1920', *Business History Review*, 65, no. 1 (1991): 91–129, at 103.

70. *Clarion* (20 April 1901), 124.

71. Elizabeth Ewing, *Fashion in Underwear: From Babylon to Bikini Briefs* (London: B. T. Batsford, 1971), 78–9.

72. *Colour* (3 April 1918), vii.

73. Jill Fields, *An Intimate Affair: Women, Lingerie, and Sexuality* (Berkeley, Los Angeles, and London: University of California Press, 2007), 102.

74. 'Eminent Surgeons Endorse the Corset', *Corsets & Lingerie* (December 1921), 32–5. See Fields, *An Intimate Affair*, 62.

75. *Westminster Gazette* (17 April 1926), 7.

76. *CL* (23 September 1939), xxv.

77. Ibid. (12 May 1977), 1212.

78. Priya Elan, 'Blackfishing: "Black is Cool Unless You Are Actually Black"', *Guardian*, 14 April 2020, https://www.theguardian.com/fashion/2020/apr/14/blackfishing-black-is-cool-unless-youre-actually-black (accessed 22 November 2023).

2 DIET AND EXERCISE

1. *London Chronicle* (20–22 April 1758), 379.

2. The Diary of Mrs Boscowan, 1763, Bodleian, MS. Eng. Misc. f. 71, p. 3 [49].

3. *Connoisseur* (30 January 1755), 316.

4. NMM COD/21/1/A, Admiral Codrington to his wife (26 May 1819).

5. *Public Advertiser* (31 May 1762), 1.

6. Cecil Aspinall-Oglander, *Admiral's Wife: Being the Life and Letters of The Hon. Mrs. Edward Boscawen from 1719 to 1761* (London: Longmans, Green and Co., 1940), 56, F. Boscawen to her husband (21 October 1747). Cf. her diary for 1763, Bodleian, MS. Eng. Misc. f. 71.

7. *Morning Chronicle* (2 May 1777), 3.

8. *The Art of Beauty, Or, A Companion for the Toilet* (London: J. Williams, 1760), 7.

9. Anna Seward, *Letters of Anna Seward: Written Between the Years 1784 and 1807*, 6 vols (Edinburgh: Archibald Constable & Co., 1811), I, 276–7.

10. *Public Advertiser* (3 November 1767), 1.

11. *The Oracle* (25 June 1799), 2.

12. George Cheyne, *An Essay of Health and Long Life* (London: George Strahan, 1724), 95.

13. William Buchan, *Domestic Medicine: Or, A Treatise on the Prevention and Cure of Diseases*, 11th edn (London: A. Strahan et al., 1790), 83.

14. *The World* (14 January 1791), 1.

15. *Whitehall Evening Post* (5–7 May 1798), 1.

16. *The Oracle* (4 November 1796), 8.

17. *ILN* (29 August 1891), 287.

18. *Morning Advertiser* (14 November 1806), 3.

19. [William Wadd], *Cursory Remarks on Corpulence* (London: J. Callow, 1810), 16–17.

20. Christopher E. Forth, 'Fat, Desire and Disgust in the Colonial Imagination', *History Workshop Journal*, 73, no. 1 (2012): 211–39, at 226.

21. William Wadd, *Cursory Remarks on Corpulence* (London: J. Callow, 1816), 53–4.

22. Lady Charlotte Bury, *The Diary of a Lady-in-Waiting*, ed. A. Francis Steuart, 2 vols (London: John Lane, 1908), I, 38–9.

23. *The Lady's Magazine* (April 1811), 169.

24. Frances Anne Kemble, *Records of Later Life*, 3 vols (London: Richard Bentley and Son, 1882), I, 52, FAK to Harriet St Leger (28 March 1836).

25. Sydney Morgan, *Lady Morgan's Memoirs, Autobiography, Diaries and Correspondence*, 2 vols (London: W. H. Allen & Co., 1862), II, 342.

26. Robert Southey, *Correspondence with Caroline Bowles* (Dublin: Hodges, Figgis & Co., 1881), 301, RS to CB (April 1834).

27. Lola Mendez, *The Arts of Beauty; Or, Secrets of a Lady's Toilet* (New York: Dick & Fitzgerald, 1858), 27–8.

28. *CLO*, 10.1215/lt-18631102-JWC-MW-01, JWC to Margaret Welsh (2 November 1863).

29. George Eliot, *The George Eliot Letters*, ed. Gordon S. Haight, 9 vols (New Haven: Yale University Press, 1954–78), VII, 328, GE to Charles Lee Lewes (19 September 1880).

30. Joseph S. Alter, 'Indian Clubs and Colonialism: Hindu Masculinity and Muscular Christianity', *Comparative Studies in Society and History*, 46, no. 3 (2004): 497–534.

31. Maud Rittenhouse, *Maud*, ed. Richard Lee Strout (London: Macmillan & Co., 1939), 488.

32. Martha Pike Conant et al., *A Girl of the Eighties at College and at Home* (Boston and New York: Houghton Mifflin Company, 1931), 78.

33. Ishbel Hamilton-Gordon, *The Canadian Journal of Lady Aberdeen*, ed. John T. Saywell (Toronto: Champlain Society, 1960), 189.

34. Elizabeth Aldrich, *From the Ballroom to Hell: Grace and Folly in 19th-Century Dance* (Evanston, IL: Northwestern University Press, 1991), 47.

35. *Beauty and Hygiene for Women and Girls* (London: Swan Sonnenschein & Co., 1893), 28; *ILN* (24 June 1871), 614.

36. *HB* (8 April 1899), 290.

37. Eliot, *The George Eliot Letters*, 43, GE to Mrs Elma Stuart (10 July 1878).
38. Naomi Wolf, *The Beauty Myth: How Images of Beauty Are Used against Women* (London: Chatto & Windus, 1990), 153, 161.
39. Katharina Vester, 'Regime Change: Gender, Class, and the Invention of Dieting in Post-Bellum America', *Journal of Social History*, 44, no. 1 (2010): 39–70.
40. William Banting, *Letter on Corpulence, Addressed to the Public*, 3rd edn (London: Harrison, 1864), 14.
41. Jaime M. Miller, ' "Do you Bant?" William Banting and Bantingism: A Cultural History of a Victorian Anti-Fat Aesthetic' (PhD thesis, Old Dominion University, Norfolk, VA, 2014), 197 ff.
42. Alice Catherine Miles, *Every Girl's Duty: The Diary of a Victorian Debutante*, ed. Maggy Parsons (London: Andre Deutsch Ltd, 1992), 103; *Beauty and How to Keep It, by a Professional Beauty* (London: Brentano's, 1889), 50.
43. Lynn Sherr, *Failure Is Impossible: Susan B. Anthony in Her Own Words* (New York: Times Books, 1995), 132.
44. *Christian Recorder* (7 January 1886), 2.
45. *Chicago Defender* (6 March 1915), 6.
46. *ILN* (19 April 1913), 532.
47. Virginia Woolf, *The Diary of Virginia Woolf*, ed. Anne Olivier Bell, 5 vols (New York: Harcourt, Brace, Jovanovich, 1980), I, 194.
48. Heloise Edwina Hersey, *To Girls: A Budget of Letters* (Boston: Small, Maynard & Co., 1901), 217.
49. *Beauty and Hygiene for Women and Girls*, 33.
50. *HB* (6 May 1899), 388.
51. *The Bystander* (26 October 1912), 176.
52. *CL* (14 August 1909), lxiv; (10 April 1897), viii.
53. Ibid. (14 April 1900), xxiii.
54. *ILN* (28 March 1896), 409.
55. Bodleian, John Johnson Collection: Patent Medicines 12 (9).
56. *Quiver* (July 1909), 25; *London* (10 January 1914), 175.
57. *The Bystander* (25 September 1912), 649.
58. *ILN* (28 February 1914), 348.
59. *Answers* (21 September 1912), 504.
60. *Woman's Health and Beauty* (May 1902), 54.
61. Ibid. (April 1902), 31.
62. *London* (13 February 1926), 4.
63. *CL* (12 April 1924), xlviii; (28 June 1924), lxxiii.
64. Ibid. (7 June 1924), cc.
65. Penny Tinkler, *Smoke Signals: Women, Smoking and Visual Culture in Britain* (Oxford: Berg, 2006), 88–90; John Hill, *Cautions against the Immoderate Use of Snuff* (London: R. Baldwin, 1761), 42–3.
66. Paula J. Martin, *Suzanne Noël: Cosmetic Surgery, Feminism and Beauty in Early Twentieth-Century France* (London: Routledge, 2014), 49.
67. *Answers* (21 February 1931), 13.
68. *The Tatler* (13 May 1925), 2.
69. Alison Bashford and Philippa Levine, eds, *Oxford Handbook of the History of Eugenics* (Oxford: Oxford University Press, 2010), 7.
70. *ILN* (19 May 1928), 887.

71. *Britannia and Eve* (May 1931), 82; *The Referee* (30 December 1900), 11.
72. *ILN* (23 May 1914), 872.
73. *The Highway* (January 1938), 76–7.
74. *Britannia and Eve* (January 1945), 37.
75. *CL* (6 March 1958), 18.
76. Ibid. (29 May 1958), 1216.
77. *Britannia and Eve* (December 1951), 46.
78. Helen Belinkie, *The Gourmet in the Low-Calorie Kitchen* (New York: David McKay Co., 1961), 204.
79. *Times Educational Supplement* (21 March 1969), 925; (19 February 1971), 12.
80. *Daily Mirror* (27 September 1979), 2.
81. *Times Educational Supplement* (12 April 1991), 8.
82. Mimi Nichter, *Fat Talk: What Girls and Their Parents Say about Dieting* (Cambridge, MA: Harvard University Press, 2000), 159 ff.
83. Vena Moore, 'Dieting While Black', *Fearless She Wrote*, 31 October 2019, tiny.cc/v5lbvz (accessed 29 September 2023).
84. Vanessa Higgins, James Nazroo, and Mark Brown, 'Pathways to Ethnic Differences in Obesity: The Role of Migration, Culture and Socio-Economic Position in the UK', *SSM – Population Health*, 7 (2019), https://doi.org/10.1016/j.ssmph.2019.100394 (accessed 28 October 2023).
85. *Forbes India* (May 2021), 13.
86. See, e.g., *Flamingo* (April 1962), 30–1.
87. Vester, 'Regime Change', 40, 44.
88. George Orwell, *The Road to Wigan Pier* (London: William Collins, 2021; 1st edn 1937), 86.

3 SKIN

1. Daniel Turner, *De Morbis Cutaneis: A Treatise of Diseases Incident to the Skin* (London: R. Bonwicke et al., 1714), 23.
2. SP diary, VIII, 584 (20 December 1667).
3. *Weekly Miscellany* (21 July 1739), 1.
4. *The Ladies' Hand-Book of the Toilet; A Manual of Elegance and Fashion* (London: H. G. Clarke, 1843), 5–6.
5. Kevin P. Siena, *Venereal Disease, Hospitals and the Urban Poor: London's 'Foul Wards', 1600–1800* (Woodbridge: Boydell Press, 2004), 10.
6. Frances Anne Kemble, *Records of a Girlhood* (New York: Henry Holt & Co., 1880; 1st edn 1879), 82.
7. *Morning Chronicle* (10 January 1793), 4.
8. *Girlhood and Wifehood, Practical Counsel and Advice* (London: The 'Family Doctor' Publishing Co., 1896), 146–7.
9. 'Elizabeth Butler's Book. Medicinal and Culinary Recipes' (1679), BL Sloane MS 3842, f. 39.
10. *Public Advertiser* (19 March 1765), 1.
11. Charlotte Brontë, *The Letters of Charlotte Brontë: With a Selection of Letters by Family and Friends, Vol. I, 1829–1847*, ed. Margaret Smith (Oxford: Clarendon Press, 1995), 184, CB to Ellen Nussey (20 January 1839).

12. *CLO*, 10.1215/lt-18560208-JWC-MR-01, JWC to Mary Russell (8 February 1856).
13. *Girlhood and Wifehood*, 34.
14. *HB* (13 June 1868), 519.
15. Boyd Laynard, *Secrets of Beauty, Health, and Long Life* (London: Hammond, Hammond & Co., 1900), 8–10.
16. Stuart Anderson, 'Travellers, Patent Medicines, and Pharmacopoeias: American Pharmacy and British India, 1857–1931', *History of Pharmacy and Pharmaceuticals*, 58, no. 3–4 (2016): 63–82.
17. The Independent … Devoted to the Consideration of Politics, Social and Economic Tendencies, History, Literature, and the Arts (15 May 1879), 15.
18. Montagu, *Letters*, I, 314, LM to Lady — (1 April 1717).
19. *The Age* (1 July 1838), 206.
20. *Dublin Medical Press* (5 February 1851), 10; Angela Rosenthal, 'Visceral Culture: Blushing and the Legibility of Whiteness in Eighteenth-Century British Portraiture', *Art History*, 27, no. 4 (2004): 563–92, at 567.
21. *The Art of Beauty, Or, A Companion for the Toilet* (London: J. Williams, 1760), 76–7.
22. *The Post-Man and the Historical Account* (10–13 May 1707), 3.
23. *Weekly Journal or Saturday's Post* (6 October 1722), 1204; *London Journal* (28 January 1727), 4.
24. OBP, 30 June 1714, Old Bailey Proceedings advertisements (a17140630-1).
25. *Public Advertiser* (2 July 1754), 4.
26. *Lloyd's Evening Post* (10–13 March 1769), 260; *Public Advertiser* (7 June 1786), 4.
27. *Gazetteer and London Daily Advertiser* (18 April 1764), 3; *St James's Chronicle or the British Evening Post* (16–19 February 1788), 2; *Public Advertiser* (3 November 1769), 3.
28. Montagu, *Letters*, I, 369, LM to Lady — (17 June 1717).
29. 'Elizabeth Butler's Book', BL Sloane MS 3842, f. 40; *The Art of Beauty*, 24–5.
30. *The Art of Beauty*, 30.
31. *HB* (13 June 1868), 519.
32. Cookery and Medical Receipts by Margaret Baker (1672), BL Sloane MS 2485, f. 33v; *Beauty and How to Keep It* (London: Brentano's, 1889), 7.
33. *Le Follet* (1 June 1891), 326; Alisa Webb, 'Constructing the Gendered Body: Girls, Health, Beauty, Advice, and the *Girls' Best Friend*, 1898–99', *Women's History Review*, 15, no. 2 (2006): 253–75, at 268.
34. *Read's Weekly Journal Or, British Gazetteer* (18 August 1733), 4.
35. *Beauty and How to Keep It*, 8.
36. Arthur Clarke, *An Essay on Diseases of the Skin* (London: Henry Colburn & Co., 1821), 31.
37. *John Bull* (14 June 1879), 382.
38. *Beauty and Hygiene for Women and Girls* (London: Swan Sonnenschein & Co., 1893), 64.
39. Mieneke te Hennepe, '"To Preserve the Skin in Health": Drainage, Bodily Control and the Visual Definition of Healthy Skin 1835–1900', *Medical History*, 58, no. 3 (2014): 397–421, at 405–6.
40. John Floyer and Edward Baynard, *The History of Cold Bathing Both Ancient and Modern* (Manchester: J. Gadsby, 1844; 1st edn 1706), 86.

41. *Girlhood and Wifehood*, 34.

42. *The Listener* (4 April 1934), 577.

43. Montagu, *Letters*, I, 407, LM to the Countess of — [May 1718].

44. *Beauty and How to Keep It*, 11.

45. *HB* (13 June 1868), 519.

46. Ibid. (7 January 1899), 8; *Beauty and Hygiene for Women and Girls*, 115.

47. *The Post-Man and the Historical Account* (9–12 June 1716), 2.

48. *Girlhood and Wifehood*, 31.

49. Lydia Huntley Sigourney, *Letters to Mothers* (Hartford, CT: Hudson and Skinner, 1838), 65.

50. Charlotte Howard Conant, *A Girl of the Eighties at College and at Home*, ed. Martha Pike Conant (Boston: Houghton, Mifflin and Co., 1931), 118–19, CHC to parents, 6 March 1881.

51. *Beauty and How to Keep It*, 15.

52. *Myra's Journal of Dress and Fashion* (1 July 1876), 142.

53. *Fashionable London, An Illustrated Journal for Ladies* (April 1892), 1.

54. *The Diary of Else Elisabeth Koren, 1853–1854*, trans. and ed. David T. Nelson (Northfield, MN: Norwegian-American Historical Association, 1955), 256.

55. Frances Anne Kemble, *Records of Later Life*, 3 vols (London: R. Bentley, 1882), I, 68–9, FAK to Harriet St Leger (5 October 1836).

56. Ibid., III, 190, FAK to Hal (31 May 1847).

57. Maria Edgeworth, *Letters from England 1813–1844* (Oxford: Clarendon Press, 1971), 607, ME to Mrs Edgeworth (2 February 1844).

58. *CL* (10 February 1872), 114.

59. *Beauty and Hygiene for Women and Girls*, 80, 138; *Girls' Own Paper* (12 July 1884), 644.

60. *The Art of Beauty*, 28–9.

61. Lindy Woodhead, *War Paint: Helena Rubinstein and Elizabeth Arden: Their Lives, Their Times, Their Rivalry* (London: Virago, 2003), 148.

62. *ILN* (17 November 1934), 32.

63. *CL* (13 September 1956), 553.

64. Ibid. (2 February 1961), 251.

65. *Aberdeen Press and Journal* (19 February 1979), 1.

66. Elizabeth Wynne, *The Wynne Diaries*, ed. Anne Fremantle, 3 vols (Oxford: Oxford University Press, 1935), II, 180.

67. *CL* (27 June 1925), lxxx.

68. *Picture Show* (4 October 1930), 21.

69. Elizabeth A. Bohls, 'The Aesthetics of Colonialism: Janet Schaw in the West Indies, 1774–1775', *Eighteenth-Century Studies*, 27, no. 3 (1994): 363–90, at 385; Jennifer L. Morgan, *Laboring Women: Reproduction and Gender in New World Slavery* (Philadelphia: University of Pennsylvania Press, 2004), 26; Charmaine A. Nelson, *Slavery, Geography and Empire in Nineteenth-Century Marine Landscapes of Montreal and Jamaica* (London and New York : Routledge, 2016), 235.

70. Controversial even at the time. See C. Melmonth [Samuel Jackson Pratt], *The New Cosmetic, Or the Triumph of Beauty, A Comedy* (London: n.p., 1790).

71. Arnold A. Sio, 'Race, Colour, and Miscegenation: The Free Coloured of Jamaica and Barbados', *Caribbean Studies*, 16, no. 1 (1976): 5–21. I am also indebted to Olivia Wyatt for several key contributions to this section.

72. Debbie Weekes, 'Shades of Blackness: Young Black Female Constructions of Beauty', in Heidi Safia Mirza, ed., *Black British Feminism: A Reader* (London and New York: Routledge, 1997), 113–27; Shirley Anne Tate, *Black Beauty: Aesthetics, Stylization, Politics* (Farnham: Ashgate, 2009), 65–6.

73. Margaret Hunter, 'The Cost of Color: What We Pay For Being Black and Brown', in Ronald E. Hall, ed., *Racism in the 21st Century: An Empirical Analysis of the Impact of Skin Color* (New York: Springer, 2008), 63–77, at 70; Steeve O. Buckridge, *The Language of Dress Resistance and Accommodation in Jamaica 1760–1890* (Kingston, Jamaica: University of the West Indies Press, 2004), 139. Cf. Laila Haidarali, *Brown Beauty: Color, Sex, and Race from the Harlem Renaissance to World War II* (New York: NYU Press, 2018), 250.

74. Ellis P. Monk Jr, 'Colorism and Physical Health: Evidence from a National Survey', *Journal of Health and Social Behavior*, 62, no. 1 (2021): 37–52.

75. Mary Rose Abraham, 'Dark is Beautiful: The Battle to End the World's Obsession with Lighter Skin', *Guardian*, 4 September 2017, https://tinyurl.com/mryv7nuh (accessed 29 September 2023).

76. E.g. Rochelle Rowe, *Imagining Caribbean Womanhood: Race, Nation and Beauty Competitions 1929–1970* (Manchester: Manchester University Press, 2013), 2.

77. *CL* (27 January 1900), 108–10.

78. *Times Magazine* (30 May 1998), 85.

79. Ljubica Cvetkovska, '45 Absolutely Astonishing Beauty Industry Statistics', 5 March 2022, https://loudcloudhealth.com/resources/beauty-industry-statistics (accessed 28 October 2023).

80. @Sellab_co23, 5 March 2021, https://twitter.com/Sellab_co23/status/136767 2613116383239?s=09 (accessed 24 November 2023).

4 MAKEUP

1. Alma Lutz, ed., *With Love, Jane: Letters from American Women on the War Fronts* (New York: John Day Co., 1945), 5.

2. John Bulwer, *Anthropometamorphosis: Man Transform'd; Or, The Artificiall Changeling Historically Presented* (London: William Hunt, 1653), 261.

3. JE diary, III, 97 (11 May 1654).

4. [John Gauden and Jeremy Taylor], *A Discourse of Artificial Beauty. In Point of Conscience, Between Two Ladies* (London: R. Royston, 1662; 1st edn 1656), 259.

5. *A Hue and Cry After Beauty and Virtue* (London: n.p., 1680), ll. 14–19.

6. *The Ladies Dictionary; Being a General Entertainment for the Fair Sex* (London: John Dunton, 1694), 55.

7. E.g. Bulwer, *Anthropometamorphosis*, 261; English school, *Portrait of Two Ladies*, c. 1650, https://tinyurl.com/u547bjzw (accessed 28 October 2023).

8. *The Art of Beauty, Or, A Companion for the Toilet* (London: J. Williams, 1760), 60; Hannah Woolley, *The Accomplish'd Lady's Delight* (London: B. Harris, 1675), 193.

9. Montagu, *Letters*, I, 327, LM to Lady — (1 April 1717).

10. *The Art of Beauty*, 53.
11. William Congreve, *The Way of the World*, ed. Diane Maybank (Oxford: Oxford University Press, 2014), 63, III.138–44.
12. Montagu, *Letters*, I, 439, LM to Lady Rich (September 1718).
13. *Universal Spectator and Weekly Journal* (20 February 1742), 1.
14. Ibid.
15. Joseph Spence, *Crito: Or, A Dialogue on Beauty* (London: R. Dodsley, 1752), 50–1.
16. Meg Cohen Ragas and Karen Kozlowski, *Read My Lips: A Cultural History of Lipstick* (San Francisco: Chronicle Books, 1998), 16.
17. Addison & Steele et al., *The Spectator*, no. 33 (7 April 1711), repr. ed. Gregory Smith, 4 vols (London: Dent, 1979) I, 100–1.
18. *The Accomplish'd Housewife; Or, the Gentlewoman's Companion* (London: J. Newbery, 1745), 71.
19. TNA L 30/14/333/100 (5 June 1778).
20. *The Morning Post, and Daily Advertiser* (23 October 1782), 4.
21. Daniel Defoe, *Roxana: The Fortunate Mistress*, ed. John Mullan (Oxford: Oxford University Press, 1996), 73.
22. [William Creech], *Letters Respecting the Mode of Living, Trade, Manners, and Literature etc of Edinburgh, in 1763, and the Present Period* (Edinburgh: n.p., 1783), 17.
23. Jessica Pallingston, *Lipstick: A Celebration of a Girl's Best Friend* (London: Simon & Schuster, 1999), 182.
24. E.g. *The Art of Beauty*, 32.
25. Bulwer, *Anthropometamorphosis*, 261.
26. Mary Delany, *The Autobiography and Correspondence of Mary Granville, Mrs Delany*, ed. Lady Llanover, 3 vols (London: Richard Bentley, 1861), III, 584, MD to Mrs Dewes (2 February 1760).
27. Frances Burney, *Diary and Letters of Madame d'Arblay*, ed. Charlotte Barrett, 6 vols (London: Macmillan & Co., 1904), I, 253 (20 July 1779).
28. *Letters to and from Henrietta, Countess of Suffolk and Her Second Husband, the Hon. George Berkeley. From 1712 to 1767*, 2 vols (London: John Murray, 1824), I, 70.
29. Elizabeth Craven, *A Journey through the Crimea to Constantinople* (London: G. G. J. & J. Robinson, 1789), 111.
30. Mary Robinson, *Memoirs of Mary Robinson*, ed. J. Fitzgerald Molloy (Philadelphia: J. B. Lippincott Co., 1895), x.
31. Mary Wollstonecraft, *Collected Letters of Mary Wollstonecraft*, ed. Ralph M. Wardle (Ithaca and London: Cornell University Press, 1979), 133. MW to Everina Wollstonecraft (*c.* 15 January 1787).
32. Alexander Pope, *The Rape of the Lock and Other Major Writings*, ed. Leo Damrosch (London: Penguin, 2011), 42, I.133–4.
33. Caroline Palmer, 'Brazen Cheek: Face-Painters in Late Eighteenth-Century England', *Oxford Art Journal*, 31, no. 2 (2008): 195–213, at 200.
34. See NMM HNL/56/8:20 (1809).
35. Elizabeth Fry, *Memoir of the Life of Elizabeth Fry, with Extracts from Her Journal and Letters*, 2 vols (London: John Hatchard & Son, 1848), I, 40.

36. *The Mirror of the Graces: Or, The English Lady's Costume* (Edinburgh: A. Black, 1830; 1st edn 1811), 40, 42.
37. Lady Charlotte Bury, *The Diary of a Lady-in-Waiting*, ed. A. Francis Steuart, 2 vols (London: John Lane, 1908), I, 382.
38. Anne Katharine Elwood, *Narrative of a Journey Overland from England*, 2 vols (London: Henry Colburn and Richard Bentley, 1830), II, 200; Frances Elliot, *Diary of an Idle Woman in Constantinople* (London: John Murray, 1893), 388.
39. *CLO*, 10.1215/lt-18430108-JWC-JW-01, JWC to Jeannie Welsh (8 January 1843).
40. *The Family Treasury*, 2 vols (London: Houlston & Stoneman, 1853–4), I, 139.
41. *The Ladies' Hand-Book of the Toilet; A Manual of Elegance and Fashion* (London: H. G. Clarke, 1843), 29–30.
42. *HB* (6 February 1869), 81–2; (24 November 1877), 738.
43. Receipt book of Jane Freestone, 1843–57, Wellcome Collection MS.8207, f. 70.
44. Frances Trollope, *Domestic Manners of the Americans* (London and New York: Whittaker, Treacher & Co., 1832), 240–1.
45. Lewis A. Sayre, *Three Cases of Lead Palsy from the Use of a Cosmetic Called 'Laird's Bloom of Youth'* (Philadephia: Collins, 1869), 3.
46. *Lancashire Evening Post* (29 December 1896), 3.
47. *HB* (7 March 1885), 166; (11 March 1882), 158.
48. *South Wales Daily News* (5 December 1896), 3.
49. *The Chemists' Annual List* (London: John Sanger & Sons, 1871), 40, Bodleian, John Johnson Collection: Patent Medicines 14 (54); L. Shaw, *How to Be Beautiful* (New York, 1883), 40, Bodleian, John Johnson Collection: Beauty Parlour 1 (52).
50. Michale Ryan, *Prostitution in London with a Comparative View of That in Paris and New York* (London: H. Bailliere, 1839), 216, 43, 120.
51. William Acton, *Prostitution, Considered in Its Moral, Social and Sanitary Aspects in London and Other Large Cities* (London: John Churchill, 1857), vi.
52. *Beauty and Hygiene for Women and Girls* (London: Swan Sonnenschein & Co., 1893), 109.
53. *Beauty and How to Keep It* (London: Brentano's, 1889), 21.
54. *ILN* (7 June 1856), 642.
55. *Leeds Times* (15 July 1882), 6.
56. *Beauty and Hygiene for Women and Girls*, 111, 142; *HB* (11 April 1874), 243.
57. *HB* (14 December 1878), 794; (22 October 1870), 685.
58. Shaw, *How to Be Beautiful*, 31.
59. Ibid., 33.
60. *HB* (20 January 1894), 58–9; (27 August 1887), 594.
61. *Beauty and Fashion – The Illustrated Journal for Women*, 1 (29 November 1890), 6.
62. *HB* (25 August 1894), 692.
63. *Yorkshire Gazette* (5 March 1887), 5; *Beauty and Hygiene for Women and Girls*, 110.
64. Montagu, *Letters*, I, 327, LM to Lady Mar (1 April 1717).
65. Morag Martin, *Selling Beauty: Cosmetics, Commerce, and French Society 1750–1830* (Baltimore: Johns Hopkins University Press, 2009), 128; OBP, 21 February 1787, trial of John Ponsarque Dubois (t17870221-6).

66. *The World* (6 August 1790), 4.
67. Martin I. Wilbert, 'Cosmetics as Drugs: A Review of Some of the Reported Harmful Effects of the Ordinary Constituents of Widely Used Cosmetics', *Public Health Reports (1896–1970)*, 30, no. 42 (1915): 3059–66, at 3060.
68. Kathy Peiss, *Hope in a Jar: The Making of America's Beauty Culture* (New York: Metropolitan Books, 1998), 134–66.
69. UKDS, 'Interview with Mrs. Talbot', https://discover.ukdataservice.ac.uk//QualiBank/Document/?id=q-99fdd095-dd8f-464d-9e53-484aded55938 (accessed 28 October 2023).
70. UKDS, 'Interview with Allen', https://discover.ukdataservice.ac.uk//QualiBank/Document/?id=q-57d93d59-d941-461e-bf1c-40b66a9fedd7; 'Interview with Mr. Williamson', https://discover.ukdataservice.ac.uk//QualiBank/Document/?id=q-efd94940-a953-482e-b8a0-028a39facd41.
71. Caitlin Davies, *Bad Girls: A History of Rebels and Renegades* (Rearsby: W. F. Howes Ltd, 2019), 185; *HB* (April 1914), 8.
72. *HB* (March 1925), 136.
73. Ibid. (June 1931), 45; (March 1932), 41.
74. *Daily Mirror* (10 November 1939), 2.
75. Erna Barschak, *My American Adventure* (New York: Ives Washburn, 1945), 130–1.
76. Jean L. Kraemer, 'African American Women, Beauty and Marketing' (MA thesis, University of Reunion Island, 2015), 18.
77. *HB* (January 1941), 16.
78. Barschak, *My American Adventure*, 129; Peiss, *Hope in a Jar*, 245.
79. *ILN* (24 December 1955), 2.
80. *HB* (July 1960), 21.
81. Geoffrey Jones, *Beauty Imagined: A History of the Global Beauty Industry* (Oxford: Oxford University Press, 2010), 363.
82. Rochelle Rowe, *Imagining Caribbean Womanhood: Race, Nation and Beauty Competitions 1929–1970* (Manchester: Manchester University Press, 2013), 168.
83. I owe this point to Olivia Wyatt.
84. India Knight, *The Thrift Book: Live Well and Spend Less* (London: Fig Tree 2008), 200.
85. Kraemer, 'African American Women, Beauty and Marketing', 149.
86. *HB* (August 2013), 160–1.
87. *CL* (31 October 1957), 951.

5 HYGIENE

1. Maria Edgeworth, *Letters from England 1813–1844*, ed. Christina Colvin (Oxford: Clarendon Press, 1971), 458, ME to Mrs Edgeworth (n.d.).
2. SP diary, V, 129 (21 April 1664).
3. *Dundee Courier* (8 August 1879), 4.
4. Virginia Smith, *Clean: A History of Personal Hygiene and Purity* (Oxford: Oxford University Press, 2007), 190.
5. *The Echo or Edinburgh Weekly Journal* (17 March 1731), 1.

6. Fanny Burney, *The Early Diary of Frances Burney, 1768–1778*, ed. Annie Raine Ellis, 2 vols (London: George Bell & Sons, 1889), II, 279.

7. Eugen Weber, *France, Fin de Siècle* (Cambridge, MA and London: Belknap Press, 1986), 59.

8. Thomas Tryon, *A Treatise of Cleanness in Meats and Drinks* (London: n.p., 1682), 12.

9. Lady Mary Coke, *The Letters and Journals of Lady Mary Coke*, ed. J. A. Home, 4 vols (Edinburgh: David Douglas, 1889–96), III, 24–5 (9 January 1769).

10. Alain Corbin, *The Foul and the Fragrant: Odor and the French Social Imagination* (Leamington Spa, Hamburg, and New York: Berg Publishers, 1986).

11. Coke, *Letters and Journals*, III, 483–4 (27 November 1771).

12. Carter, *Letters*, III, 254–5 (24 November 1785).

13. Thomas Turner, *The Diary of Thomas Turner*, ed. David Vaisey (Oxford: Oxford University Press, 1984), 319.

14. A. W. Thibaudeau, ed., *The Hamilton and Nelson Papers* (The Collection of Autograph Letters and Historical Documents formed by Alfred Morrison, 2nd series), 2 vols ([London], 1893–4), I, 109.

15. C. P. Moritz, *Travels in England in 1782* (London: Cassell & Co., 1886), 25.

16. *The World* (24 September 1793), 1.

17. *The Ladies' Hand-Book of the Toilet; A Manual of Elegance and Fashion* (London: H. G. Clarke and Co., 1843), 19.

18. Corbin, *The Foul and the Fragrant*, 178.

19. Philip Hamerton, *French and English: A Comparison* (Boston: Roberts Brothers, 1889), 269.

20. Blanche Butler Ames, *Chronicles from the Nineteenth Century: Family Letters of Blanche Butler and Adelbert Ames, Married July 21st 1870*, 2 vols (Clinton, MA: privately issued, 1957), I, 91, BBA to Sarah Hildreth Butler (15 September 1860).

21. *Manchester Evening News* (11 June 1873), 2.

22. Elizabeth Grant, *Memoirs of a Highland Lady*, ed. Lady Strachey (London: John Murray, 1898), 168.

23. Metropolitan Working Classes' Association for Improving the Public Health, *Bathing and Personal Cleanliness* (London: John Churchill and B. Wertheim, 1847), 8–9.

24. *CLO*, 10.1215/lt-18460929-JWC-HW-01, JWC to Helen Welsh (29 September 1846); 10.1215/lt-18450628-JWC-JWE-01, JWC to John Welsh (28 June 1845).

25. *The World* (2 December 1793), 1.

26. Frances Anne Kemble, *Records of Later Life*, 3 vols (London: R. Bentley, 1882), II, 13, FAK to Harriet St Leger (23 March 1840).

27. *Cleanliness—Bathing—Ventilation*, 5–9, in *Chambers's Miscellany of Useful and Entertaining Tracts*, vol. III (Edinburgh: William and Robert Chambers, 1854), no. 51.

28. *First [and Second] Report of the Commissioners for Inquiring into the State of Large Towns and Populous Districts*, vol. II (London: William Clowes and Sons, 1845), 128.

29. Antony S. Wohl, *Endangered Lives: Public Health in Victorian Britain* (London: J. M. Dent & Sons Ltd, 1983), 62; Corbin, *The Foul and the Fragrant*, 119.

30. R. D. Grainger, *Unhealthiness of Towns, Its Causes and Remedies* (London: Charles Knight & Co., 1845), 20, 18.
31. *Monmouthshire Merlin* (21 July 1855), 2.
32. *Girlhood and Wifehood, Practical Counsel and Advice* (London: The "Family Doctor" Publishing Co., 1896), 16.
33. *ILN* (18 December 1858), 584.
34. Marie Schultz, *Hygiène générale de la femme* (Paris: O. Doin, 1903), 6.
35. Rachel Henning's diary, 24 February 1861, SS Great Britain Trust, 2015.00034.
36. *The Lady's Magazine* (April 1811), 170.
37. *HB* (30 May 1868), 490.
38. *Beauty and How to Keep It* (London: Brentano's, 1889), 11.
39. *Girlhood and Wifehood*, 32.
40. *Albion and Evening Advertiser* (27 November 1800), 4.
41. *CL* (8 September 1906), lii.
42. *Chicago Defender* (3 September 1910), 5.
43. *HB* (May 1916), 83; https://repository.duke.edu/dc/adaccess/BH1056 (accessed 24 November 2023).
44. *CL* (23 January 1904), xliii.
45. *Christian Recorder* (3 January 1900), 3; (17 January 1901), 8.
46. Hildi Hendrickson, ed., *Clothing and Difference: Embodied Identities in Colonial and Post-Colonial Africa* (Durham, NC, and London: Duke University Press, 1996), 12; Timothy Burke, *Lifebuoy Men, Lux Women: Commodification, Consumption, and Cleanliness in Modern Zimbabwe* (Durham, NC, and London: Duke University Press, 1996), 20.
47. Mobeen Hussain, 'Combining Global Expertise with Local Knowledge in Colonial India: Selling Ideals of Beauty and Health in Commodity Advertising (c. 1900–1949)', *South Asia: Journal of South Asian Studies*, 44, no. 5 (2021): 926–47, at 930.
48. *Berkshire Chronicle* (23 February 1861), 7.
49. *HB* (28 April 1900), 370.
50. Laila Haidarali, *Brown Beauty: Color, Sex, and Race from the Harlem Renaissance to World War II* (New York: NYU Press, 2018), 87.
51. *Belfast News-letter* (22 January 1878), 3; *Rochdale Times* (4 April 1874), 2; *HB* (30 June 1900), 564–5.
52. Lambeth Palace Library Collections, MQ766.H9a.
53. *HB* (26 February 1898), 182.
54. Ibid. (December 1904), 1231–3; *CL* (29 September 1906), lxii; *CL* (19 December 1925), lii.
55. *Huddersfield Chronicle* (22 July 1865), 3.
56. *Irish Times* (7 November 1873), 7.
57. *Deal, Warmer and Sandwich Mercury* (4 March 1882), 7.
58. *The Leisure Hour: An Illustrated Magazine for Home Reading* (September 1894), 740.
59. *The Times* (18 June 1914), 5.
60. *CLO*, 10.1215/lt-18580712-JWC-TC-01, JWC to Thomas Carlyle (12 July 1858); 10.1215/lt-18601230-JWC-MR-01, JWC to Mary Russell (30 December 1860).

61. Gustav Jaeger, *Health-Culture*, trans. and ed. Lewis R. S. Tomalin (London: Adams Bros, 1903), 149–50.

62. John J. Bigsby, *The Sea-side Manual for Invalids and Bathers* (London: Whittaker & Co., 1841), 84.

63. UKDS, 'Interview with Mrs. Giles', https://discover.ukdataservice.ac.uk//QualiBank/Document/?cid=q-5d11fac9-8745-49df-b911-14a7e630903b (accessed 28 October 2023).

64. *The Sketch* (1 December 1958), 39.

65. Geoffrey Jones, *Beauty Imagined: A History of the Global Beauty Industry* (Oxford: Oxford University Press, 2010), 88.

66. *HB* (June 1931), 102.

67. *Chicago Defender* (20 February 1937), 8; (31 January 1942), 15; (14 June 1952), 14.

68. Margherita Karo, *Financial Analysts Journal*, 24, no. 5 (1968): 34–44, at 38; Smith, *Clean*, 338.

69. Roseann M. Mandziuk, ' "Ending women's greatest hygienic mistake": Modernity and the Mortification of Menstruation in Kotex Advertising, 1921–1926', *Women's Studies Quarterly*, 38, no. 3–4 (2010): 42–62, at 47, 49.

70. *HB* (June 1960), 86.

71. Corbin, *The Foul and the Fragrant*, 62.

72. *Christian Recorder* (23 February 1899), 4.

73. *HB* (September 1953), 151.

74. Ibid. (September 1974), 133, 165.

75. Acumen Research and Consulting, 'Feminine Hygiene Products Market Analysis' (July 2022), https://rb.gy/h08is3 (accessed 15 December 2023).

76. *The Scotsman* (21 March 1950), 6; Peter Ward, *The Clean Body: A Modern History* (Montreal, Kingston, London, and Chicago: McGill-Queens University Press, 2019), passim.

77. Winston James, 'Migration, Racism and Identity Formation: The Caribbean Experience in Britain', in Winston James and Clive Harris, eds, *Inside Babylon: The Caribbean Disaspora in Britain* (London and New York: Verso, 1993), 231–87, at 242.

78. 'Moins se laver pour la planète?', 13 February 2022, https://www.radiofrance.fr/franceinter/podcasts/social-lab/social-lab-du-dimanche-13-fevrier-2022-8434394 (accessed 28 October 2023).

79. *Women's Wear* (28 March 1922), 47.

80. *West London Observer* (9 September 1932), 8.

6 TEETH

1. *Scientific American*, 25, no. 10 (September 1871): 145.

2. E. G. Kelley, *A Popular Treatise on the Human Teeth and Dental Surgery* (Boston: James Munroe and Co., 1843), 55.

3. Thomas Baker, *Tunbridge-Walks: Or, the Yeoman of Kent; A Comedy* (London: Barnard Lintott, 1703), 45.

4. Clive Ponting, *World History: A New Perspective* (London: Chatto & Windus, 2000), 510.

5. Anna Eliza Bray, *Traditions, Legends, Superstitions, and Sketches of Devonshire on the Borders of the Tamar and the Tavy*, 3 vols (London: John Murray, 1838), II, 291–2.

6. *Female Tatler* (12–14 September 1709), 2.

7. SP diary, II, 53 (11 March 1661); VIII, 583 (19 December 1667).

8. Montagu, *Letters*, II, 460–1, LM to Lady Oxford (23 June [1750]).

9. William Roberts, *Memoirs of the Life and Correspondence of Mrs. Hannah More*, 3 vols (London: R. B. Seeley and R. Burnside, 1834), III, 369, HM to the Misses Roberts (February 1813).

10. Sarah E. Andrews, *Postmarked Hudson: The Letters of Sarah A. [sic, E] Andrews to Her Brother*, ed. Willis Harry Miller (Hudson, WI: Star-Observer Publishing Co., 1955), 100 (21 June 1865).

11. Nicolas Dubois de Chémant, *A Dissertation on Artificial Teeth in General* (London: J. Barker, 1797), 11; Roberts, *Memoirs of Mrs. Hannah More*, III, 319, HM to Mrs Kennicott (1810); *CLO*, 10.1215/lt-18530809-JWC-MR-01, JWC to Mary Russell (9 August 1853).

12. Michael le Maitre, *Advice on the Teeth: With Some Observations and Remarks* (London: B. Law, 1782), 62–3; R. Wooffendale, *Practical Observations on the Human Teeth* (London: J. Johnson, 1783), 59–60.

13. Maria Edgeworth, *Letters from England 1813–1844*, ed. Christina Colvin (Oxford: Clarendon Press, 1971), 128, ME to Mrs Edgeworth (23 October 1818).

14. Sarah Cowper's Commonplace Book, 1673, Hertfordshire Archives and Local Studies, D/EP F37, 4.

15. Kelley, *A Popular Treatise*, 171.

16. Lady Mary Coke, *The Letters and Journals of Lady Mary Coke*, ed. J. A. Home, 4 vols (Edinburgh: David Douglas, 1889–96), IV, 93 (3 July 1772).

17. *CLO*, 10. 1215/lt-18470929-TC-JWC-01, TC to JWC (29 September 1847).

18. *CLO*, 10.1215/lt-18501115-TC-AC-01, TC to AC (15 November 1850).

19. SP diary, V, 293 (10 October 1664).

20. Bartholomew Ruspini, *A Treatise on the Teeth* (London: the author, 1779), 105.

21. *Morning Chronicle* (19 December 1800), 4.

22. Mary Delany, *The Autobiography and Correspondence of Mary Granville, Mrs Delany*, ed. Lady Llanover, 2nd series, 3 vols (London: Richard Bentley, 1862), II, 206, MD to Mrs Port of Ilam (9 April 1776).

23. Colin Jones, *The Smile Revolution in Eighteenth-Century Paris* (Oxford: Oxford University Press, 2014), passim.

24. Frances Eleanor Trollope, *Frances Trollope: Her Life and Literary Work from George III to Victoria*, 2 vols (London: R. Bentley & Son, 1895), II, 201.

25. Coke, *Letters and Journals*, IV, 26, fn 2.

26. Le Maitre, *Advice on the Teeth*, 47.

27. Mary Wollstonecraft, *Letters Written During a Short Residence in Sweden, Norway, and Denmark*, ed. Tone Brekke and Jon Mee (Oxford: Oxford University Press, 2009; 1st edn 1796), 34, 85.

28. Hugh Symthson, *The Compleat Family Physician; Or, Universal Medical Repository* (London: Harrison & Co., 1781), 274.

29. *The Ladies' Hand-Book of the Toilet; A Manual of Elegance and Fashion* (London: H. G. Clarke and Co., 1843), 17; *HB* (15 November 1884), 731.

30. *Chester Courant* (11 February 1806), 4; *Reading Mercury* (28 March 1840), 4; *Birmingham Journal* (19 September 1840), 3.

31. Catharine Macaulay, *Letters on Education; With Observations on Religious and Metaphysical Subjects* (Dublin: H. Chamberlaine and Rice, 1790), 26.

32. *Morning Chronicle, and London Advertiser* (22 October 1776), 1; *Public Advertiser* (23 August 1785), 2.

33. *Norfolk Chronicle* (28 August 1779), 1.

34. *The World* (10 September 1791), 3; Rachel Bairsto, *The British Dentist* (Oxford: Shire, 2015), 13.

35. Robert D. Hume, 'The Value of Money in Eighteenth-Century England: Incomes, Prices, Buying Power – and Some Problems in Cultural Economics', *Huntington Library Quarterly*, 77, no. 4 (2015): 373–416.

36. Edwin Saunders, *Mineral Teeth: Their Merits & Manufacture* (London: Henry Renshaw, 1841), 46.

37. Amanda McDowell Burns, *Fiddles in the Cumberlands*, ed. Amanda McDowell and Lela McDowell Blankenship (New York: Richard R. Smith, 1943), 148.

38. Marie Bayard, *The Art of Beauty or Lady's Companion to the Boudoir* (London: Weldon & Co., 1876), 31.

39. Dorothy Atkinson Robinson, *It's All in the Family: A Diary of an American Housewife, Dec. 7, 1941–Dec. 1, 1942* (New York: William Morrow and Company, 1943), 47.

40. G. P. B. Naish, ed., *Nelson's Letters to His Wife and Other Documents 1785–1831* (London: Routledge and Keegan Paul for the Naval Records Society, 1958), 265 (7 December 1794).

41. See British Dental Association Museum, LDBDA: 1168; Helena Whitbread, ed., *The Secret Diaries of Miss Anne Lister 1791–1840* (London: Virago, 2010), 207 (23 June 1822).

42. Fanny Burney, *The Early Diary of Frances Burney, 1768–1778*, ed. Annie Raine Ellis, 2 vols (London: George Bell & Sons, 1889), I, 316.

43. *HB* (2 May 1868), 418.

44. *Hampshire Chronicle* (13 May 1776), 4.

45. Quoted in N. A. M. Rodger, *The Wooden World: An Anatomy of the Georgian Navy* (London: Fontana Press, 1988), 102.

46. NMM COD 21/1/A (4 August 1810); MDT/3/1 (28–29 September 1805).

47. Naish, ed., *Nelson's Letters*, 265 (7 December 1794).

48. Frances Anne Kemble, *Records of Later Life*, 3 vols (London: Richard Bentley, 1882), I, 172, FAK to Harriet St Leger (13 November 1838).

49. John Gray, *Preservation of the Teeth* (London: Richard and John E. Taylor, 1840; 1st edn 1838), 29.

50. *Daily Gazette for Middlesbrough* (18 June 1914), 5.

51. *HB* (November 2019), 178.

52. *Leeds Intelligencer* (11 September 1787), 1.

53. *Drewry's Derby Mercury* (12 August 1774), 4. See also *Morning Chronicle, and London Advertiser* (5 December 1776), 3.

54. *HB* (19 August 1899), 701.

55. Gray, *Preservation of the Teeth*, 14–15.

56. *West Kent Guardian* (6 March 1847), 5.

57. *Tyrone Courier* (24 February 1898), 1. See also *Woman's Herald* (7 January 1893), 15.
58. *Hackney and Kingsland Gazette* (7 June 1871), 3.
59. *Freeman's Journal* (12 January 1859), 4; *Hampshire Advertiser* (5 February 1873), 3; *Manchester Evening News* (1 May 1914), 4; *Northampton Chronicle and Echo* (3 January 1924), 5.
60. *HB* (28 November 1874), 73; Hiram Preston, *Hints for the Multitude: Relative to Teeth* (Hartford: Press of the Fountain, 1848), 80.
61. *HB* (14 March 1896), 205.
62. Ibid. (January 1930), 9.
63. *Public Advertiser* (27 August 1790), 1.
64. Betty Bentley Beaumont, *A Business Woman's Journal* (Philadelphia: T. B. Peterson & Bros., 1888), 33, 39.
65. *Vote* (16 April 1910), 2.
66. *The People* (15 April 1900), 15; *Leamington Spa Courier* (4 September 1914), 4.
67. Louise Raw, *Striking a Light: The Bryant and May Matchwomen and Their Place in Labour History* (London: Continuum, 2009), 91.
68. *HB* (January 1904), 21.
69. *CL* (16 April 1910), 543.
70. Richard Meckel, 'Health and Science', in Colin Heyward, ed., *A Cultural History of Childhood and Family in the Age of Empire* (London: Bloomsbury Publishing, 2012), 168.
71. LMA CLA/042/IQ/02/01/018/137; see also CLA/042/IQ/02/01/013/175; *The Ladies' Physician* (London: Cassell & Company Ltd., 1895), 227.
72. George Orwell, *The Road to Wigan Pier* (London: Victor Gollancz Ltd., 1937), 97.
73. *Sunderland Daily Echo and Shipping Gazette* (5 May 1937), 3.
74. *Christian Recorder* (3 August 1861), 120; Laurie A. Wilkie and John M. Chenoweth, eds, *A Cultural History of Objects in the Modern Age* (London: Bloomsbury Academic, 2020), 113.
75. *CL* (19 May 1906), xlvi.
76. *Chicago Defender* (14 July 1928), A3; (21 February 1931), A; (26 July 1947), 14; (11 October 1947), 14.
77. *Sheffield Independent* (19 May 1916), 3.
78. T. S. Eliot, *The Waste Land, and Other Poems* (London: Faber and Faber, 1999), 32 (ll. 148–9).
79. Edith E. Johnson, *Leaves from a Doctor's Diary* (Palo Alto, CA: Pacific Books, 1954), 242.
80. Suzanne Stutman, ed., *My Other Loneliness: Letters of Thomas Wolfe and Aline Bernstein* (Chapel Hill and London: University of North Carolina Press, 1983), 370, AB to TW (19 February 1934).
81. *Aberdeen Press and Journal* (2 April 1935), 6.

7 HAIR

1. *Old Maid* (3 July 1756), 203.
2. *The Diary, or, Woodfall's Register* (18 March 1793), 7.

3. Emma Dabiri, *Don't Touch My Hair* (London: Allen Lane, 2019), 47.

4. [John Shirley], *The Accomplished Ladies Rich Closet of Rarities, or, the Ingenious Gentlewoman and Servant-Maids Delightfull Companion* (London: W. W. for N. Bodington and J. Blare, 1687), 57.

5. *The Westmorland Gazette* (2 March 1872), 8.

6. George Cheyne, *The English Malady* (London: G. Strahan and J. Leake, 1733), 101; *HB* (21 November 1868), 882.

7. Montagu, *Letters*, I, 265, LM to Lady Mar (14 September 1716).

8. E. M. Sewell, *A Journal Kept During a Summer Tour, for the Children of a Village School* (London: Longman, Brown, Green, and Longmans, 1852), Part III, 27.

9. Elizabeth Way, 'Race and Ethnicity: Strands of the Diaspora', in Sarah Heaton, ed., *A Cultural History of Hair* (London: Bloomsbury Academic, 2019), 117–38.

10. Elizabeth Craven, *A Journey through the Crimea to Constantinople* (London: C. C. J. and J. Robinson, 1789), 63.

11. *Salisbury Times* (8 December 1888), 3.

12. *Bombay Gazette* (8 March 1828), 13.

13. David G. Ritchie, ed., *Early Letters of Jane Welsh Carlyle* (London: Swan Sonnenschein & Co., 1889), 203 fn 8.

14. William Hogarth, *The Analysis of Beauty. Written with a View of Fixing the Fluctuating Ideas of Taste* (London: J. Reeves, 1753), 35.

15. Alice Catherine Miles, *Every Girl's Duty: The Diary of a Victorian Debutante*, ed. Maggy Parsons (London: Deutsch, 1992), 15.

16. Harriot Georgina Blackwood, Marchioness of Dufferin and Ava, *Our Viceregal Life in India*, 2 vols (London: John Murray, 1890), II, 44.

17. *HB* (September 1966), 145.

18. *Sunday Reformer and Universal Register* (30 June 1793), 1.

19. Anna Green Winslow, *Diary of Anna Green Winslow: A Boston School Girl of 1771*, ed. Alice Morse Earle (Westminster: Archibald Constable & Co., 1895), 71.

20. Mary Frampton, *The Journal of Mary Frampton from . . . 1779, until . . . 1846*, ed. Harriot Georgiana Mundy (London: Sampson Low, Marston, Searle & Rivington, 1886), 36.

21. *Derby Mercury* (17 February 1785), 1.

22. *Kentish Gazette* (17 August 1768), 4.

23. Peter Gilchrist, *A Treatise on the Hair* (London: n.p., 1770), 12.

24. [Eliza Haywood], *The Wife* (London: T. Gardner, 1756), 54.

25. Francis Place, *The Autobiography of Francis Place*, ed. Mary Thrale (Cambridge: Cambridge University Press, 1972), 78.

26. *The Diary, or, Woodfall's Register* (16 December 1790), 2.

27. Susan Sibbald, *The Memoirs of Susan Sibbald 1783–1812*, ed. F. P. Hett (London: John Lane, 1926), 14.

28. *Shrewsbury Chronicle* (18 January 1777), 3.

29. Edward Cocker, *Cocker's English Dictionary* (London: T. Norris et al., 1715), 98, 213.

30. Marianne Baillie, *Lisbon in the Years 1821, 1822 and 1823*, 2 vols in 1 (London: John Murray, 1824), II, 89.

31. Jane Austen, *Jane Austen's Letters*, ed. Dierdre Le Fay (Oxford: OUP, 1995), 211, JA to Cassandra Austen (20 May 1813).

32. Maria Edgeworth, *Letters from England 1813–1844*, ed. Christina Colvin (Oxford: Clarendon Press, 1971), 379, ME to Mrs Edgeworth (3 April 1822).

33. *ILN* (3 November 1886), 513.

34. George Eliot, *The George Eliot Letters*, ed. Gordon S. Haight, 9 vols (New Haven: Yale University Press, 1954–78), IV, 293, John Blackwood to GE (2 August 1866).

35. Austen, *Letters*, 14, JA to Cassandra Austen (1–2 December 1798); 72, JA to Cassandra (20 November 1800).

36. Lady Maria Nugent, *A Journal of a Voyage to, and Residence in, the Island of Jamaica, from 1801 to 1805, and of Subsequent Events in England from 1805 to 1811*, 2 vols (London: n.p., 1839), II, 199.

37. *Glasgow Evening Post* (26 May 1887), 4.

38. Robert Southey, *The Correspondence of Robert Southey with Caroline Bowles*, ed. E. Dowden (Dublin: Hodges, Figgis & Co., 1881), 138, CB to RS (3 April 1828).

39. Edgeworth, *Letters*, 448, ME to Mrs Edgeworth (15 December 1830).

40. Emma Willard, *Journal and Letters, from France and Great Britain* (Troy, NY: N. Tuttle, 1833), 178.

41. *CLO*, 10.1215/lt-18590214-JWC-DD-01, JWC to David Davidson (14 February 1859).

42. E.g. *HB* (July 2002), 96.

43. *Public Advertiser* (17 September 1760), 4.

44. L. Shaw, *How to Be Beautiful* (New York: Russell Brothers, 1883), 39, Bodleian, John Johnson Collection: Beauty Parlour 1 (52).

45. Alexie Geers, 'A Magazine to Make You Beautiful: *Votre Beauté* and the Cosmetics Industry in the 1930s', *Clio. Women, Gender, History*, no. 40 (2014): 189–204, at 191.

46. *Lichfield Mercury* (15 December 1893), 7.

47. *The Suffragist* (5 October 1909), 24.

48. *The New London Toilet* (London: Richardson & Urquhart, 1778), 98; *HB* (24 June 1882), 836.

49. Galia Ofek, *Representations of Hair in Victorian Literature and Culture* (Aldershot: Ashgate, 2009), 37.

50. Maria Stanley, *The Early Married Life of Maria Josepha, Lady Stanley*, ed. J. H. Adeane (London: Longmans, Green & Co., 1899), 231, MJS to Louisa Dorothea Clinton (7 March 1802).

51. *CL* (2 July 1904), lxvi; (10 July 1909), xlv.

52. *Sheffield Daily Telegraph* (2 October 1884), 7.

53. *Liverpool Journal of Commerce* (27 December 1875), 5; *North British Advertiser & Ladies' Journal* (31 October 1891), 6.

54. Elizabeth Grant, *Memoirs of a Highland Lady*, ed. Lady Strachey (London: John Murray, 1898), 106; Amelia Murray, *Recollections from 1803–1837. With a Conclusion in 1868* (London: Longmans, Green, and Co., 1868), 10.

55. *Bell's Weekly Messenger* (19 August 1798), 260.

56. Frances Anne Kemble, *Records of a Girlhood* (New York: Henry Holt & Co., 1880), 415.

57. Gilchrist, *A Treatise on the Hair*, 30, 38.

58. Grant, *Memoirs of a Highland Lady*, 189.

59. Marie Bayard, *The Art of Beauty, or Lady's Companion to the Boudoir* (London: Weldon & Co., 1876), 17, 22; Arnold J. Cooley, *The Toilet and Cosmetic Arts* (London: Robert Hardwicke, 1866), 248.

60. Helen Follett Stevans, *The Woman Beautiful* (Chicago: Stevans & Handy, 1899), 50.

61. *Beauty and How to Keep It, by a Professional Beauty* (London: Brentano's, 1889), 36–8.

62. *Falkirk Herald* (14 August 1889), 7; *HB* (2 July 1898), 574.

63. *Beauty and How to Keep It*, 36–8.

64. *Drogheda Conservative* (27 August 1892), 3.

65. *CLO*, 10.1215/lt-18421225-JWC-JW-01, JWC to Jeannie Welsh (25 December 1842).

66. *ILN* (15 March 1884), 243; *CL* (22 April 1905), xxxviii.

67. *The Globe* (14 October 1909), 4.

68. *Christian Recorder* (3 May 1900), 7.

69. Tanisha Ford, *Liberated Threads: Black Women, Style, and the Global Politics of Soul* (Chapel Hill: University of North Carolina Press, 2015), 130.

70. *Chicago Defender* (26 July 1947), 19. See also Laila Haidarali, *Brown Beauty: Color, Sex, and Race from the Harlem Renaissance to World War II* (New York: NYU Press, 2018), 100–1.

71. Kim Smith, 'Strands of the Sixties: A Cultural Analysis of the Design and Consumption of the New London West End Hair Salons *c.* 1954–1975' (PhD thesis, University of East London, 2014), 222.

72. Frances Burney, *Diary and Letters of Madame d'Arblay (1778–1840)*, ed. Charlotte Barrett, 6 vols (London: Macmillan & Co., 1904–5), II, 457–8 (13 August 1786).

73. Ibid., IV, 104 (4 September 1788).

74. Austen, *Letters*, 220, JA to Cassandra Austen (15–16 September 1813).

75. Edgeworth, *Letters*, 26, ME to Honora Edgeworth (26 April 1813).

76. Harriet Martineau, *Household Education* (London: Edward Moxon, 1849), 280.

77. *HB* (2 July 1898), 574.

78. *Ballymena Advertiser* (15 August 1885), 7.

79. *HB* (22 August 1874), 537–8.

80. *CL* (21 December 1907), xxxvii.

81. Kemble, *Records of a Girlhood*, 415.

82. Frampton, *Journal*, 3.

83. *Public Advertiser* (26 July 1764), 3.

84. Steeve O. Buckridge, *The Language of Dress Resistance and Accommodation in Jamaica 1760–1890* (Kingston, Jamaica: University of the West Indies Press, 2004), 86–96.

85. Eliot, *Letters*, VII, 334, GE to Mrs Elma Stuart (15 November 1880).

86. Frances Anne Kemble, *Further Records 1848–1883: A Series of Letters* (London: Henry Holt & Co., 1891), 103, 111, FAK to Harriet St Leger (29 June and 28 July 1875).

87. *Worcestershire Chronicle* (17 October 1896), 8.

88. *CL* (3 June 1916), 52.

89. Anna Daly Morrison, *Diary of Anna Daly Morrison* (Boise, ID: Em-Kayan Press, 1951), 140.

90. *HB* (November 1940), 34.
91. 'Help End Afro Hair Discrimination', *Procter & Gamble*, 2023, https://tinyurl.com/4sneew9u (accessed 29 September 2023).

8 SPA TOWNS AND SEA BATHING

1. *Elizabeth Ham, By Herself, 1783–1820*, ed. Eric Gillett (London: Faber & Faber, 1945), 29.
2. Mary Cowper, *Diary of Mary, Countess Cowper*, ed. Charles Spencer Cowper (London: John Murray, 1864), 208, Duchess of Marlborough to MC (3 September 1716).
3. Gladys Scott Thomson, ed., *Letters of a Grandmother, 1732–1735. Being the Correspondence of Sarah, Duchess of Marlborough with Her Granddaughter Diana, Duchess of Bedford* (London: Jonathan Cape, 1943), 46, LSC to Lady Russell (11 July 1732).
4. *The Ladies Dispensary: Or Every Woman Her Own Physician* (London: James Hodges, 1734), 3, 18; *Letters to and from Henrietta, Countess of Suffolk and Her Second Husband, the Hon. George Berkley; From 1712 to 1767*, 2 vols (London: John Murray, 1824), II, 5, Dr Arbuthnot to Lady Suffolk (6 July 1731).
5. Frances Burney, *Diary and Letters of Madame d'Arblay (1778–1840)*, ed. Charlotte Barrett, 6 vols (London: Macmillan & Co., 1904–5), I, 117 (4 November 1782).
6. LMA CLC/427/MS03041/4/63; E. Montagu, *Letters*, IV, 272–3, EM to Lord Lyttelton (7 August 1760).
7. LMA CLC/427/MS03041/6 (i).
8. E. Smith, *The Compleat Housewife: Or, Accomplish'd Gentlewoman's Companion* (London: H. Pemberton, 1747; 1st edn 1728), 240.
9. Amanda E. Herbert, 'Gender and the Spa: Space, Sociability and Self at British Health Spas, 1640–1714', *Journal of Social History*, 43, no. 2 (2009): 361–83, at 373.
10. Ralph Davies, *The Rise of the English Shipping Industry in the Seventeenth and Eighteenth Centuries* (Newton Abbot: David & Charles, 1962), 139.
11. LMA CLC/427/MS03041/4/37.
12. LMA CLC/427/MS03041/4/39.
13. E. Montagu, *Letters*, III, 9, EM to Duchess of Portsmouth (27 [August] 1745).
14. Elizabeth Carter, *Memoirs of the Life of Mrs. Elizabeth Carter*, ed. Montagu Pennington, 2 vols (London: F. C. and J. Rivington, 1808), I, 287, EC to Catherine Talbot (14 July 1763); I, 305 (25 July 1765).
15. E. Montagu, *Letters*, I, 72–3, EM to Duchess of Portland (27 December 1740).
16. BARS, Wrest Park (Lucas) Archive L 30/9a/5, f. 153, Jemima, Marchioness Grey to Catherine Talbot (3 October 1749).
17. Ibid., L 30/9a/2, f. 78, Jemima, Marchioness Grey to Lady Mary Gregory (10 July 1752).
18. E. Montagu, *Letters*, III, 121, EM to her husband (1749).
19. Ibid., III, 94, EM to Mrs Donellan (26 [September] 1749).
20. Ibid., III, 82, EM to Mrs Anstey (1749).
21. Carter, *Letters*, III, 231 (9 November 1784).

22. BARS, Wrest Park (Lucas) Archive L 30/9a/5, f. 148, Jemima, Marchioness Grey to Catherine Talbot (24 September 1749).

23. Mary Jepp Clarke, *Clarke Family Letters* (Alexandria, VA: Alexander Street, 2002), 407, MJC to Edward Clarke (24 June 1700).

24. E. Montagu, *Letters*, IV, 270, EM to Lord Lyttelton ([July] 1760).

25. Maria Josepha Stanley, *The Girlhood of Maria Josepha Holroyd, Lady Stanley of Alderley*, ed. J. H. Adeane (London: Longmans, Green, and Co., 1896), 83, Miss Moss to MJS (21 September 1791).

26. Lady Louisa Stuart, *Gleanings from an Old Portfolio* (Correspondence of Lady Louisa Stuart), ed. Mrs Godfrey Clark, 3 vols (Edinburgh: privately published, 1895–8), II, 89, LS to Duchess of Buccleuch (1 October 1787).

27. G. P. B. Naish, ed., *Nelson's Letters to His Wife and Other Documents 1785–1831* (London: Routledge and Kegan Paul for the Naval Records Society, 1958), 360–1, Frances Nelson to Nelson (10 April 1797).

28. *CL* (21 December 1961), 1596.

29. *Round Table. A Saturday Review of Politics, Finance, Literature, Society and Art* (19 June 1869), 389.

30. *Beauty and Hygiene for Women and Girls* (London: Swan Sonnenschein & Co., 1893), 107.

31. *ILN* (8 August 1903), 214.

32. *CL* (19 June 1897), xiii.

33. Ibid. (16 May 1925), lxxiii.

34. Ibid. (13 February 1909), lxiii.

35. T. Maude, *Viator, A Poem: Or, A Journey from London to Scarborough* (London: B. White, T. Becket, and J. Walter, 1732), 39; Thomson, ed., *Letters of a Grandmother*, 64, Lady Marlborough to Lady Russell (8 August 1732).

36. *Lloyd's Evening Post* (2–4 March 1763), 211.

37. *General Evening Post* (16–19 August 1783), 5.

38. Ibid. (15–17 August 1751), 1; E. Montagu, *Letters*, IV, 239, EM to Lord Lyttelton (16 September [1759]).

39. *St James's Chronicle or the British Evening Post* (19–21 May 1761), 1.

40. Fanny Burney, *The Early Diary of Frances Burney, 1768–1778*, ed. Annie Raine Ellis, 2 vols (London: George Bell & Sons, 1889), I, 245.

41. Hester Thrale, *Thraliana: The Diary of Mrs. Hester Lynch Thrale (Later Mrs Piozzi) 1776–1809*, ed. Katharine C. Balderston, 2nd edn, 2 vols (Oxford: Clarendon Press, 1951), I, 367 (10 February 1779).

42. Burney, *Diary and Letters*, II, 128 (20 November 1782).

43. Carter, *Letters*, III, 263 (21 July 1786).

44. Burney, *Diary and Letters*, IV, 296–7, FB to Dr Burney (8 and 13 July 1789).

45. *The Listener* (17 August 1932), 218.

46. Ham, *Elizabeth Ham, By Herself*, 49.

47. 'Scarborough. A Poem' in *The Scarborough Miscellany ... By Several Hands* (London: J. Roberts, 1732), 7.

48. Allan Brodie, 'Scarborough in the 1730s: Spa, Sea and Sex', *Journal of Tourism History*, 4, no. 2 (2021): 125–53, at 153.

49. *Public Advertiser* (19 June 1767), 4.

50. *Ipswich Journal* (3 October 1801), 2.

51. John Travis, 'Continuity and Change in English Sea-Bathing 1730–1900: A Case of Swimming with the Tide', in Stephen Fisher, ed., *Recreation and the Sea* (Exeter: Exeter University Press, 1997), 8–35, at 15.
52. *The Observer* (28 August 1859), 5.
53. Ibid. (16 July 1865), 5.
54. Philip Hamerton, *French and English: A Comparison* (Boston: Roberts Brothers, 1889), 317.
55. Frances Anne Kemble, *Records of Later Life*, 3 vols (London: Richard Bentley and Son, 1882), I, 158–9, FAK to Harriet St Leger (10 August 1838).
56. *ILN* (31 August 1895), 278.
57. Carter, *Letters*, II, 155 (5 August 1772).
58. Lady Charlotte Bury, *The Diary of a Lady-in-Waiting*, ed. A. Francis Steuart, 2 vols (London: John Lane, 1908), II, 61.
59. Allan Brodie, *The Seafront* (Swindon: Historic England, 2018), 216.
60. Ham, *Elizabeth Ham, By Herself*, 147.
61. Diaries of Catherine Paget, Bodleian, MS. Eng. misc. f. 655, 43 (26 August 1870).
62. *CLO*, 10.1215/lt-18610806-JWC-TC-01, JWC to TC (6 August 1861).
63. *CLO*, 10.1215/lt-18650815-JWC-TC-01, JWC to TC (15 August 1865).
64. Mary Ann Radcliffe, *The Memoirs of Mrs. Mary Ann Radcliffe: In Familiar Letters to Her Female Friend* (Edinburgh: privately published, 1810), 526.
65. Burney, *The Early Diary*, I, 204, Maria to Fanny Burney (25 April 1773).
66. Burney, *Diary and Letters*, V, 19 (16 August 1791).
67. *Morning Herald* (4 August 1785), 1.
68. *Bow Bells: A Magazine of General Literature and Art for Family Reading* (15 August 1890), 154.
69. *The World* (13 January 1790), 4; *ILN* (4 September 1875), 233; *Bow Bells* (1 September 1893), 234; *ILN* (23 September 1911), 494.
70. Bodleian, John Johnson Collection: Beauty Parlour 5 (24+).

EPILOGUE

1. Sally Meeson, 'Why Plastic-Surgery Demand Is Booming Amid Lockdown', *BBC Worklife*, 17 September 2020, https://www.bbc.com/worklife/article/20200909-why-plastic-surgery-demand-is-booming-amid-lockdown (accessed 28 October 2023).
2. Emily Gerstell et al., 'How Covid-19 Is Changing the World of Beauty', McKinsey & Company, May 2020, https://tinyurl.com/4msvc33y (accessed 29 September 2023).
3. Sophie Marchessou and Emma Spagnuolo, 'Taking a Good Look at the Beauty Industry', McKinsey & Company, 22 July 2021, https://tinyurl.com/2p8feyr4 (accessed 29 September 2023).
4. Katalin Medvedev, 'Social Class and Clothing', in Valerie Steele, ed., *The Berg Companion to Fashion* (Oxford: Berg, 2010), 646.
5. Rachel Moss, 'Miriam Margolyes on Body-Acceptance at 78', *Huffpost*, 9 March 2020, https://tinyurl.com/4kfp6pbj (accessed 29 September 2023).

6. Lotte Van Eijk, 'Tough As You', drmartins.com, 2020, https://tinyurl.com/pushv3j6 (accessed 29 September 2023).

7. Modern Girl Around the World Research Group, *The Modern Girl Around the World: Consumption, Modernity, and Globalization* (Durham, NC, and London: Duke University Press, 2008); Sharon Block, 'Early American Bodies: Creating Race, Sex, and Beauty', in Jennifer Brier, Jim Downs, and Jennifer L. Morgan, eds, *Connexions: Histories of Race and Sex in North America* (Urbana, Chicago, and Springfield: University of Illinois Press, 2016), 107.

8. Frame, 'Fact or Fiction? Mapping Perceptions of Animal Testing', frame.org.uk, summer 2020, https://tinyurl.com/5ekmftcj; 'Animal Testing Licences for Makeup Banned', BBC News, 17 May 2023 https://tinyurl.com/228mdk8n (accessed 29 September 2023).

9. Cuthbert Collingwood, *The Private Correspondence of Admiral Lord Collingwood*, ed. Edward Hughes (London: Navy Records Society, 1957), 262.

10. *CLO*, 10.1215/lt-18500930-TC-JWC-01, TC to JWC (30 September 1850).

11. Charlotte Charke, *A Narrative of the Life of Mrs. Charlotte Charke* (London: W. Reeve, A. Dodd, and E. Cook, 1755), 273.

12. Elizabeth Cady Stanton, *Elizabeth Cady Stanton as Revealed in Her Letters, Diary and Reminiscences*, ed. Theodore Stanton and Harriot Stanton Blatch, 2 vols (New York and London: Harper & Brothers, 1922), I, 344, and II, 53, ECS to Elizabeth Smith Miller (20 June 1853).

13. Frances Anne Kemble, *Further Records 1848–1883: A Series of Letters*, 2 vols (London: R. Bentley & Son, 1890), I, 197, FAK to Harriet St Leger (1 October 1875).

14. David Ritchie, *A Treatise on the Hair* (London: printed for the author, 1770), 92.

15. *Prospect* (June 2022), 86; *London Review of Books* (16 March 2023), 40.

FURTHER READING

This list is intended for those interested in a broader, contextual guide to the material covered in this book. What follows is not exhaustive, and there is some overlap between categories.

GENERAL

Baker, Nancy C., *The Beauty Trap: Exploring Women's Greatest Obsession*. New York: Franklin Watts, 1984

Bindman, David and Henry Louis Gates, Jr, eds, *The Image of the Black in Western Art*. 4 vols. Cambridge, MA: Belknap Press, Harvard University Press, 2009–12

Black, Paula, *The Beauty Industry: Gender, Culture, Pleasure*. London: Routledge, 2004

Bradstock, Lillian and Jane Condon, *The Modern Woman: Beauty, Physical Culture, Hygiene*. London: Associated Newspapers [1936]

Bressey, Caroline, 'Looking for Work: The Black Presence in Britain 1860–1920', in Caroline Bressey and Hakim Adi, eds, *Belonging in Europe: The African Diaspora and Work*. London: Routledge, 2011

Buckridge, Steeve O., *The Language of Dress Resistance and Accommodation in Jamaica 1760–1890*. Kingston, Jamaica: University of the West Indies Press, 2004

Clark, Jessica P., *The Business of Beauty*. London: Bloomsbury, 2019

Craig, Maxine Leeds, *Ain't I a Beauty Queen? Black Women, Beauty, and the Politics of Race*. Oxford: Oxford University Press, 2002

———, ed., *The Routledge Companion to Beauty Politics*. Abingdon and New York: Routledge, 2021

Cunningham, Patricia A., *Reforming Women's Fashion, 1850–1920: Politics, Health, and Art*. Kent, OH: Kent State University Press, 2003

Dabiri, Emma, *Disobedient Bodies: Reclaim Your Unruly Beauty*. London: Profile Books, 2023

Eger, Elizabeth and Lucy Peltz, *Brilliant Women: 18th-Century Bluestockings*. London: National Portrait Gallery, 2008

Entwistle, Joanne, *The Fashioned Body: Fashion, Dress and Modern Social Theory*. Cambridge: Polity Press, 2000

Entwistle, Joanne and Elizabeth Wilson, eds, *Body Dressing: Dress, Body, Culture*. London: Bloomsbury, 2001

Furman, Frida Kerner, *Facing the Mirror: Older Women and Beauty Shop Culture*. New York and London: Routledge, 1997

Gill, Tiffany M., *Beauty Shop Politics: African American Women's Activism in the Beauty Industry*. Urbana and Chicago: University of Illinois Press, 2010

Haidarali, Laila, *Brown Beauty: Color, Sex, and Race from the Harlem Renaissance to World War II*. New York: NYU Press, 2018

Hall, Kim F., *Things of Darkness: Economies of Race and Gender in Early Modern England*. Ithaca: Cornell University Press, 1996

Kalof, Linda and William Bynum, eds, *A Cultural History of the Human Body*. Oxford and New York: Berg, 2010, vols 4–6

Jones, Geoffrey, *Beauty Imagined: A History of the Global Beauty Industry*. Oxford: Oxford University Press, 2010

Lakoff, Robin Tolmach and Raquel L. Scheer, *Face Value: The Politics of Beauty*. London: Routledge & Kegan Paul, 1984

McClintock, Anne, *Imperial Leather: Race, Gender and Sexuality in the Colonial Contest*. New York: Routledge, 1995

Myers, Sylvia Harcstark, *The Bluestocking Circle: Women, Friendship, and the Life of the Mind in Eighteenth-Century England*. Oxford: Clarendon Press, 1990

Otele, Olivette, *African Europeans: An Untold History*. London: Hurst & Company, 2020

Qureshi, Sadiah, *Peoples on Parade: Exhibitions, Empire, and Anthropology in Nineteenth-Century Britain*. Chicago: University of Chicago Press, 2011

Reischer, Erica and Kathryn S. Koo, 'The Body Beautiful: Symbolism and Agency in the Social World', *Annual Review of Anthropology*, 33 (2004): 297–317

Ribeiro, Aileen, *Facing Beauty: Painted Women and Cosmetic Art*. New Haven and London: Yale University Press, 2011

Rowe, Rochelle, *Imagining Caribbean Womanhood: Race, Nation and Beauty Competitions 1929–1970*. Manchester: Manchester University Press, 2013

Tate, Shirley Anne, *Black Beauty: Aesthetics, Stylization, Politics*. Farnham: Ashgate, 2009

Vigarello, Georges, *Histoire de la beauté. Le corps et l'art d'embellir de la Renaissance à nos jours*. Paris: Seuil, 2004

Wolf, Naomi, *The Beauty Myth: How Images of Beauty Are Used against Women*. London: Vintage, 1991

BODY SCULPTURE

Crais, Clifton and Pamela Scully, *Sara Baartman and the Hottentot Venus: A Ghost Story and a Biography*. Princeton: Princeton University Press, 2009

Davis, Kathy, *Reshaping the Female Body: The Dilemma of Cosmetic Surgery*. New York and London: Routledge, 1995

Ewing, Elizabeth, *Dress and Undress: A History of Women's Underwear*. London: B. T. Batsford, 1978

Fontanel, Béatrice, *Support and Seduction: The History of Corsets and Bras*. Translated by Willard Wood. New York: Abrams, 1997

Forth, Christopher E., 'Fat, Desire and Disgust in the Colonial Imagination', *History Workshop Journal*, 73, no. 1 (2012): 211–39

Geertsen, Lauren, *The Invisible Corset: Break Free from Beauty Culture and Embrace Your Radiant Self*. Boulder, CO: Sounds True, 2021

Gimlin, Debra L., *Body Work: Beauty and Self-Image in American Culture*. Berkeley: University of California Press, 2002

Hobson, Janell, *Venus in the Dark: Blackness and Beauty in Popular Culture*. New York: Routledge, 2005

Lynn, Eleri, *Underwear: Fashion in Detail*. London: V&A Publishing, 2014

Magubane, Zine, 'Which Bodies Matter? Feminism, Poststructuralism, Race, and the Curious Theoretical Odyssey of the "Hottentot Venus"', in Deborah Willis, ed., *Black Venus 2010: They Called Her 'Hottentot'*, Philadelphia: Temple University Press, 2010, 47–61

Qureshi, Sadiah, 'Displaying Sara Baartman, the "Hottentot Venus"', *History of Science*, 42, no. 2 (2004): 233–57

Steele, Valerie, ed., *The Berg Companion to Fashion*. Oxford: Berg, 2010

————, *The Corset: A Cultural History*. New Haven and London: Yale University Press, 2001

Vigarello, Georges, *The Silhouette: From the 18th Century to the Present Day*. Translated by Augusta Doerr. London: Bloomsbury, 2016

Vincent, Susan J., ed., *A Cultural History of Dress and Fashion*. London: Bloomsbury Academic, 2016, vols 4–6

Waugh, Norah, *Corsets and Crinolines*. New York: Routledge/Theatre Arts, 2004; first published 1954

DIET AND EXERCISE

Braziel, Jana Evans and Kathleen LeBesco, eds, *Bodies out of Bounds: Fatness and Transgression*. Berkeley and Los Angeles: University of California Press, 2001

Brumberg, Joan Jacobs, *Fasting Girls: The History of Anorexia Nervosa*. New York: Vintage, 2000

Day, Carolyn, *Consumptive Chic: A History of Beauty, Fashion, and Disease*. London: Bloomsbury, 2017

Foxcroft, Louise, *Calories and Corsets: A History of Dieting over Two Thousand Years*. London: Profile Books, 2012

Friedman, Danielle, *Let's Get Physical: How Women Discovered Exercise and Reshaped the World*. New York: G. P. Putnam's Sons, 2022

Haslam, David and Fiona Haslam, *Fat, Gluttony and Sloth: Obesity in Literature, Art and Medicine*. Liverpool: Liverpool University Press, 2009

Kennedy, Eileen and Pirkko Markula, eds, *Women and Exercise: The Body, Health and Consumerism*. New York and Abingdon: Routledge, 2012

Oddy, Derek J., Peter J. Atkins and Virginie Amilien, eds, *The Rise of Obesity in Europe: A Twentieth Century Food History*. Farnham: Ashgate, 2009

Orbach, Susie, *Fat Is a Feminist Issue*. London: Arrow, 2016; first published 1978

Petrzela, Natalia Mehlman, *Fit Nation: The Gains and Pains of America's Exercise Obsession*. Chicago: University of Chicago Press, 2022

Radford, Peter, *They Run with Surprising Swiftness: The Women Athletes of Early Modern Britain*. Charlottesville, VA: UVA Press, 2023

Schwartz, Hillel, *Never Satisfied: A Cultural History of Diets, Fantasies and Fat*. New York: Free Press, 1986

Strings, Sabrina, *Fearing the Black Body: The Racial Origins of Fat Phobia*. New York: New York University Press, 2019

Vigarello, Georges, *The Metamorphoses of Fat: A History of Obesity*. Translated by C. Jon Delogu. New York: Columbia University Press, 2013

Walvin, James, *Sugar: The World Corrupted: From Slavery to Obesity*. London: Robinson, 2017

Zweiniger-Bargielowska, Ina, *Managing the Body: Beauty, Health, and Fitness in Britain 1880–1939*. Oxford: Oxford University Press, 2010

SKIN

Barron, Lee, *Tattoo Culture: Theory and Contemporary Contexts*. London: Rowman & Littlefield International Ltd, 2017

Benthien, Claudia, *Skin: On the Cultural Border Between Self and the World*. Translated by Thomas Dunlap. New York and Chichester: Colombia University Press, 2002

Brown, Tina, *Tattoos: An Illustrated History*. Stroud: Amberley Publishing, 2018

Connor, Steven, *The Book of Skin*. Ithaca: Cornell University Press, 2004

David, Alison Matthews, *Fashion Victims: the Dangers of Dress Past and Present*. London: Bloomsbury, 2015

DeMello, Margo and Gayle S. Rubin, *Bodies of Inscription: A Cultural History of the Modern Tattoo Community*. Durham, NC, and London: Duke University Press, 2000

Glenn, Evelyn Nakano, ed., *Shades of Difference: Why Skin Color Matters*. Stanford: Stanford University Press, 2009

Hunter, Margaret L., *Race, Gender, and the Politics of Skin Tone*. New York and London: Routledge, 2005

Leader, Karen, 'On the Book of My Body', *Feminist Formations*, 28, no. 3 (2016): 174–95

Lyman, Monty, *The Remarkable Life of Skin*. London: Bantam Press, 2019

Mifflin, Margot, *Bodies of Subversion: A Secret History of Women and Tattoo*. New York: Juno Books, 1997

Mohammed, Patricia, '"But most of all mi love me browning": The Emergence in Eighteenth and Nineteenth-Century Jamaica of the Mulatto Woman as the Desired', *Feminist Review*, 65, no. 1 (2000): 22–48

Rappaport, Helen, *Beautiful for Ever: Madame Rachel of Bond Street*. London: Vintage, 2012

Rees, Michael, 'From Outsider to Established: Explaining the Current Popularity and Acceptability of Tattooing', *Historical Social Research*, 41, no. 3 (2016): 157–74

Thomas, Lynn M., *Beneath the Surface: A Transnational History of Skin Lighteners*. Durham, NC: Duke University Press, 2020

Wheeler, Roxann, *The Complexion of Race: Categories of Difference in Eighteenth-Century British Culture*. Philadelphia: University of Pennsylvania Press, 2000

MAKEUP

De Castelbajac, *The Face of the Century: 100 Years of Makeup and Style*. London: Thames and Hudson, 1995

Eldridge, Lisa, *Face Paint: The Story of Make-Up*. New York: Abrams Image, 2015

Fetto, Funmi, *Palette: A Black Beauty Bible*. London: Hodder & Stoughton, 2019

Hankir, Zahra, *Eyeliner: A Cultural History*. London: Harvill Secker, 2023

Lennox, Sarah, 'The Beautified Body: Physiognomy in Victorian Beauty Manuals', *Victorian Review*, 42, no. 1 (2016): 9–14

Little, Claire Douglass, ed., *Makeup in the World of Beauty Vlogging: Community, Commerce, and Culture*. Lanham: Lexington Books, 2020

Martin, Morag, *Selling Beauty: Cosmetics, Commerce, and French Society 1750–1830*. Baltimore: Johns Hopkins University Press, 2009

Pearl, Sharrona, *About Faces: Physiognomy in Nineteenth-Century Britain*. Cambridge, MA: Harvard University Press, 2010

Peiss, Kathy, *Hope in a Jar: The Making of America's Beauty Culture*. New York: Metropolitan Books, Henry Holt & Company, 1998

Shuker, Nancy, *Elizabeth Arden: Cosmetics Entrepreneur*. Englewood Cliffs, NY: Silver Burdett Press, 1989

Woodhead, Lindy, *War Paint: Miss Elizabeth Arden and Madame Helena Rubinstein: Their Lives, Their Rivalry*. London: Virago, 2003

HYGIENE

Brown, Kathleen M., *Foul Bodies: Cleanliness in Early America*. New Haven: Yale University Press, 2009

Burke, Timothy, *Lifebuoy Men, Lux Women: Commodification, Consumption, and Cleanliness in Modern Zimbabwe*. Durham, NC: Duke University Press, 1996

Corbin, Alain, *The Foul and the Fragrant: Odor and the French Social Imagination*. Translated by Miriam L. Kochan. Cambridge, MA: Harvard University Press, 1986

Hendrickson, Hildi, ed., *Clothing and Difference: Embodied Identities in Colonial and Post-Colonial Africa*. Durham, NC: Duke University Press, 1996

Hussain, Mobeen, 'Combining Global Expertise with Local Knowledge in Colonial India: Selling Ideals of Beauty and Health in Commodity Advertising (c. 1900–1949)', *South Asia: Journal of South Asian Studies*, 44, no. 5 (2021): 926–47

Smith, Virginia, *Clean: A History of Personal Hygiene and Purity*. Oxford: Oxford University Press, 2007

Vigarello, Georges, *Concepts of Cleanliness: Changing Attitudes in France since the Middle Ages*. Translated by Jean Birrell. Cambridge: Cambridge University Press, 1988

Woods, Walter V., *Health: How to Get and Keep It. The Hygiene of Dress, Food, Exercise, Rest, Bathing, Breathing, and Ventilation*. Philadelphia: Penn Publishing Co., 1905

TEETH

Barnet, Richard, *The Smile Stealers: The Fine and Foul Art of Dentistry*. London: Thames & Hudson, 2017

Hillam, Christine, *Brass Plate and Brazen Impudence: Dental Practice in the Provinces 1755–1855*. Liverpool: Liverpool University Press, 1991

Jones, Colin, *The Smile Revolution in Eighteenth-Century Paris*. Oxford: Oxford University Press, 2014

Trevers, John and Martin Orskey, *Open Wide! A Series of Eighteenth & Nineteenth Century Caricatures on Dentistry*. Stow on the Wold: Wychwood Books, 2009

Woodforde, John, *The Strange Story of False Teeth*. London: Routledge & Kegan Paul, 1968

Wynbrandt, James, *The Excruciating History of Dentistry*. New York: St Martin's Press, 1998

HAIR

Banks, Ingrid, *Hair Matters: Beauty, Power, and Black Women's Consciousness*. New York and London: New York University Press, 2000

Biddle-Perry, Geraldine, ed., *A Cultural History of Hair*. London: Bloomsbury Academic, 2022, vols 4–6

Dabiri, Emma, *Don't Touch My Hair*. London: Allen Lane, 2019

Ford, Tanisha, *Liberated Threads: Black Women, Style, and the Global Politics of Soul*. Chapel Hill: University of North Carolina Press, 2015

Ofek, Galia, *Representations of Hair in Victorian Literature and Culture*. Farnham: Ashgate, 2009

Sagay, Esi, *African Hairstyles: Styles of Yesterday and Today*. Oxford: Heinemann International, 1983

Sherrow, Victoria, *Encyclopedia of Hair: A Cultural History*. Westport, CT: Greenwood Press, 2006

Thompson, Cheryl, *Beauty in a Box: Detangling the Roots of Canada's Black Beauty Culture*. Waterloo: WLU Press, 2019

SPA TOWNS AND SEA BATHING

Brodie, Allan, *The Seafront*. Swindon: Historic England, 2018

Corbin, Alain. *The Lure of the Sea: The Discovery of the Seaside in the Western World, 1760–1840*. Translated by Jocelyn Phelps. Cambridge: Polity Press, 1994

Herbert, Amanda E., 'Gender and the Spa: Space, Sociability and Self at British Health Spas, 1640–1714', *Journal of Social History*, 43, no. 2 (2009): 361–83

McCormack, Rose Alexandra, 'Leisured Women and the English Spa Town in the Long Eighteenth Century: A Case Study of Bath and Tunbridge Wells'. PhD thesis, Aberystwyth University, 2015

Ritchie, Robert C., *The Lure of the Beach: A Global History*. Oakland, CA: University of California Press, 2021

Rotherham, Ian D., *Spas and Spa Visiting*. Oxford: Shire Publications, 2014

INDEX